Futures at Stake

The Gambling Studies Series

Futures at Stake

Youth, Gambling, and Society

Edited by

Howard J. Shaffer
Matthew N. Hall
Joni Vander Bilt
Elizabeth George

Foreword by

Thomas N. Cummings

University of Nevada Press ▲▲ Reno / Las Vegas

The Gambling Studies Series

Series Editor: William R. Eadington

University of Nevada Press

Reno, Nevada 89557 USA

Copyright © 2003 by

University of Nevada Press

Manufactured in the

United States of America

The paper used in this book meets the
requirements of American National
Standard for Information Sciences—
Permanence of Paper for Printed Library
Materials, ANSI Z39.48-1984. Binding
materials were selected for strength and
durability.

First Printing

12 11 10 09 08 07 06 05 04 03

5 4 3 2 1

Library of Congress

Cataloging-in-Publication Data

Futures at stake : youth, gambling, and
society / edited by Howard J. Shaffer . . .
[et al.].

   p. cm. — (The gambling studies
series)

Includes bibliographical references (p.   )
and index.

   ISBN 0-87417-368-X (hardcover : alk.
paper)

   1. Teenage gamblers—United States.
2. Teenage gamblers—Canada.   3.
Compulsive gambling—United States—
Prevention.   4. Compulsive gambling—
Canada—Prevention.   I. Shaffer, Howard,
1948– II. Series.

HV6715 .F87 2003

363.4'2'0835097—dc21

2002156590

We dedicate this book to the children in our lives

and to the lives of children throughout the world.

Contents

Illustrations

Figures

Tables

Foreword

I begin this foreword with a look backward. It is said, after all, that those who do not learn from history are doomed to repeat it. So I first look to my own experiences. Had this been a book about adult compulsive gambling, I would have readily shared my views and experiences. I know what it is to be a compulsive gambler. I also could have described what it took to change and escape this difficult circumstance. I could have told you how these changes came about. I might even have suggested that my personal odyssey certifies me as an expert in matters of recovery.

However, this book is not about adult gambling; it is about adolescent gambling. Consequently, it is reasonable to ask, Are my experiences with adult gambling and gamblers relevant? Do my views on the initiation and development of risk-taking and gambling among adolescents have value? And if these ideas are useful, for whom are they useful? In spite of these questions, I will press on and raise some "big picture" questions that the other contributors have not asked. For example, if the problem gambler begins the journey to that state very early in life, should the book be titled "Child and Adolescent Gambling"?

During the 1990s, Americans started to focus more attention on adolescent gambling issues. For the first time, at least in this country, a generation of young people reached adulthood within a context of approval and endorsement of gambling as a source of entertainment and recreation. The State and the Church, traditional opponents of gambling, are now unlikely bedfellows in their use of gambling as a source of revenue.

To date, only a handful of states have addressed the issue of problem gambling with the commitment of resources appropriate to the task. This struggle to obtain the funds necessary to study and treat gambling-related concerns will continue in the twenty-first century. Perhaps the burgeoning scope of problem gambling among adolescents will spark a dedicated response, similar to the attention devoted to adolescent alcohol and drug use. For this to happen, we need everyone with a stake (direct or indirect) in legalized gambling, its benefits and its costs, to work together. This book represents only a small portion of those workers who have been, are, and should be involved in this issue.

Contributors to this volume include some of the usual suspects: theorists, researchers, treatment providers, and prevention specialists. Some observers may think that this book also provides a forum for those whose self-interest conflicts with those working to find ways to mitigate problem gambling. However, input from the gambling industry about its role and responsibility is a welcome perspective.

Massachusetts, which everyone should consider a significant part of the gambling industry through its monopoly of the state lottery, is represented on two levels: by the elected incumbent with legislative and programmatic responsibility, State Treasurer Joseph Malone, and by the manager of the lottery's day-to-day business, director Eric Turner.[1] This lottery remains the most efficient in the nation. By presenting a review of youth gambling and policy in Canada, this book tries to show that adolescent gambling is not limited to the United States but concerns North America as a whole. We hope to include our South American neighbors in a subsequent book.

The interdisciplinary character of the contributors represents the multifaceted nature of the problems related to youth gambling. Psychiatrists, psychologists, sociologists, and social workers are joined by experts in law and economics, probability and mathematics. These contributors stand with executives from the public and private sectors who have a stake in legalized gambling. The diversity of the contributors to this volume seems in tune with the times. At this stage of our knowledge and level of commitment, varied perspectives seem most appropriate. We do not know which road to take. The past can teach us much and provide needed direction. Nevertheless, we must view adolescent gambling as an entity with its own character and identity.

This book was inspired by the first North American Think Tank on Youth Gambling Issues. The final report—a testimony to the pioneers who were sufficiently bold to participate in this watershed event—is included as a special appendix to this volume. Just the list of those attending is worth inspecting: One learns which parts of society saw a need to address the many issues that surround adolescent gambling. It is in this same spirit of coming together, despite the many differences in perspectives and values, that we offer this book. We are looking forward to attending the first international conference on risk-taking and gambling among children and adolescents. We can achieve good things if we work together.

Thomas N. Cummings, CAS
Boston, Massachusetts

Preface

The stakes are high for our young people.

Convening the North American Think Tank on Youth Gambling Issues was a major step toward keeping them out of harm's way.

Forty-two public and private sector leaders from the United States and Canada came together in April 1995 at Harvard Medical School, Division on Addictions, with a common vision: to seek solutions to what is fast becoming a leading social-health problem across the continent.

Experts from education, finance, government, and the gambling industry collaborated with specialists from law enforcement, the judiciary, health care, and research communities to develop public policy strategies to cope with this emerging health-care issue.

All of the think tank collaborators invested considerable time, energy, and talent in advancing the issues surrounding this symposium. Not one of the presenters, keynote speakers, or participants was compensated for attending.

We gratefully acknowledge those donors who provided think tank funding: gaming operators, the banking industry, tribal governments, and insurance executives in Minnesota and Mississippi. Thomas J. Brosig, former executive vice-president of Grand Casinos Inc., led the fund-raising effort.

I would like to give a special tribute to visionary Howard J. Shaffer, director of the Harvard Medical School Division on Addictions, who kindly offered Harvard Medical School as the North American Think Tank's academic partner. His leadership provided the impetus needed to move this entire symposium forward.

The results of the North American Think Tank has helped define public policy at the federal, provincial, state, and local levels. We are confident that the think tank recommendations and this resulting thoughtful book will serve as the blueprint for developing a responsible, and responsive, binational approach to managing youth gambling.

Elizabeth M. George
Executive Director
North American Training Institute

Acknowledgments

This book is evidence of a continuity of vision and commitment on the part of numerous individuals and organizations throughout North America. Initiated at the first North American Think Tank on Compulsive Gambling, held in 1988, the vision of addressing the spectrum of issues surrounding compulsive gambling was extended at the 1995 think tank to focus on youth gambling.

We would like to thank all those who steadfastly held the thread that enabled this work to expand and develop. In particular, we would like to thank all of the participants and speakers at the 1995 think tank, many of whom are contributors to this book. We appreciate the hard work of the Think Tank Planning Committee members, who made the think tank possible: Linda Berman, Tom Brosig, Watson Butts, Colin Campbell, Stanley Crooks, Tom Cummings, William Eadington, Johan Finley, William Fisher, Durand Jacobs, Henry Lesieur, I. Nelson Rose, and Chrissy Thurmond. A special thank-you is extended to North American Training Institute staff Lorraine Grymala, Jeanne Schroeder, and Lynn John Rambeck, who worked tirelessly on this project. Special thanks also go to Marsha Kelly, who, in addition to being a terrific colleague, is an energetic, efficient, competent, and creative facilitator. The think tank and, by extension, this book, would not have been possible without her efforts.

Tom Brosig, one of the contributors to this volume, deserves special recognition as the chairman of the think tank's fund-raising task force and the provider of much of the enthusiasm necessary to support the think tank. In addition, Tom has been an inspirational and devoted proponent of proactive attention to the issues of youth gambling and compulsive gambling. We wish to thank the other members of the fund-raising task force, Nick Roberts, Watson Butts, Johan Finley, John Sneed, and William Fisher. We also thank the task force volunteers, Earl Yanase, Rob Wyre, Tim Moncur, and Chris Boone, and all the contributors who made the think tank possible.

We want to extend our gratitude to every contributor to this book. Each worked long and hard over the many months it took to complete the process of compiling and revising this volume. We greatly appreciate their diligent efforts and contributions.

A special word of thanks to Tom Cummings, Kathy Scanlan, Reingard Heller, Mary Kadaras, and David Gagne at the Massachusetts Council on Compulsive Gambling. This remarkable team has developed and sustained one of the most productive state councils on compulsive gambling in the country. They have offered consistent personal and financial support for gambling research. Sadly, during the preparation of this volume, Tom Cummings passed away, but his spirit, generosity, and wisdom continue to guide the Massachusetts Council on Compulsive Gambling and all of us who were lucky enough to have known him. His foreword is testimony to the richness of his thought and the character of his remarkable being. Tom, we miss you.

We would also like to express our special thanks to Carolyn Howard, Emily McNamara, Greg O'Donohue, and Chrissy Thurmond at Harvard Medical School's Division on Addictions for the patience, support, and intellectual guidance they provided in their efforts to make the think tank and this volume come to life.

Finally, we would like to acknowledge and thank our families, especially Linda Shaffer, Sarah Hall, Anne Tilley, and Dale Sola, as well as our colleagues, who sacrificed time and made the space in their lives that afforded us the time to undertake this venture.

Futures at Stake

Youth and Gambling
Creating a Legacy of Risk

Howard J. Shaffer, Matthew N. Hall, Joni Vander Bilt, and Lisa Vagge

> *Each child is an adventure into a better life—an opportunity to change the old pattern and make it new.*
>   Hubert H. Humphrey (1911–1978), former vice-president of the United States[1]

> *"Children have never been very good at listening to their elders, but they have never failed to imitate them."*
>   James Baldwin (1924–1987), U.S. author[2]

Background

Futures at Stake: Youth, Gambling, and Society represents only one of the many products of a think tank held at Harvard Medical School on April 3 and 4, 1995. The think tank was a watershed event in the history of North American gambling. For the first time a diverse group of professionals gathered to investigate the multiplicity of factors specifically associated with youth gambling. The purpose of this event was to design a blueprint for social policy—an action plan for determining how the gaming industry, health-care providers, the criminal justice system, and institutions of higher learning should respond to youth gambling and gambling's influence on youth. This book represents an important step toward recognizing the significant impact that gambling has on children. By understanding the response of children to this phenomenon, we can begin to understand the influence of gambling on the fabric of contemporary society.[3]

We are now in the midst of the third wave of widespread legal gambling in the United States (Rose, 1995). During the past two decades the opportunity to gamble has exploded across America. Between 1974 and 1995, the total amount of money legally wagered annually in the United States increased from $17.3 billion to $550 billion (Christiansen, 1996; National Council on Problem Gambling, 1993). Between 1975 and 1985, annual national per capita sales of lottery products alone increased from $20 to $97 per year (Clotfelter & Cook, 1989). By the end of 1995, annual national per capita lottery sales had surpassed $130 per year (North American Gaming Report, 1996; U.S. Census Bureau, 1996).

The majority of state legislators and governors have decided that gambling provides an economic solution to diminished revenue streams. For example, when U.S. Senator David Durenberger (R-Minn.) chaired the October 3, 1984, hearing on the legalization of state lotteries before the Senate Subcommittee on Intergovernmental Relations of the Committee on Governmental Affairs during the 98th Congress, he opened the meeting by noting:

> For large segments of the American public, gambling—whether promoted openly by the State or conducted outside the law—is, and has always been, a moral question. That's why it's against the law in most States—against the law, unless the lawmaking body of that State finds itself pressed for funds. The recent advent of government-supported lotteries thus raises the question of whether it is appropriate for States now to promote an activity which for most of our history the States punished as a vice. . . . Whether it is a tax or not, we can agree that it raises revenue. It's for a good cause. States are, in some sense, like public charities that have been allowed to use raffles to raise money because the money goes for a good cause. So we are asked to ignore our discomfort over the means, and to focus on the ends. (Subcommittee on Intergovernmental Relations of the Committee on Governmental Affairs, 1985, pp. 1–2)

There are few parents who would accept for their children the value system endorsed by an "ends justify the means" strategy. Yet when Senator Durenberger opened the 1984 Senate hearing on state lotteries, no one objected to this characterization of state economics. Since these 1984 hearings on state lotteries, most states no longer find gambling illicit or immoral. As this book goes to press, thirty-seven states and the District of Columbia have legalized lotteries and thirty states have endorsed the presence of land- or water-based casino gambling (International Game Technology, 1995). All states, with the exception of Utah and Hawaii, have legalized some form of gambling.

Eadington has noted, "what is presently occurring to legal commercial gaming activities in America can only be described as a veritable avalanche of proliferation" (Eadington, 1992, p. 1). The increase in gambling opportunities for adults, along with the advertising and other hyperbole associated with gambling promotions, has not bypassed children. From church bingo to state-sponsored lotteries, America is exposing its young to a variety of gambling-related events. The evening news, which used to lead with the weather, now often begins by reporting lottery numbers. There is no shortage of stories about lottery winners, implying that gambling holds the potential for enormous wealth. These stories are neither public service announcements nor advertising; when the television media tell about gambling winners, the information is presented as *news*.

State-sponsored advertising for lotteries often suggests—both purposefully and inadvertently—that gambling provides the path to financial independence. One recent advertising campaign in Massachusetts, for example, suggested that young people could earn a living the "hard way" by going to college, or the "easy way" by playing the lottery. While this advertising was short-lived, it did represent the way gambling is often portrayed to young people. Advertising phrases used to promote the New York lottery have included "A dollar and a dream," and "Hey, you never know" (Hernandez, 1996). While contemporary North American society is coming to grips with the impact of alcohol and tobacco advertising on young people, it has not yet determined what to do about gambling advertisements and youth.

As gambling spread rapidly across the country during the late twentieth century, offering adolescents a variety of opportunities to begin gambling, there has been relatively little supervision of adolescents' involvement in this activity. In previous eras, children's access to gambling opportunities was more limited, and most games of chance required a process of negotiation, odds-setting, and communication that demanded time before the actual wager could take place. These factors provided informal social protection from excessive gambling. Contemporary gambling, however, is more readily available, and with the new technology used to produce, distribute, and market games of chance, there is little natural social control to protect young people. For example, adolescents need not negotiate to purchase a lottery ticket from a vending machine. Although states have established some formal controls, such as laws prohibiting minors from purchasing lottery tickets, today's young people have been raised in an environment of informal social acceptance and approval of gambling. Until relatively recently, there have been few societal messages expressing concern over problem and youth gambling from a society whose churches and state governments are among the most prominent providers and promoters of gambling opportunities.

Futures at Stake will explore the nature of adolescents' involvement in gambling by examining issues related to youth-gambling research, treatment, education, economics, and policy. Initially, it is important that we develop a set of concepts—we must be precise in our language so that we share common ground. Therefore, we will begin our introduction to youth gambling by defining concepts.

Defining Terms

YOUTH

Some people may think of children as only those young people who have yet to reach adolescence. Indeed, preadolescent children often gamble, and pathological gamblers often begin gambling before they attain adolescence (Shaffer, LaBrie, Scanlan, & Cummings, 1994). To fully explore underage gambling, however, we consider it more accurate to think of *youth* as those who have yet to reach the legal age of majority.

GAMBLING

For our purposes, the term *gambling* will refer to any form of wagering or betting, such as playing casino games, lottery games (that is, buying a lottery ticket, pull-tab game, or scratch-off ticket), slot machines, or video gambling machines, or participating in parimutuel betting or charitable gaming activities. In addition to these established and legal forms of gambling, which are legally prohibited for minors, the term *gambling* also includes informal betting (betting on card games and activities involving personal skill) and more organized but illegal activities such as sports betting. *Gambling* can also refer to wagering personal belongings on the outcome of games or activities, such as pogs. Finally, *gambling* includes any computerized wagering activities, including any such activity conducted over the Internet.[4]

PATHOLOGICAL GAMBLING

Researchers, clinicians, and organizations have defined *pathological gambling* in a variety of ways. Gamblers Anonymous, for example, has its own criteria, and researchers have devised a number of scales to classify pathological gamblers, including the South Oaks Gambling Screen (SOGS) and the Massachusetts Gambling Screen (MAGS). The American Psychiatric Association's definition of pathological gambling, listed in the *Diagnostic and Statistical Manual, Fourth Edition* (DSM-IV), is currently considered the "gold standard" among clinicians. According to the DSM-IV definition, pathological gambling is a persistent and recurrent maladaptive gambling behavior as indicated by five (or more) of the following:

1. The person needs to gamble with increasing amounts of money in order to achieve the desired excitement.
2. The person, after losing money gambling, often returns another day to get even.
3. The person is restless or irritable when attempting to cut down or stop gambling.
4. The person has repeated unsuccessful efforts to control, cut back, or stop gambling.
5. The person gambles as a way of escaping from problems or of relieving a dysphoric mood.

6. The person is preoccupied with gambling.
7. The person lies to family members, therapist, or others to conceal the extent of involvement with gambling.
8. The person has committed illegal acts such as forgery, fraud, theft, or embezzlement to finance gambling.
9. The person has jeopardized or lost a significant relationship, job, or educational or career opportunity because of gambling.
10. The person relies on others to provide money to relieve a desperate financial situation caused by gambling.

In addition, to fit the criteria for pathological gambling, the individual's gambling behavior cannot be the result of a manic episode (American Psychiatric Association, 1994).

Like criteria from other instruments measuring pathological gambling (e.g., SOGS, MAGS) the DSM-IV criteria imply that pathological gambling affects the gambler's place in society. Not only does gambling behavior preoccupy and control the gambler, but excessive gambling behaviors adversely influence interpersonal relationships.

Currently, the DSM-IV classifies pathological gambling as an impulse-control disorder. The decision to classify pathological gambling in this way is probably related to the fact that despite its recognition of substance abuse and dependence, the DSM-IV has no classification for addiction. However, the DSM-IV criteria for pathological gambling were modeled on the preexisting DSM criteria for substance-use disorders (Lesieur, 1988), implying an underlying construct of addictive process common to both substance dependence and pathological gambling. Numerous research studies have supported this concept and show similarities between pathological gambling and substance-use disorders (McCormick, Russo, Ramirez, & Taber, 1984; Ramirez, McCormick, Russo, & Taber, 1983), including the presence of tolerance and physical symptoms of withdrawal among abstinent problem gamblers (Shaffer, Hall, Walsh, & Vander Bilt, 1995; Wray & Dickerson, 1981). Despite the lack of conceptual clarity in clinical diagnoses, the research and treatment communities tend to recognize pathological gambling as an addictive behavior. This recognition is not universal, however, and professional and lay people alike often misuse the construct of addiction (Shaffer, 1999). Researchers and theorists have expanded the notion of addiction to include addictive behaviors related to activities (process addictions) as well as those related to substances. Although a full discussion of this topic is beyond the scope of this introduction, these concepts are discussed in more detail in several papers by Shaffer (1997a, 1997b, 1999).

Estimating the Prevalence of Youth Gambling Problems

In an effort to integrate all of the prevalence studies of gambling problems among youth in North America, Shaffer and Hall (1996) developed a generic classification scheme for distinguishing the various levels of gambling problem severity. The first level of this system, Level 0, includes those who have never gambled. Level 1 represents those who have gambled but do not have any problems associated with gambling. Level 2 gamblers, sometimes called "at-risk" or "in-transition" gamblers, are those who have some problems associated with their gambling but whose problems are not sufficient for a clinical diagnosis. This group is often considered "subclinical." Level 3 gamblers are those whose behavior meets a level of pathology according to one of the many diagnostic coding systems, such as DSM-IV. Level 4 gamblers are those who display interest in entering treatment for their gambling problems. Table 0.1 illustrates the proposed standard gambling nomenclature.

Using these levels, Shaffer and Hall (1996) completed the first meta-analysis of all available youth-gambling prevalence studies done in North America. By aggregating all of the different methods and all of the different criteria used to classify respondents, this study generated estimates of the gambling problems among adolescents throughout North America.

Level 1 gamblers, those who experience no symptoms, range from 77.9 percent to 83 percent of young people.[5] This estimate uses a variety of diagnostic criteria and includes data from several regions of North America. These data reveal that the majority of adolescents do not experience psychological or social symptomatology.

Level 2 gamblers represent a group of young people who rarely gain the attention of the general population. Level 2 gamblers—who have some symptomatology but do not meet diagnostic code—can be moving toward or away from more severe gambling problems. This group consists of 9.9 percent to 14.2 percent of young people. It is reasonable to assume that young people who have some gambling problems but are not identified by a diagnostic screen are nevertheless distracted from their homework, family chores, or social activities because of their gambling; they are not fully engaged in the kinds of things that ultimately would lead them to make scientific, professional, or other contributions to society. Consequently, Level 2 gamblers are emerging as an important and understudied segment of the population. We must not restrict our attention only to the minority of people diagnosed as pathological gamblers; we must begin to recognize the range of effects gambling has on gamblers and attend to nonpathological gamblers who have symptoms that compromise their ability to experience productive and satisfying lives.

Finally, this study revealed that between 4.4 percent and 7.4 percent of adolescents can be classified as Level 3 gamblers, that is, compulsive or pathological gamblers. No studies to date have investigated Level 4 gambling, but one report (Shaffer, LaBrie, Scanlan, & Cummings, 1994) indicates that approximately 4 percent of the

Table 0.1 *Classifications of Gambling Involvement*

Levels of Gambling Involvement and Experience	Operational Definition	Possible Education, Prevention, and Treatment Opportunities
0: Non-gambling	Individual never gambled	Educational awareness Primary prevention programs
1: Non-problem gambling	Individual gambled recreationally and does not experience any signs or symptoms of gambling-related disorder	Secondary prevention
2: In-transition gambling	Individual experiences symptoms or displays signs of problems related to gambling activity; may be progressing either *toward* more serious or intense symptoms (i.e., progression) or *away* from these symptoms (i.e., during recovery)	Tertiary prevention Early treatment to arrest progression Relapse-prevention activities to facilitate and sustain recovery
3: Gambling-related disorder with impairment	Individual meets diagnostic criteria (e.g., DMS-IV, MAGS, SOGS) for biologic, sociologic, or psychologic impairment	Tertiary prevention to minimize harm Treatment
4: Gambler who displays willingness to enter treatment	Individual displays interest in entering the health care domain (with or without existing obstacles)	Treatment Relapse prevention

Source: Shaffer & Hall, 1996.

adolescents studied had sought help for gambling-related problems. This estimate likely includes adolescents who do not meet Level 3 diagnostic criteria. Future studies should investigate Level 4 gambling further, since this information will allow policymakers and treatment providers to estimate the treatment costs associated with underage problem gambling.

Why Be Concerned about Youth Gambling?

Once initiated, many patterns of behavior are difficult to stop. For example, people who began smoking as adolescents represent the majority of adult smokers. Prevention efforts reveal that by reducing the onset of certain behaviors, the economics of health care can be improved greatly (Botvin, Baker, Dusenbury, Botvin, & Diaz, 1995). To minimize the difficulties that problematic behaviors pose for society— drinking, substance use, smoking, or gambling-related problems—we must either *prevent or delay the onset* of these behavior patterns or *minimize the negative consequences* of involvement. To accomplish either of these objectives for gambling-related problems, it is essential to understand how young people begin to gamble.

INITIATION TO GAMBLING

Knowing how children begin gambling can provide clues to when, where, and how society should direct efforts to educate children about gambling. For example, recent research (Vagge, 1996) shows that many young people have their first gambling experience with friends, indicating that the peer group plays a vital role in the development of gambling behavior. Attempts to curb gambling among adolescents must address the issue of peer pressure and the general attitude of acceptance that young people seem to have toward gambling among their friends. Yet even more children begin gambling with a family member than with a friend, so family education must become the centerpiece of any prevention effort.

Most youths are initiated to gambling through sports betting, card playing, or the state lottery (Vagge, 1996). Research also suggests that most children generally start betting with relatively small amounts of money. Although many people may feel that such activities are harmless, educators should be aware that these situations provide children with their first exposure to the world of gambling. Any attempts to teach young people about the dangers of gambling must be realistic and take into account the methods by which children learn to gamble.

Educational programs must also consider how children view their initial gambling experience. Research indicates that young people tend to think very positively about their first few experiences with gambling. Most believe that they won the first few times they placed a bet (Vagge, 1996). Therefore, educational programs about gambling must make an effort to inject a dose of statistical reality into young people's thinking about gambling and risk taking. In comparison with other areas of youth behavior, little research has been conducted on how children become involved in gambling. More information about what first attracts children to the world of financial risk taking will prove helpful in determining the factors that make this world attractive to children.

PSYCHOSOCIAL CONSEQUENCES OF EXCESSIVE GAMBLING

Gambling is neither financially nor psychologically risk free. In addition to the possibility of losing their money, gamblers also risk experiencing a variety of psychological, social, and biological consequences. Given the increasing exposure and access to gambling in general and state lotteries in particular, public health researchers, clinicians, and policymakers should continue to expand their investigations of the impact of legalized gambling on the development of children and adolescents. Although gambling is still seen as an entertaining recreational activity, numerous studies show the serious consequences of addiction to gambling (Frank, Lester, & Wexler, 1991; Lesieur & Rosenthal, 1991; Jacobs et al., 1989). As the popularity of legalized gambling grows, greater attention is being directed to the public health risks and the economic, legal, and social costs of expanded gambling (Eadington, 1994).

Shaffer, Hall, Walsh, and Vander Bilt (1995) examined some of the adverse consequences often faced by young people who gamble. Their study revealed a wide range of detrimental social and emotional consequences of gambling among its student sample. The pathological gamblers experienced a variety of problems: 89 percent were preoccupied with gambling; 85 percent chased their losses; 83 percent increased the amount they were gambling to get the same effect as they experienced at a lower level of betting; 79 percent gambled to escape problems or relieve feelings of helplessness, guilt, anxiety, or depression; 79 percent lied to conceal the extent of their gambling; 79 percent engaged in illegal behaviors to finance gambling; 71 percent had problems at home, work, or school because of gambling; 71 percent got in trouble because of gambling; 68 percent neglected their home, work, or school obligations for at least two consecutive days because of gambling; 68 percent jeopardized or lost a significant relationship, job, or educational or career opportunity because of gambling; 64 percent felt pressure to gamble when they did not gamble; 64 percent were unable to stop gambling when they wanted; 61 percent felt pressure to increase the amount they gamble; 54 percent were arrested for gambling; 43 percent felt guilty about their gambling; and 39 percent sought help for their gambling problem.

However, pathological gamblers are not the only people who experience problems as a result of their gambling. These same problems exist among young people who are not pathological gamblers. For example, Shaffer et al. (1995) reported that 28 percent of youthful gamblers who failed to meet diagnostic code admitted to "chasing" their losses, and an alarming 16 percent of these young people reported having experienced some physiological symptoms (i.e., tolerance) related to their gambling. For nonpathological gamblers (adolescents who fail to satisfy diagnostic criteria), the prevalence of psychological distress related to gambling is similar to the rates of alcohol dependence—yet the resources allocated to gambling-related problems are sparse by comparison.

PHYSIOLOGICAL ELEMENTS OF PATHOLOGICAL GAMBLING

Recent physiological theories of gambling are beginning to support the psychosocial patterns identified among pathological gamblers. Recent research found preliminary evidence for the hypothesis that significantly more pathological gamblers than controls had a variant of the dopamine D2 receptor gene (DRD2), suggesting that pathological gambling may have an important genetic component (Comings et al., 1994). Empirical evidence also supports the notion that regular gamblers experience arousal when they are engaged in gambling, and studies have demonstrated that arousal may be the prime reinforcer for gamblers (Griffiths, 1995).

In another study, male pathological gamblers had significantly lower platelet MAO (monoamine oxidase) activity than a comparison group (Blanco, Orensanz-Muñoz, Blanco-Jerez, & Saiz-Ruiz, 1996). These researchers speculated that changes in platelet MAO activity may be a sign of serotonergic dysfunction. Other preliminary research indicates the possibility of a direct connection between brain serotonin levels and pathological gambling (Carlton & Manowitz, 1987). In addition, preliminary research suggests that certain subgroups of pathological gamblers, such as horse-race gamblers, have significantly lower levels of B-endorphin (a combination of endogenous opiates) than other gamblers and controls (Blaszczynski, McConaghy, & Winter, 1986; Pratt, Maltzman, Hauprich, & Ziskind, 1982). These studies offer preliminary evidence of the physiological (genetic, neurochemical, and hormonal) elements of compulsive gambling.[6]

GAMBLING AS AN OBJECT OF ADDICTION

We can advance our conceptual understanding of addiction by considering the objects of addiction to be those things or activities that reliably and robustly shift subjective experience. The most reliable and robust "shifters" hold the greatest potential to stimulate the development of addictive disorders. Psychoactive drugs, gambling, and certain other activities correlate highly with addictive behaviors because these activities reliably shift subjective states. The strength and consistency of any activity's capacity to shift subjective states will vary across individuals. In spite of this variation, psychoactive drug use and gambling are sufficiently reliable shifters of subjective states that this model of addiction will continue to rank these experiences high among addiction objects. Epstein (1989) described the subjective experience of neurochemical shifts, that is, dopamine release, stimulated by gambling:

> Gambling is personal. It is associated with our status in life. No activity has
> been more rationalized than gambling—odds figured, probabilities worked

out, point spreads meticulously established—and no activity, surely, is finally more irrational. In this essentially irrational activity, the first item that must be fixed, and with some precision, is the stake. Above all, it cannot be too little; *it must be enough to stimulate whatever those spiritual glands are that gambling calls into action* [emphasis added]. The punishment must fit the crime; the agony of losing must be roughly equivalent to the ecstasy of winning. In this sense, it becomes clear that no bet can ever be too large; and herein lies the madness inherent in gambling, for the more you have, the more you need to risk. (p. 100)

Shaffer (1994) reports that of six illicit activities investigated among a sample of Massachusetts students in grades seven through twelve, the lifetime prevalence of gambling activity was exceeded only by the lifetime rate of alcohol use. Gambling may be one contemporary way that young people initiate shifts in consciousness. While shifting subjective states is a common phenomenon, particularly among young people, gambling and drugs pose significant risk to those who engage in these activities. For example, Shaffer et al. (1995) report that 69 percent of students who satisfied the DSM-IV criteria for pathological gambling reported that the same amount of gambling had less effect on them than it had previously; 83 percent increased the amount they were gambling to get the same effect as they experienced at a lower level of betting; 77 percent got restless, irritable, and had difficulty concentrating when they stopped gambling; and 54 percent continued to gamble to make withdrawal symptoms go away. These symptoms represent neuro-adaptive patterns much like those observed among people with substance dependence disorders. In a process similar to withdrawal among the chemically dependent, pathological gamblers can make their symptoms go away by gambling again. Like psychoactive stimulant abuse, gambling can influence the central nervous system in powerful ways.

Conceptual Problems with Measuring Pathological Gambling

One of the first matters of business is to determine the prevalence of gambling disorders. However, identifying rates of problems that evidence relatively low base rates in the population, like problem gambling, poses a challenging research task. Gambling prevalence studies measure the percentage of a population that fit certain gambling-related criteria for a specific period of time. Both household surveys and school surveys may underestimate the prevalence of problem gambling because of the likelihood that people with gambling problems will not be at home to answer the phone or in school to complete the survey at the time chosen to conduct the study. That is, individuals with gambling problems are likely to be out gambling or engaging in behaviors that are associated with gambling, for example, drinking, skipping

school, trying to get funds to support gambling. People ravaged by gambling problems may not even have working telephones at their disposal. Adequate estimates
of the prevalence of intemperate gambling require a family of special studies in addition to the traditional telephone surveys. For example, it is time to begin studying
homeless, incarcerated, mentally ill, and other special populations to determine their
rates of gambling problems.

Gambling incidence studies describe the frequency of occurrence of new problem
gambling cases during a specified time period. Almost all of the extant disordered
gambling studies are prevalence rather than incidence studies (National Research
Council, 1999), perhaps because incidence studies require a greater investment of
time and resources. Thus, little is known about the rate at which problem gambling
is increasing (or decreasing). Prevalence studies that sample the same population at
two distinct points in time, for example, now and two years from now, most often
use two different samples from the same population because of the difficulty of
tracking the original respondents for the second study. Although the use of two different samples is more practical, this method results in an inability to be confident
that the measured change in prevalence accurately reflects any changes in the existing estimates.

All our efforts to measure the prevalence and incidence of gambling-related disorders require a multi-trait multi-method strategy (Campbell & Fiske, 1959). Researchers must employ several methods and different instruments to determine if
these techniques yield similar or different results. As these various methods narrow
the range of estimates, we can become more confident that these estimates reflect
valid prevalence and incidence rates (e.g., Shaffer, Hall, & Vander Bilt, 1997, 1999).

SENSITIVITY AND SPECIFICITY OF GAMBLING SCREEN MEASURES

The degree to which any screening instrument correctly classifies those with gambling problems as "cases" (sensitivity) and those without gambling problems as
"noncases" (specificity) depends on where the researchers draw the line for classification. That is, if the criteria that a respondent needs to meet to qualify as a "case"
are very stringent (8 out of 10 criteria), the sensitivity will be decreased and the
specificity will be increased. If the criteria are relaxed (4 out of 10 criteria), sensitivity will increase and specificity will decrease. Thus, making decisions about criteria for case definition has important implications for estimates of problem gambling.

DRAWING THE CONCEPTUAL LINE: MORE SENSITIVE INSTRUMENTS
FOR YOUTHFUL GAMBLERS

Problem gambling exists on a continuum. Unlike some biological conditions that are
either present or absent, such as pregnancy, problem gambling is syndromal and
manifests an array of problems that can vary in severity from minor to severe. Thus,
before a diagnosis of pathological gambling can be made, clinicians and researchers

establish cutoff points that separate at-risk gamblers from pathological gamblers. The placement of this cutoff point is determined, in part, by issues related to sensitivity and specificity. To illustrate: While a *less* sensitive measure would reduce the number of adolescents who might be stigmatized by a pathological gambler label, it would also reduce the opportunity for early identification of gambling problems. Restricting early identification compromises the opportunity for primary and secondary prevention as well as treatment efforts.

Conversely, a *more* sensitive measure of gambling problems would increase the magnitude of the observed difficulties among adolescent gamblers and give advance warning of these developing problems, creating the opportunity for more focused education, prevention, and treatment programs. The decision to employ a more- or less-sensitive measure should take into account the purposes of the prevalence estimate. An appropriate estimate of problem gambling among youth, who are more vulnerable to gambling-related problems than are their adult counterparts, would capture more than only the most severe problems. Thus, screening measures for youthful gamblers, while being careful not to exaggerate the nature of existing problems, should aim for moderately high sensitivity by relaxing the criteria used to distinguish a pathological gambler from a problem gambler.

Prospects for Gambling Prevention and Education Programs

To best develop and apply prevention and education programs that will protect young people from gambling-related problems, it is essential to avoid some of the obstacles that have limited the efficacy of similar programs in the drug and alcohol field (Ellickson, 1995). For example, school systems currently deliver most alcohol and other drug prevention programs. By locating prevention programs only in school systems, already overburdened school faculty are faced with the demands of learning about new topics beyond their areas of specialization. Furthermore,

> current health promotion strategies focus primarily on specific individual lifestyle practices that are known risk factors for disease and attempt to change these practices with the goal of decreasing morbidity and mortality. The main responsibility for behavior change is placed solely upon the individual. The rationale for this approach is that individuals, once informed of their risk, will adopt or modify behaviors to lower that risk. Although the expansion in recent years of health promotion efforts to include families, peer groups, work groups, and to some extent communities, is encouraging, the dominant focus continues to be on providing individuals with information, knowledge or skills so they can avoid or modify high-risk characteristics. This individual approach is limited because it is expensive, does little to address those factors in the environment that contribute to disease risk, and is

ineffective with diseases having high prevalences. (Wallack & Winkleby, 1987, p. 925)

To be effective, gambling prevention programs must move beyond the individual intervention strategy Wallack described and gain broad-based community support. Parents, government, criminal justice, sports organizations, media, religious organizations, and other community groups provide important opportunities for prevention intervention. By integrating all of the available community resources, gambling prevention programs can become more effective than current research has shown other addiction prevention efforts to be.

In large part, communities have not rallied around prevention efforts because there is insufficient scientific research identifying prevention programs that produce convincing positive effects. However, new work (Botvin, Baker, Dusenbury, Botvin, & Diaz, 1995) has identified characteristics of successful prevention programs. For example, prevention programs must implement activities guided by models that are relevant to the specific needs of the program's target population. When decision-makers select a proper model for their prevention program, they often fail to implement the model as it was designed. When a properly matched program is implemented adequately, Botvin et al. suggest that the positive effects may only be moderate and short-lived. Therefore, effective community prevention programs will require a long-term commitment—not just an effort when gambling trends are high or begin to move upward. There must be an ongoing effort to deliver an adequate "dose" of prevention and then an ongoing program of "booster" sessions that will sustain the positive dose-related effects at least through the high school years.

Specific characteristics of effective drug and alcohol prevention programs (Botvin et al., 1995; Ellickson, 1995) are also essential to gambling prevention programs. Successful prevention efforts are multifaceted, repetitive, include both information and skills, and are matched both to young people's developmental stage and to their place within the natural history of addiction. In addition, effective prevention programs match activities to the specific objects of addiction and integrate the educational information and program activities with both the immediate and more-distant social setting, that is, social policies, mores, and folkways. Finally, successful programs recognize the importance of using appropriate outcome measures—not simply whether young people ever gamble during their lifetime. Measuring efficacy is of great importance; the following discussion considers this issue in more detail.

PREVENTION AND OUTCOME MEASURES

Prevention programs can achieve a variety of positive objectives. However, to achieve this array of objectives, prevention programs require a set of outcome measures rather than a single outcome index. For example, effective gambling prevention programs should fulfill the following fundamental objectives: First, they should prevent or delay the onset of gambling behaviors; second, if gambling has occurred, the program should delay the onset of any harms that may result from gambling; and third, if gambling-related harms are present, the program should arrest or delay these harms in progression and scope. Prevention programs that focus on these objectives can be implemented across a variety of community institutions such as prisons and schools. By weaving these programs into the fabric of a community, we can prevent the development of some gambling patterns, help limit relapse when gambling-related problems have been effectively treated, and encourage early recovery, that is, tertiary prevention, when gambling has been excessive.[7]

However, we must recognize that, like efforts to treat alcohol and drug abuse, efforts to prevent the onset of gambling—as well as efforts to prevent the harms associated with gambling and arrest the progression of adversity once a pattern of problem gambling has been established—can have advantages as well as disadvantages. Under every circumstance, communities must be wary and watchful that prevention efforts do not inadvertently stimulate gambling behavior or the potential harms associated with gambling activities. Although the array of prevention programs designed to limit the development of drug and alcohol use has increased during the past two decades, there remains a paucity of rigorous community program evaluation. In some cases, programs designed to prevent drug use have stimulated such use instead (Ellickson, 1995). Therefore, in spite of any existing face validity, prevention programs always require careful evaluation. Absent careful monitoring, communities risk violating the first principle of medical ethics to "do no harm." A commitment to ongoing program evaluation is one essential mechanism in this effort.

EDUCATION: CONSIDERING THE MATHEMATICS OF GAMBLING

One potentially important component of youth education in the area of gambling is instruction on the mathematics of gambling. Probability and number sense are two important requirements for contemporary living. The National Research Council stresses the importance of these areas: "To function in today's society, mathematical literacy (of which number sense is a component) is as essential as verbal literacy. [But] numeracy requires more than just familiarity with numbers. To cope confidently with the demands of today's society, one must be able to grasp the implications of many mathematical concepts—for example, chance" (National Research Council, 1989, as cited in Crites, 1994, p. 203).

Adolescents confronted with increasing opportunities to gamble often lack the skills necessary to apply mathematical reasoning to existing and new gambling situations. In addition, research has indicated that adolescents who believe gambling involves a high degree of skill are more likely to be pathological gamblers than those who correctly identify gambling as being mostly chance related (Vagge, 1996). Innovative curricula can provide young people with the critical thinking and mathematical skills necessary to make informed decisions and choices about gambling activities. Examples of this type of curriculum can be found in chapter 4, "What Are My Chances? Using Probability and Number Sense to Educate Teens About the Mathematical Risks of Gambling," by Terry Crites, as well as in Shaffer, Hall, & Vander Bilt (2000) and Svendsen & Griffin (1994).

In addition to educating adolescents about important mathematical topics such as probability and statistics, these curricula may have the potential to improve students' knowledge about gambling and decrease the likelihood of problem gambling behaviors. Well-designed program evaluations, as described previously, must be conducted to identify the full range of effects these curricula have on adolescents. For example, evaluation research must determine if any iatrogenic effects emerge from exposure to these programs. Iatrogenic effects result when programs designed to reduce or prevent a particular problem—in this case, excessive gambling—inadvertently increase the target behavior instead.

Identifying the Stakeholders: Getting Everyone to the Table
YOUTH AND PROBLEM GAMBLING HURT THE FABRIC OF SOCIETY
Problem gambling is not simply an emotional, physical, or economic problem for the individual. Problem gambling strains the economy of society. Distracted from many of the tasks of daily living, problem gamblers—adolescent and adult—are less productive students, workers, and family members. In every aspect of daily living, problem gamblers have less to give because some part of their being is preoccupied with gambling or recovering from gambling-related debts. The result can be lost productivity and increased emotional distress, physical illness, family problems, and crime. Problem gamblers lose the precious time of their lives. Lessons remain unlearned, projects unfinished, relationships unfulfilled. The result is that society loses its most valuable assets, the fruits of human creativity and productivity.

YOUTH AND PROBLEM GAMBLING HURT THE GAMING INDUSTRY
While it seems obvious that a social problem like excessive gambling is destructive for society, it is not readily apparent to most observers that underage and disordered gambling also hurt the gaming industry. The presence of these problems produces an unpleasant environment for other patrons, diminishes customers' unstated sense of trust in the gaming facility that is necessary for patrons to believe they have an honest chance to win, and increases the likelihood of legal sanctions and legal fees that unnecessarily inflate the cost of doing business. Like any business, particularly any business associated with entertainment, a negative and uncomfortable experience diminishes consumer satisfaction and participation. Gambling in the presence of minors or intemperate gamblers is disquieting and disturbing. It can lead recreational gamblers to question the nature of their behavior. The result can be diminished gambling.

Furthermore, if consumers identify a specific setting or purveyor of gambling as untrustworthy, they will also be less likely to participate in games of chance. Similarly, the vast majority of adult gamblers will be distracted—if not preoccupied—by the presence of minors during their gambling experience. Finally, legal sanctions against gambling establishments that permit participation by minors are likely to increase as gaming proliferates and regulatory bodies become more attentive to the problems associated with underage gambling. Extensive legal battles become a cost of doing business that few industries can endure. Furthermore, problem gamblers are not reliable customers. They sometimes engage in illicit activities that can stimulate bad press and ill will among the public. Self-destructive gamblers do not encourage gambling among recreational gamblers. Ultimately, underage and problem gamblers will hurt the gaming industry.

New Social Policies

The federal government, acting on a growing concern over the societal impacts of the ever-expanding opportunities to gamble, established the National Gambling Impact Study Commission. Over a period of two years, the nine-member commission conducted "a comprehensive legal and factual study of the social and economic impacts of gambling in the United States on federal, state, local, and Native American tribal governments and on communities and social institutions generally, including individuals, families, and businesses within such communities and institutions" (National Gambling Impact and Policy Commission Act of 1996). The commission assessed pathological or problem gambling, including its effect on individuals, families, businesses, social institutions, and the economy (National Gambling Impact Study Commission, 1999). The work of this commission holds the promise of new awareness, research, and social policies that will help us better address and guide the impact of gambling on American society.

On the Nature and Organization of this Book

This volume represents an important historical moment. For the first time, researchers in the field of adolescent gambling, clinicians, lawyers, politicians, and representatives of the gambling industry collectively recognize and address the issue of youth gambling in a single volume. The contributors to this work are diverse; readers may experience these voices as inconsistent. While edited volumes present a challenge to editors and readers alike, in this instance, the richness, depth, and intellectual stimulation of this collection far outweighs the variations of contributor style and perspective. We think that these differences are best thought of as the collaborative architecture from which a stable design emerges.

Section and Chapter Introductions

In the first chapter, Howard Shaffer discusses the emergence of gambling behavior among youth and some of the consequences of this behavior. The author describes the prevalence of illicit substance use and lottery involvement among a sample of adolescents and shows the similarities between the patterns of involvement in these two activities. The author then reviews data revealing the current social pressures that encourage gambling and the social and emotional consequences of gambling experiences. Finally, Shaffer considers some recent studies that reveal the factors associated with the initiation of gambling behavior.

Darryl Zitzow reviews the unique situation of American Indian populations with respect to gambling. He discusses the positive as well as the negative consequences of gambling for American Indians. Finally, Zitzow presents the research conducted on risk factors for problem and pathological gambling among American Indians, as well as the findings of preliminary prevalence studies among these populations.

Wayne Yorke provides an overview of gambling in Canada and discusses the ways in which gambling has affected Canadian society and Canadian youth. After presenting a history of gambling in Canada, Yorke discusses the current levels of gambling expenditures by Canadian citizens and compares these figures with the corresponding figures from the United States. Yorke then reviews the literature on the nature and prevalence of gambling problems in Canada, focusing on studies of adolescents. The chapter concludes with a list of recommendations for increasing our understanding of gambling and its effects, improving public awareness of potential problems that may emerge as a consequence of gambling, and implementing programs to prevent gambling-related problems.

Terry Crites approaches gambling as an opportunity to educate children in the area of probability. Using mathematical principles, Crites demonstrates how to calculate the probability of winning the lottery, keno, roulette, and craps. In addition, Crites discusses some common myths and misperceptions about gambling and probability and concludes by presenting a range of specific hands-on activities related to probability and gambling, which teachers can use in the classroom.

Sirgay Sanger directs his attention to treatment issues for adolescents with gambling problems. Sanger provides an in-depth discussion and analysis of specific clinical concepts and techniques related to the treatment of adolescents with gambling problems. Sanger covers a wide range of topics related to therapy for youth problem gamblers, focusing his discussion on dissociation—the psychological process that is prevalent among adolescents and precedes problem gambling. In addition, Sanger provides a practical guide to broader mental health treatment for adolescents, including topics such as creating a therapeutic alliance, providing motivation for therapy, addressing family patterns of guilt and shame, and handling ambivalence and resistance.

Joni Vander Bilt and Joanna Franklin examine the impact of problem gambling on the family of the problem gambler. In addition, these authors discuss a range of issues related to therapy for problem gamblers and their family members. This chapter begins by examining the consequences of youth problem gambling for adolescents and the consequences of adult problem gambling for the partner/spouse and children. The authors then review the literature on family violence and discuss gambling-related studies that suggest a possible connection between problem gambling and family violence. The potential similarities between pathological gambling and violence as impulse-control disorders and the possible links among pathological gambling, violence, and substance abuse are examined. The authors conclude their literature review with a discussion of the range of research questions that require future research.

The second half of the chapter discusses a range of issues related to the treatment of disordered gamblers and their families. The authors present specific strategies and techniques for therapy and discuss treatment of problem-gambling youths, treatment of children of problem gamblers, family therapy, and common mistakes made by counselors providing youth and family therapy. The authors conclude the chapter with suggestions for the direction of future research on youth and the family.

I. Nelson Rose, one of the country's leading experts on gambling law, presents a comprehensive discussion of the law as it relates to underage gambling. Rose begins by discussing the philosophy of setting age limits for potentially dangerous activities and the benefits and problems inherent in creating a discrete cutoff point for these activities. He then outlines the history of age limits for potentially dangerous activities in the United States, comparing gambling with other activities such as drinking alcohol. In this discussion, Rose outlines the role played by politics and major societal events in changing the age limits for activities like drinking. Rose concludes the chapter with a discussion of the enforcement of age minimums for gambling, and recommends age limits for gambling. The chapter includes a detailed, state-by-state analysis of age restrictions for gambling.

William Eadington discusses some of the economic, social, and psychological aspects of gambling that make it attractive to youths. Eadington presents the theory that children become involved in gambling as a result of the desire to extend the "fantasy principle" and omnipotence of childhood into adulthood. Eadington further hypothesizes that the economic environment confronting contemporary adolescents—including diminished career opportunities, Social Security and Medicare crises, and mounting taxes—makes this group less likely to pursue goals through education, hard work, and saving and more likely to pursue pleasure recklessly and hedonistically. This chapter ends by suggesting that educators take advantage of youths' interest in gambling by using this topic to teach probability and statistics.

Joe Malone, Eric Turner, Tom Brosig, and Phil Satre represent the public and the private gaming industries' perspectives on the issue of youth gambling. Joe Malone, former Massachusetts State Lottery Commission chairman, and Eric Turner, former executive director of the Massachusetts State Lottery Commission, present two public-gaming perspectives on youth-gambling issues. Both authors begin with discussions of how their personal backgrounds have affected their outlooks on gambling in general and youth gambling in particular. The authors then discuss the conflicting aims of raising money for the state and protecting the state's citizens from gambling-related problems. Both authors also discuss the range of initiatives the Common-wealth of Massachusetts has taken to prevent lottery sales to youths, to educate youths, and to raise public awareness. Malone and Turner conclude with a discussion of their goals for the state's role in preventing youth problem gambling in the future.

Phil Satre presents his views on the industry's responsibility in the area of under-age gambling and discusses the initiatives designed by Harrah's casinos to prevent underage gambling and its associated problems. Satre discusses the role casinos and other members of the gambling industry must play in preventing underage gambling, as well as the responsibility that parents, educators, and policymakers have to address this problem. Satre describes Project 21, Harrah's innovative program to prevent underage gambling in its casinos and to raise public awareness on the issues related to youth gambling. Satre discusses the success of this program and its growth into a multistate initiative. In addition, Satre discusses Harrah's efforts to involve other companies in this initiative and cites examples of other casino companies that recently have made similar successful efforts. Satre concludes by recommending four specific commitments that all members of the casino industry should make.

In chapter 10, Tom Brosig, former president of Grand Casinos Inc., describes the history of Grand Casino's involvement with initiatives to prevent problem gambling. Brosig begins by discussing the process by which he and Grand Casinos Inc. first became aware of problem gambling within its casinos and the first steps the company took to address these issues. Brosig describes his own increasing involvement in these initiatives, from consulting the North American Training Institute[8] and helping to plan the Minnesota Public Policy Think Tank, to raising funds for the North American Think Tank on Youth Gambling Issues and acting as chairman of the Policy Board on Youth Gambling Issues. Throughout the chapter, Brosig presents his thoughts on the role the casino industry should play in addressing problem gambling.

Henry Lesieur reviews the existing literature on youth gambling, examines the gaps that exist in the field, and makes suggestions for future research. Lesieur emphasizes studies of youth problem gambling, the range of gambling problems, risk factors, definitional issues, and related topics. In addition, Lesieur reviews the existing investigations into the prevention and treatment of problem gambling among teens. He concludes by outlining the areas of needed research and suggesting a more inclusive multifactorial model of inquiry.

In the epilogue, Durand Jacobs reviews trends in youth gambling during the past decade and discusses the issues that must be addressed in the future. The appendix presents the final report of the proceedings of the North American Think Tank on Youth Gambling Issues. This report summarizes the issues identified during the think tank and the recommendations made by think tank participants in the areas of policy, funding, law enforcement, research, treatment, education, and public awareness.

Notes

1. Speech in Detroit, Mich., July 27, 1965. Cited in Andrews (1993).

2. "The Precarious Vogue of Ingmar Bergman" (first published in *Esquire* April 1960; reprinted in *Nobody Knows My Name,* 1961). Cited in Andrews (1993).

3. This book, like the think tank from which it was derived, is limited to youth gambling in North America. For an excellent discussion of youth gambling that focuses on the United Kingdom, see Griffiths (1995).

4. Adapted from National Gambling Impact and Policy Commission Act of 1996, Pub. L. No. 104–69.

5. This range represents a 95 percent confidence interval; in addition, the ranges corresponding to Levels 2 and 3 also represent a 95 percent confidence interval.

6. For an broad overview of physiological as well as other theories of gambling and pathological gambling, see Griffiths (1995).

7. See Korn and Shaffer (in press) for a detailed account of how public health strategies can influence prevention and treatment efforts.

8. In 1995, the board of the Minnesota Council on Compulsive Gambling changed the organization's name to the North American Training Institute to better reflect its services.

References

American Psychiatric Association. (2000). *Diagnostic and statistical manual of mental disorders*—text revision. 4th edition. Washington, DC: American Psychiatric Association.

American Psychiatric Association. (1994). *Diagnostic and statistical manual of mental disorders.* 4th edition. Washington, DC: Author.

Andrews, R. (Ed.). (1993). *The Columbia dictionary of quotations.* [Microsoft Bookshelf '95 CD-ROM]. New York: Columbia University Press.

Blanco, C., Orensanz-Muñoz, L., Blanco-Jerez, C., & Saiz-Ruiz, J. (1996). Pathological gambling and platelet MAO activity: A psychobiological study. *American Journal of Psychiatry, 153,* 119–21.

Blaszczynski, A. P., McConaghy, N., & Winter, S. W. (1986). Plasma endorphin levels in pathological gambling. *Journal of Gambling Behavior, 2,* 3–14.

Botvin, G. J., Baker, E., Dusenbury, L., Botvin, E. M., & Diaz, T. (1995). Long-term follow-up results of a randomized drug abuse prevention trial in a white middle-class population. *Journal of the American Medical Association, 273* (14), 1106–12.

Campbell, D. T., & Fiske, D. W. (1959). Convergent and discriminant validation by the multitrait-multimethod matrix. *Psychological Bulletin, 56,* 81–105.

Carlton, P. L., & Manowitz, P. (1987). Physiological factors as determinants of pathological gambling. *Journal of Gambling Behavior, 3,* 274–85.

Christiansen, E. M. (1996). The United States '95 gross annual wager. *Gaming & Wagering Business, 17* (8), 55–92.

Clotfelter, C. T., & Cook, P. J. (1989). *Selling hope: State lotteries in America.* Cambridge: Harvard University Press.

Comings, D. E., Rosenthal, R. J., Lesieur, H. R., Rugle, L. J., Muhleman, D., Chiu, C., Dietz, G., & Gade, R. (1994, June). The molecular genetics of pathological gambling: The DRD2 gene. Paper presented at the Ninth International Conference on Gambling and Risk Taking, Las Vegas, NV. (Cited in Griffiths, 1995.)

Crites, T. (1994). Using lotteries to improve students' number sense and understanding of probability. *School Science and Mathematics, 94,* 203–7.

Eadington, W. R. (1992, October 27). Emerging public policy challenges from the proliferation of gaming in America. Paper presented at the Second Annual Australian Conference on Casinos and Gaming, Sydney, Australia.

Eadington, W. R. (1994, May). Understanding gambling. Keynote address, Ninth International Conference on Gambling and Risk Taking, Las Vegas, NV.

Ellickson, P. L. (1995). Schools. In R. H. Coombs & D. Ziedonis (Eds.), *Handbook on drug abuse prevention* (pp. 93–120). Boston: Allyn & Bacon.

Epstein, J. (1989). Confessions of a low roller. In R. Atwan (Ed.), *The best American essays 1989* (pp. 98–113). New York: Ticknor & Fields.

Frank, M. L., Lester, D., & Wexler, A. (1991). Suicidal behavior among members of Gamblers Anonymous. *Journal of Gambling Studies, 7,* 249–54.

Griffiths, M. (1995). *Adolescent gambling.* London: Routledge.

Hernandez, R. (1996, April 18). Pataki finds lottery ads too rich for good taste. *New York Times,* p. 5, col. 5.

International Game Technology. (1995). *Gaming in the United States.* [Brochure.] Las Vegas, NV: Author.

Jacobs, D. F., Marston, A. R., Singer, R. D., Widaman, K., Little, T., & Veizades, J. (1989). Children of problem gamblers. *Journal of Gambling Behavior, 5,* 261–68.

Korn, D., & Shaffer, H. J. (in press). Gambling and the health of the public: Adopting a public health perspective. *Journal of Gambling Studies.*

Lesieur, H. R. (1988). Altering the DSM-III criteria for pathological gambling. *Journal of Gambling Behavior, 4,* 38–47.

Lesieur, H. R., & Rosenthal, R. J. (1991). Pathological gambling: A review of the literature. (Prepared for the American Psychiatric Association Task Force on DSM-IV Committee on Disorders of Impulse Control Not Elsewhere Classified.) *Journal of Gambling Studies, 7,* 5–40.

McCormick, R. A., Russo, A. M., Ramirez, L. F., & Taber, J. I. (1984). Affective disorders among pathological gamblers seeking treatment. *American Journal of Psychiatry, 141,* 215–18.

National Council on Problem Gambling, Inc. (1993, November 1). *The need for a national policy on problem and pathological gambling in America.* New York: Author.

National Gambling Impact Study Commission. (1999). *National Gambling Impact Study Commission report.* Washington, DC: Author.

National Gambling Impact and Policy Commission Act of 1996, Pub. L. No. 104–169.

National Research Council. (1999). *Pathological gambling: A critical review.* Washington DC: National Academy Press.

North American Gaming Report 1996. (1996, July). *International Gaming & Wagering Business, 17* (7), S3–S38.

Pratt, M., Maltzman, I., Hauprich, W., & Ziskind, E. (1982). Electrodermal activity of sociopaths and controls in the pressor test. *Psychophysiology, 19,* 342.

Ramirez, L. F., McCormick, R. A., Russo, A., & Taber, J. I. (1983). Patterns of substance abuse in pathological gamblers undergoing treatment. *Addictive Behaviors, 8,* 425–28.

Rose, I. N. (1995). Gambling and the law: Endless fields of dreams. *Journal of Gambling Studies, 11,* 15–33.

Shaffer, H. J. (1994). *The emergence of youthful addiction: The prevalence of underage lottery use and the impact of gambling* (Technical Report No. 011394-100). Boston: Massachusetts Council on Compulsive Gambling.

Shaffer, H. J. (1997a). The most important unresolved issue in the addictions: Conceptual chaos. *Substance Use & Misuse, 32,* 1573–80.

Shaffer, H. J. (1997b). Understanding the means and objects of addiction: Technology, the Internet, and gambling. *Journal of Gambling Studies, 12,* 461–69.

Shaffer, H. J. (1999). Strange bedfellows: A critical view of pathological gambling and addiction. *Addiction, 94* (10), 1445–48.

Shaffer, H. J., & Hall, M. N. (1996). Estimating the prevalence of adolescent gambling disorders: A quantitative synthesis and guide toward standard gambling nomenclature. *Journal of Gambling Studies, 12,* 193–214.

Shaffer, H. J., Hall, M. N., & Vander Bilt, J. (2000). *Probability, statistics & number sense in gambling and everyday life: A contemporary mathematics curriculum.* Boston: Harvard Medical School Division on Addictions.

Shaffer, H. J., Hall, M. N., & Vander Bilt, J. (1997). *Estimating the prevalence of disordered gambling behavior in the United States and Canada: A meta-analysis.* Boston: Presidents and Fellows of Harvard College.

Shaffer, H. J., Hall, M. N., & Vander Bilt, J. (1999). Estimating the prevalence of disordered gambling behavior in the United States and Canada: A research synthesis. *American Journal of Public Health, 89,* 1369–76.

Shaffer, H. J., Hall, M. N., Walsh, J. S., & Vander Bilt, J. (1995). The psychosocial consequences of gambling. In R. Tannenwald (Ed.), *Casino development: How would casinos affect New England's economy. Special Report No. 2* (pp. 130–41). Boston: Federal Reserve Bank of Boston.

Shaffer, H. J., LaBrie, R., Scanlan, K. M., & Cummings, T. (1994). Pathological gambling among adolescents: Massachusetts Gambling Screen (MAGS). *Journal of Gambling Studies, 10,* 339–62.

Subcommittee on Intergovernmental Relations of the Committee on Governmental Affairs. (1985). *State lotteries: An overview.* Washington DC: United States Printing Office.

Svendsen, R., & Griffin, T. (1994). *Improving your odds: A curriculum about winning, losing, and staying out of trouble with gambling.* Anoka, MN: Minnesota Institute of Public Health.

U.S. Census Bureau. (1996). *U.S. Census Bureau: The official statistics.* [http://www. census.gov].

Vagge, L. M. (1996). The development of youth gambling. Unpublished honors thesis, Harvard-Radcliffe Colleges, Cambridge, MA.

Wallack, L., & Winkleby, M. (1987). Primary prevention: A new look at basic concepts. *Social Science and Medicine, 25,* 923–30.

Wray, I., & Dickerson, M. (1981). Cessation of high frequency gambling and "withdrawal" symptoms. *British Journal of Addiction, 76,* 401–5.

Chapter One

The Emergence of Gambling Among Youth

The Prevalence of Underage Lottery Use and the Impact of Gambling

Howard J. Shaffer

Introduction

During the past decade, the proliferation of American gambling has been extraordinary. In addition to the recent availability of riverboat, Native American, and urban casinos, the lottery has become a staple of American gambling. In spite of warnings from both scholars (Eadington, 1992; Shaffer, Stein, Gambino, & Cummings, 1989) and social policymakers regarding the potential adverse consequences of the spread of gambling, the lure of state-sponsored gambling's capacity to generate revenue without imposing a tax has shifted American morality not only to tolerate but to endorse legalized gambling.

Between 1974 and 1995, the total amount of money legally wagered nationwide increased from $17.3 billion to $550 billion (Commission on the Review of the National Policy Toward Gambling, 1976; Christiansen, 1996). Between 1975 and 1985, the national per capita sales of lottery products alone increased from $20 to $97 per year (Clotfelter & Cook, 1989). By 1995, the national per capita expenditure on the lottery had surpassed $130 per year (North American Gaming Report, 1996; U.S. Census Bureau, 1996). As of 1995, thirty-eight states had established lotteries and 33 states had established or approved tribal, riverboat, or other types of casinos (International Game Technology, 1995). Only two states had not legalized some form of gambling (McQueen, 1995).

Given the increasing access to gambling in general and state lotteries in particular, public health researchers, clinicians, and policymakers have the opportunity to study the impact of legalized gambling on the development of children and adolescents. Currently, there is a paucity of scientific research focusing on the effects on youth of the spread of gambling (National Research Council, 1999). The National Gambling Impact Study Commission (1999) has encouraged increased attention to the scientific study of gambling in general and youthful gamblers in particular. This chapter will provide basic information about the extent of gambling activities among adolescents, some of the social and psychological consequences experienced by children who gamble, and the process of initiation to gambling activities.

BACKGROUND: RECOGNIZING YOUTH GAMBLING AS A PROBLEM

Youth have gambled at a variety of activities throughout history. During the twentieth century, pitching coins, playing cards, betting on sporting events, and other forms of gambling were common among young people. In most jurisdictions that have lotteries, the sale of lottery tickets to anyone under the age of 18 is prohibited by state law, yet more young people are gambling now than ever before. Perhaps young people are encouraged to gamble by the increased access to gaming provided by the development and popularity of state-sponsored lotteries. Maybe adolescents are encouraged to gamble by the explicit endorsements promulgated by government and church advertising and product promotions. Possibly young people gamble as a consequence of the absence of warnings from public health officials, who may feel political conflicts of interest because some of their revenues derive from lottery income. Regardless of the reasons, contemporary adolescents now represent a unique generation of Americans: These young people are the first constituency to experience gambling that has been both state sponsored and culturally approved throughout their entire lifetime.

Gambling has become an average and expectable activity among adolescents (Zinberg, 1984). Young people now gamble just as they smoke and drink, in spite of the illicit status of these activities. However, teenage gambling has received relatively little attention from researchers and the media. As Jacobs (1989) noted, "Teenage gambling was not yet conceptualized as an issue fifteen years ago, even though teenage involvement with potentially addictive substances such as alcohol, prescription, and illicit drugs were matters of serious concern and have remained the subject of systematic nationwide evaluation since 1975. Potentially harmful effects of teenage gambling simply had not been a matter for professional, scientific, governmental, or lay scrutiny, as attested to by the virtually silent literature on this topic before 1980" (pp. 263–64).

In a review of five studies of gambling by high school students, Jacobs reported that the levels of probable pathological gambling among high school students are more than 3 times higher than the prevalence rates for adults. Based on this research, Jacobs estimated that 7 million American children gamble regularly and 1 million experience serious gambling problems. In a study of pathological gambling among college students, Lesieur et al. (1991) found that the rates of problematic and pathological gambling among college students were 4 to 8 times higher than the rates reported for adults.

In a more recent examination of this problem, Shaffer, Hall, and Vander Bilt (1997, 1999) reported that adolescents and college students were at significantly greater risk for gambling disorders than were adults. For example, college students were almost 3 times more likely to experience serious gambling-related problems during their lifetime compared to their adult counterparts. Further, these young people were about 2.4 times more likely to experience subclinical gambling problems during their lifetime than were adults from the general population. Similarly, precollege adolescents were about 2.5 times more likely to experience subclinical or clinical levels of a gambling disorder than were adults.

Arcuri, Lester, and Smith (1985) shed more light on adolescents by examining a random sample of 332 students from an Atlantic City high school. They found that 64 percent of these students had gambled at the local casinos. Casino gambling among these students was illicit.[1] Slot machines accounted for 66 percent of these students' wagers and blackjack accounted for about 25 percent. Arcuri et al. reported that 42 percent of the 14-year-olds, 49 percent of the 15-year-olds, 63 percent of the 16-year-olds, 71 percent of the 17-year-olds, 76 percent of the 18-year-olds, and 88 percent of the 19-year-olds had gambled. Seventy-nine percent of the students said their parents knew that they gambled. Arcuri et al. argue that through acceptance of legalized gambling, there is danger that society will unwittingly shape compulsive gambling behavior. Arcuri et al. also suggested that because teenagers often fantasize about the material goods that large sums of money can buy, casinos present a temptation for them. They desire to become rich quickly, and gambling is seen as the means to this end. However, Arcuri et al. did not discuss the meaningfulness of the teenagers' fantasies, or whether these fantasies were, in fact, directly associated with gambling behavior.

GAMBLING AND DRUG ABUSE

There is considerable clinical evidence suggesting that drug abuse and compulsive gambling overlap (Lesieur, Blume, & Zoppa, 1986; Shaffer, Hall, & Vander Bilt, 1997, 1999). For example, among Minnesota adolescents who participated in a 1990 survey, 62.3 percent of those classified as "problem gamblers" also admitted to at least a monthly use of illegal substances (Winters, Stinchfield, & Fulkerson, 1993). Similarly, in one of the first clinical research investigations of gambling and drug abuse, Ramirez, McCormick, Russo, and Taber (1983) examined 51 successive admissions to the inpatient gambling treatment unit at the Cleveland Veterans Administration medical center. Fifty percent of these patients reported substance abuse problems in one or more of their biological parents. Thirty-six percent of those patients with siblings reported these problems among their biological siblings.

Of the patients who occasionally used alcohol or other substances to relax or for

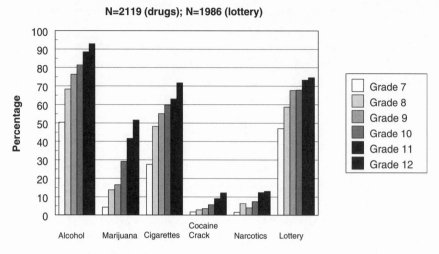

N=2119 (drugs); N=1986 (lottery)

Fig. 1.1. *Lifetime Drug- and Lottery-Use Patterns*

whom such use interfered with their life in more serious ways, 97 percent met the research diagnostic criteria for major depressive disorder or (one patient) schizo-affective disorder. Twenty-three percent reported biological parents who had gambling problems; 14 percent reported gambling problems in one or more sibling. There was a statistically significant correlation between gambling and substance abuse problems among siblings. Ramirez et al.'s results support the common observation that addictive behaviors often coexist. They concluded, "It is imperative that a thorough assessment of a potentially substance abusing patient include careful analysis of gambling behavior. Clinicians working with pathological gamblers need to be aware of the potential for a concomitant substance abuse problem. Clinicians working with the cross-addicted population of pathological gamblers need also to be aware of the likelihood of significant affective disorder, as well as suicide" (p. 428).

The Prevalence and Consequences of Underage Gambling[2]
ADOLESCENT LOTTERY USE
Shaffer (1994) reported data on underage lottery participation and substance use collected from a proportional stratified random sample of seventh- through twelfth-grade public school classes in Massachusetts. This sample represented 2,127 students from 97 schools. This survey of Massachusetts in-school[3] youth revealed that significant numbers of underage adolescents regularly buy lottery tickets. Specifically, 47.1 percent of seventh-grade children had purchased lottery tickets during their lifetime (fig. 1.1). At the senior-year level, 74.6 percent of the students reported having purchased a lottery ticket.

A better indicator of potential disordered gambling prevalence among youth is

N=2119 (drugs); N=1986 (lottery)

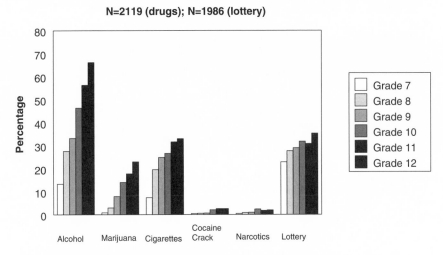

Fig. 1.2. *Current (Past Thirty Days) Drug and Lottery-Use Patterns*

the index of current, or past thirty-day, lottery use. Shaffer (1994) revealed that among Massachusetts school children in the seventh grade, 22.9 percent had purchased lottery tickets illicitly during the past thirty days. Of the seventh-grade students who had ever played the lottery, 2.9 percent had purchased lottery tickets between 6 and 19 times during the past month.

Among twelfth-grade students, 35.3 percent had purchased lottery tickets illegally during the past thirty days, and 5.5 percent of these seniors had purchased lottery tickets between 6 and 19 times during the past month. Therefore, this current-use index reveals that the trend toward growing levels of lottery play increases in frequency as well as prevalence. Overall, 7.5 percent of Massachusetts youth under the age of 17 purchased one or more lottery tickets every week; 2.7 percent of these young people reported buying twenty or more lottery tickets during the past month.

The prevalence of lottery use among youth increases with age and is widespread in this sample of students. More research is necessary to clarify the precise patterns of youthful entree and lottery use. In addition, future research may demonstrate that high-frequency lottery use among adolescents stimulates gambling to pathological levels that exceed estimates of pathological gambling in the adult community. Finally, for children, use of the lottery—though illicit—does not necessarily represent a pattern of pathological gambling. However, Lesieur (1989) noted that studies of high school and college students revealed higher rates of probable pathological gambling prevalence than those found among adults. Compared with the 1.4 percent to 1.9 percent rates of lifetime probable pathological gambling among adults, rates of pathological gambling among adolescents are estimated to be between 2.3 percent and 5.4 percent in most areas of the country; rates among college students have been

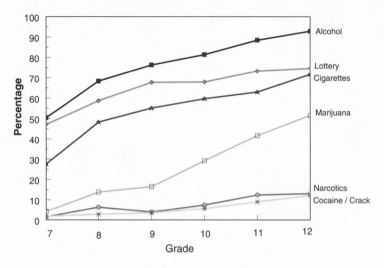

Fig. 1.3. Emerging Drug- and Lottery-Use Trends

estimated to be between 3.4 percent and 5.9 percent (Shaffer, Hall, & Vander Bilt, 1999).

COMPARING CHILDHOOD LOTTERY AND DRUG USE

To compare the association between childhood lottery use and a variety of drug use patterns, the prevalence data for each grade, partitioned for substance and lottery use, were examined using a trend analysis. Figure 1.3 illustrates the lifetime use relationship between the lottery and each of several drug categories.

The lifetime use prevalence patterns that emerge during grades seven through twelve for lottery use and use of the five drugs reveal a pattern of increasing trends. Lifetime use trends of any activity tend to increase as a direct function of time; correlations between these activities are very high but misleading, since lifetime rates of an activity with a population can only increase or remain the same over time. This pattern diminishes when prevalence rates for lottery and drug use during the past thirty days are compared. The only correlations larger than .50 represent the relationships between the lottery and alcohol (r = .74) and the lottery and marijuana (r = .80).

A trend analysis reveals that the shape of emerging lifetime patterns of using alcohol ($F = 54.42$, $p < .086$, $r^2 = .982$), marijuana ($F = 261.33$, $p < .039$; $r^2 = .996$), and cocaine ($F = 1408.33$, $p < .017$; $r^2 = .999$) most accurately reflect significant linear trends. Adolescent patterns of lottery participation also reflect a linear trend component ($F = 8.01$, $p < .216$; $r^2 = .889$) through high school as youth become involved with the lottery, though this trend is not statistically significant.

The data derived from this survey reveal that patterns of emerging drug and lottery use are remarkably similar. During the period between grades seven and twelve, students tend to explore a variety of risk-taking experiences in an increasing cycle (Jessor & Jessor, 1977). This study found that drug use escalates in a linear pattern until young adulthood; it also appears that, although there is no statistically significant trend, lottery use increases in a linear pattern through grade eleven in high school.

Absent a significant linear trend, we can only speculate that students who begin playing the lottery may switch to other gambling activities or even to more potent psychoactive experiences that include substance abuse. Furthermore, while drug-using patterns among youth peak during their 20s (Johnston, O'Malley, & Bachman, 1993), lottery use may peak much earlier. The present findings must be considered uncertain on this matter, and additional research is necessary to clarify these important trends and relationships among potentially addictive behaviors.

Figure 1.1 reveals that lifetime lottery use among this sample of adolescents begins earlier and at a higher level than does the use of all substances except alcohol. This trend may be the result of (1) the current social perception that gambling is culturally approved and (2) the low level of awareness of the risks and hazards of gambling among both parents and children. Furthermore, current levels of lottery use suggest that young people in the seventh grade use the lottery more frequently than any psychoactive substance. This finding suggests that using the lottery may be a "gateway" risk-taking activity.[4]

More investigation is necessary to determine whether early lottery-using patterns predict a younger "maturing out" (Winick, 1962) among lottery players. However, clinical evidence gathered from members of Gamblers Anonymous and from pathological gamblers who enter treatment for this disorder suggests that younger lottery-using patterns are probably associated with more problematic psychosocial consequences. Youthful gamblers are more vulnerable emotionally than adult gamblers and may integrate excessive gambling into their lifestyle as a regular and repetitive pattern (Jacobs, 1989).

SOCIAL AND EMOTIONAL CONSEQUENCES OF GAMBLING

To further clarify the implications of gambling among youth, Shaffer (1994) conducted a study of three Greater Boston suburban public schools. This study used the Massachusetts Gambling Screen (MAGS) to identify social and emotional consequences of gambling. The results of the MAGS revealed widespread and significant consequences for youthful gamblers. Seventy-seven percent of this high school student sample (N = 801) reported they had gambled on any activity during their lifetime.

This prevalence rate for gambling among adolescents represents a slightly more conservative finding than reported in the lottery survey above and suggests that the findings reported below may also depict conservative estimates of the social and emotional consequences of gambling. Among the high school student sample, the prevalence of gambling-related problems is significant, even among those students who do not gamble. For example, 32 percent of the students who do not gamble feel that their nongambling behavior is not "normal." These young people are reporting extraordinary pressure to begin gambling.

Of all the students surveyed, 11.1 percent had a relative who worries about their gambling, 9 percent felt guilty about their gambling, 13 percent were unable to stop gambling when they wanted, 10 percent experienced family problems because of their gambling, 8 percent had been in trouble at school or work because of their gambling, and 8 percent had neglected their school or work obligations for two or more consecutive days because of gambling. Furthermore, this survey found that 4 percent of the students had sought help for gambling, 4 percent had been to Gamblers Anonymous, and 5 percent had been arrested for gambling-related problems.

As others have previously identified, the prevalence of gambling-related problems differs for males and females (Jacobs, 1989). A Hotellings multivariate analysis of variance revealed that adolescent males experience significantly more social and emotional problems than adolescent females as measured on the MAGS (F = 5.17, d.f. = 14, 433, p < .001). Table 1.1 summarizes the significant univariate differences between male and female high school students who reported they had gambled at least once during their lifetime.

Although students reported the social and emotional problems described above in direct response to researchers asking if a problem was the result of gambling behavior, it is possible that these problems accrue to adolescents in general and not just to those young people who gamble (Jessor, 1975). Consequently, researchers analyzed relevant MAGS items to confirm that students who reported gambling more than most other people also showed more social and emotional problems. Of those who reported that they gambled more than most other people, 33 percent had been in trouble at school or work because of their gambling, compared with only 1 percent of those who reported gambling less than others and 16 percent of those who reported gambling as much as others. The results of a multivariate analysis (on MAGS measures of trouble, complaints, ability to stop, neglected obligations, and arrests) confirms this relationship: A Hotellings multivariate analysis reveals that adolescents who report gambling more do indeed also reveal significantly more social problems (F = 6.16, d.f. = 10, 926, p < .001).

THE IMPACT AND CONSEQUENCES OF YOUTHFUL GAMBLING

As opportunity and social approval for gambling increase, the adverse consequences among young people may be growing. One of the main questions now facing researchers is whether illicit gambling among young people is increasing at a rate proportional to the expansion of opportunities to gamble legally. As access to lottery games and other forms of legal gambling proliferates and receives (1) implicit endorsement, that is, legal status with no prevention or educational programs, and (2) explicit encouragement, for example, state-sponsored advertising and occasional promo-

Table 1.1 *Gender Differences and the Impact of Gambling*

Problem Area	Male Prevalence (%)	Female Prevalence (%)	Univariate F (d.f. = 1, 446)	Significance Level of Difference Between Prevalence Rates
Feels pressure to start gambling	20.6	9.6	$F = 9.77$	$p < .002$
Amount of gambling is abnormal	18.1	9	$F = 7.14$	$p < .008$
Friends or relatives view amount of gambling as abnormal	49.4	35	$F = 9.19$	$p < .003$
Feels guilty about gambling	11.4	5	$F = 5.36$	$p < .02$
Relatives complain about gambling	14	2.8	$F = 15.92$	$p < .001$
Feels pressure to gamble when not gambling	15.9	5.1	$F = 12.41$	$p < .001$
Thought about reducing gambling	19	9	$F = 8.69$	$p < .003$
Experiencing family problems	12	4.5	$F = 7.64$	$p < .006$
Gotten in trouble at school or work	11	2.8	$F = 10.29$	$p < .001$
Neglected obligations for 2 or more consecutive days	10.7	1.7	$F = 13.43$	$p < .001$
Cannot stop gambling when wants to stop	14.7	9.6	$F = 2.57$	$p < .11$
Sought help about gambling	5.2	1.7	$F = 3.55$	$p < .06$
Been arrested for gambling	5.5%	2.3	$F = 2.83$	$p < .09$

Source: Shaffer (1994).

tional lottery coupons mailed to homes, it is reasonable to expect that gambling among young people will continue to increase. Consider, for example, this observation from Gene McLean, president of Kentucky Off-Track Betting: "If we are going to keep this business viable we have to find a way to entice the younger generation into the game. The only way to do that is to expose them to the sport" (Doocey, 1993, p. 68).

In addition to the direct consequences of excessive gambling, research has identified some unexpected consequences of legalized and normalized gambling. Specifically, the finding that almost one-third of nongambling high school students felt their behavior was not normal implies that, like those who gamble too much, those who participate in very few or no gambling activities feel increasing social pressure to change their behavior to comply with convivial mores and customs.

Teenagers are very attuned to their self-concept and sensitive to the views of others. In the sample investigated by Shaffer (1994), students who had not yet gambled were very clear about their experience of social pressure to gamble. Although this study did not attempt to separate the adverse consequences associated with the legalized lottery from the consequences associated with other illicit forms of gambling, the prevalence of meaningful social and emotional problems that derive from gambling cannot be discounted. Additional research is necessary to clarify the influence of legal and illegal gambling on young people as well as the social impact of legal gambling promotion on those who do not participate in gambling activities.

INITIATION TO GAMBLING ACTIVITIES

Few studies have examined in detail the factors associated with adolescents' initiation to gambling. However, two studies (Shaffer et al., 1995a; Vagge, 1996) offer some insights into this area. In a study of 1,549 middle school (fifth through eighth grade) students randomly selected from the Merrimack Valley region of Massachusetts, Shaffer et al. (1995a) investigated lifetime, past-year, and past-month prevalence rates of participation in the lottery, participation in gambling activities other than the lottery, and use of six illicit substances. This study revealed that for all three time frames, rates of gambling on activities other than the lottery—sports events, card games—exceeded the rates of all of the other illicit activities, including lottery gambling, alcohol use, and tobacco use.

The second most prevalent activity was lottery gambling, which exceeded the prevalence of all activities except nonlottery gambling in the lifetime time frame and all activities except nonlottery gambling and alcohol use in the past-year and past-month time frames. These results suggest that informal gambling, such as betting on sports events or card games, plays an important role in the initiation of gambling activities among youth. Furthermore, this study indicates that gambling in general, and informal gambling in particular, may be the first "consciousness-shifting," potentially addictive activity that youths participate in and may lead the way to other potentially addictive activities such as substance use.

In a study of 466 sixth- through eleventh-grade Massachusetts students, Vagge (1996) investigated in greater detail some of the factors associated with the initiation of gambling activity. Specifically, this study investigated respondents' first gambling experiences. The most common first gambling activity among this sample was betting on sports, followed by betting on cards and playing the lottery. This study also revealed that these adolescents were most likely to have first gambled with friends, followed by family members other than parents or siblings. The mean age at which these respondents first gambled was 10.36 years. These results support the hypothesis that gambling begins at an early age and that informal gambling with friends and family leads the way to other gambling experiences.

THE POTENTIAL ROLE OF EDUCATION IN PREVENTION

The results of these studies also suggest that education is a potentially valuable tool in the effort to prevent the development of gambling problems among youth. Data derived from Shaffer et al. (1995b) reveal that there is a significant relationship between students' interest in mathematics and their level of involvement in gambling. Students in this study who had high levels of interest in mathematics evidenced lower levels of gambling involvement, had fewer friends who gambled, and perceived gambling to be more dangerous, compared with students who had lower levels of interest in mathematics. In addition, Vagge (1996) revealed that pathological gambling among middle school students was significantly correlated with students' perceptions of the amount of skill involved in gambling: Higher levels of perceived skill were associated with higher levels of gambling pathology. Furthermore, students who believed that gambling involved larger degrees of skill had gambled significantly more frequently during the week and the year prior to the survey and had placed significantly higher bets, compared with those who believed that gambling involved lower amounts of skill.

These studies suggest the potentially important role educators can play in preventing problem gambling among youth. The integration of the topic of gambling into existing probability and statistics curriculum units could both (1) increase students' interest in mathematics by incorporating an interesting, "real-world" topic and (2) teach students through lessons in probability and statistics that gambling is usually a losing proposition. Both of these areas hold the potential to improve students' critical-thinking skills and decrease their interest in potentially addictive behaviors.[5]

TOWARD SOLUTIONS

Since the government appears eager to endorse and promote new opportunities to gamble (Eadington, 1992), it is equally vital that government agencies, for example, departments of public health, recognize the potential negative consequences of gambling. Domestic, mental health, and substance abuse problems stimulated by gambling demand recognition (Korn & Shaffer, 1999). The youthful gamblers represented in this chapter reveal that the breadth and adversity of gambling is indeed socially and emotionally significant. Consequently, as Korn and Shaffer (1999) suggest, communities must begin to establish gambling education and prevention programs. Mental health professionals must acquire the knowledge and skills associated with the treatment of gambling disorders. In addition, it is time to prepare legislation that regulates the advertising and promoting of gambling to young people. Just as policymakers regulate tobacco and alcohol advertising, social policy should reflect the potential dangers associated with gambling.

As gambling became normalized during the past three decades, the moral prohibitions that historically served to regulate betting excesses diminished. With increasing economic need, moral restraint was discarded by both policymakers and the public. Social policymakers have decided that America will gamble. It seems essential that we begin to determine how that will happen. Culturally endorsed gambling has not and will not come without a price. Will (1993) notes, "when life for most Americans is without risk, gambling may be a way of infusing life with stimulating uncertainty. But by now, with a deepening dependency of individuals and governments on gambling, we are gambling with our national character, forgetting that character is destiny" (p. A).

Notes

1. As Satre and Brosig reveal in their chapters in this volume, much has changed since the early 1980s in the way casino executives regulate and exclude young people from gaining access to gambling activities.

2. This section reports data that were reported originally in Shaffer (1994). Readers interested in learning more about the sampling strategy and survey methodology are referred to this report.

3. These results reflect data obtained from students who were in school. Although voluntary, no student declined to participate in any aspect of the data-collection process. In-school surveys of this type are biased by the absence of those students who were truant or ill during the data collection. In general, in-school surveys tend to yield conservative estimates of deviant behavior patterns because of these respondent biases (e.g., Mosher & Yanagisako, 1991).

4. Epidemiologists hypothesize that certain drugs (e.g., cigarettes) act as gateways to more pervasive illicit drug-use patterns (Kandel, 1993). In this new era of state-sponsored gambling, it is also possible to theorize that lottery playing—as a socially endorsed risk-taking behavior—provides the experience that encourages young people to engage in other risk-taking activities, such as illicit drug use. More research is necessary to clarify this point.

5. For more information about an innovative method of integrating gambling and mathematics education, see chap. 4, "What Are My Chances? Using Probability and Number Sense to Educate Teens About the Mathematical Risks of Gambling," by Terry W. Crites.

References

Arcuri, A. F., Lester, D., & Smith, F. O. (1985). Shaping adolescent gambling behavior. *Adolescence, 20,* 935–38.

Christiansen, E. M. (1996). The United States '95 gross annual wager. *Gaming & Wagering Business, 17* (8), 55–92.

Clotfelter, C. T., & Cook, P. J. (1989). *Selling hope: State lotteries in America.* Cambridge: Harvard University Press.

Commission on the Review of the National Policy Toward Gambling. (1976). *Gambling in America.* Washington, DC: U.S. Government Printing Office.

Doocey, P. (1993). A new breed of off-track betting for Kentucky. *International Gaming & Wagering Business, 14* (1), 68.

Eadington, W. R. (1992, October 27). Emerging public policy challenges from the proliferation of gaming in America. Paper presented at the Second Annual Australasian Conference on Casinos and Gambling, Sydney, Australia.

International Game Technology. (1995). *Gaming in the United States.* [Brochure.] Las Vegas, NV: Author.

Jacobs, D. F. (1989). Illegal and undocumented: A review of teenage gamblers in America. In H. Shaffer, S. Stein, B. Gambino, & T. Cummings (Eds.), *Compulsive gambling: Theory, research, and practice* (pp. 249–92). Lexington, MA: Lexington Books.

Jessor, R. (1975). Predicting time of onset of marijuana use: A developmental study of high school youth. In D. Lettieri (Ed.), *Predicting adolescent drug abuse: A review of issues, methods, and correlates* (DHEW Publication No. ADM-76-299). Washington, DC: National Institute on Drug Abuse, U.S. Government Printing Office.

Jessor, R., & Jessor, S. L. (1977). *Problem behavior and psychosocial development: A longitudinal study of youth.* New York: Academic Press.

Johnston, L. D., O'Malley, P. M., & Bachman, J. G. (1993). *National survey results on drug use from monitoring the future study, 1975–1992* (NIH Publication 93-3597). Washington, DC: U.S. Government Printing Office.

Kandel, D. (1993, March 5). Initiation into addictions: The adolescent experience. Paper presented at Harvard Medical School Continuing Education Conference, Boston.

Korn, D., & Shaffer, H. J. (1999). Gambling and the health of the public: Adopting a public health perspective. *Journal of Gambling Studies, 15* (4), 289–365.

Lesieur, H. R. (1989). Current research into pathological gambling and gaps in the literature. In H. Shaffer, S. Stein, B. Gambino, & T. Cummings (Eds.), *Compulsive gambling: Theory, research, and practice* (pp. 225–48). Lexington, MA: Lexington Books.

Lesieur, H. R., Blume, S., & Zoppa, R. (1986). Alcoholism, drug abuse, and gambling. *Alcoholism: Clinical and Experimental Research, 10,* 33–38.

Lesieur, H. R., Cross, J., Frank, M., Welch, M., White, C. M., Rubenstein, G., Moseley, K., & Mark, M. (1991). Gambling and pathological gambling among university students. *Addictive Behaviors, 16,* 517–27.

McQueen, P. A. (1995, July 1). *North American gaming report 1995*. (Supplement to *International Gaming & Wagering Business*.) New York: BMT Communications, Inc.

Mosher, J. F., & Yanagisako, K. L. (1991). Public health, not social warfare: A public health approach to illegal drug policy. *Journal of Public Health Policy, 12*, 278–323.

National Gambling Impact Study Commission. (1999). *National Gambling Impact Study Commission report*. Washington, DC: Author.

National Research Council. (1999). *Pathological gambling: A critical review*. Washington DC: National Academy Press.

North American Gaming Report 1996. (1996, July). *International Gaming & Wagering Business, 17* (7), S3–S38.

Ramirez, L. F., McCormick, R. A., Russo, A. M., & Taber, J. I. (1983). Patterns of substance abuse in pathological gamblers undergoing treatment. *Addictive Behaviors, 8*, 425–28.

Shaffer, H. J. (1994). *The emergence of youthful addiction: The prevalence of underage lottery use and the impact of gambling* (Technical Report No. 011394-100). Boston: Massachusetts Council on Compulsive Gambling.

Shaffer, H. J., Hall, M. N., & Vander Bilt, J. (1997). *Estimating the prevalence of disordered gambling behavior in the United States and Canada: A meta-analysis*. Boston: Presidents and Fellows of Harvard College.

Shaffer, H. J., Hall, M. N., & Vander Bilt, J. (1999). Estimating the prevalence of disordered gambling behavior in the United States and Canada: A research synthesis. *American Journal of Public Health, 89*, 1369–76.

Shaffer, H. J., Stein, S. A., Gambino, B., & Cummings, T. N. (Eds.). (1989). *Compulsive gambling: Theory, research, and practice*. Lexington, MA: Lexington Books.

Shaffer, H. J., Walsh, J. S., Howard, C. M., Hall, M. N., Wellington, C. A., & Vander Bilt, J. (1995a). *Science and substance abuse education: A needs assessment for curriculum design* (SEDAP Technical Report No. 082595-300). Cambridge, MA: Harvard Medical School Division on Addictions.

Shaffer, H. J., Walsh, J. S., Howard, C., Hall, M. N., Wellington, C., & Vander Bilt, J. (1995b). (Harvard/Billerica Addiction Science Education Project.) Unpublished raw data. Boston: Harvard Medical School Division on Addictions.

U.S. Census Bureau. (1996). *U.S. Census Bureau: The official statistics*. [http://www.census.gov].

Vagge, L. M. (1996). The development of youth gambling. Unpublished honors thesis, Harvard-Radcliffe Colleges, Cambridge, MA.

Will, G. F. (1993, February 8). By institutionalizing gambling, states foment mass irrationality. *Providence Journal-Bulletin*, p. A.

Winick, C. (1962). Maturing out of narcotic addiction. *United Nations Bulletin on Narcotics, 14*, 1–7.

Winters, K. C., Stinchfield, R., & Fulkerson, J. (1993). Patterns and characteristics of adolescent gambling. *Journal of Gambling Studies, 9*, 371–86.

Zinberg, N. E. (1984). *Drug, set, and setting*. New Haven: Yale University Press.

Chapter Two

American Indian Gaming

Darryl Zitzow

Background

Although American Indian gaming has expanded dramatically since 1988, historical documentation shows that gambling was part of the traditional activities of
American Indians' games prior to the 1800s, in the forms of shell games, hand
games, and moccasin games. In addition, some reservations have a recent legacy of
gambling and have operated bingo and pull-tabs for twenty-five or more years.
Video gambling machines have been available in some reservation communities for
more than fifteen years.

Recently, however, federal legislation has brought about dramatic changes in
American Indian gaming within the United States. In the 1970s, American Indian
tribes provided unregulated gambling alternatives in the forms of traditional games,
backroom poker, blackjack, sports betting similar to that available in many neigh-
boring non-Indian communities, and charity gambling based on state laws, largely
through bingo games or pull-tabs. Tribal gaming appeared largely unimportant and
unrecognized until the Seminole Tribe of Hollywood, Florida, established the nation's first tribal high-stakes bingo. The operation was upheld by a federal court,
which defined the tribe's right to own and manage the bingo operation (Gaming &
Wagering Business, 1990). This new source of revenue captured the attention of
American Indian tribes elsewhere.

Following this federal court decision, the U.S. Congress sought to "provide a
statutory basis for the regulation of gaming by an Indian tribe" through the Indian
Gaming Regulatory Act (IGRA) of 1988 (Public Law 100-497 25 USC). The inten-
tion was to promote "tribal economic development, tribal self-sufficiency, strong
tribal governments," and the protection of American Indian gaming rights (25 USC,
2702, Sec. 3).

Many American Indian tribes did not see the IGRA as supportive of Indian rights;
to the contrary, some tribes perceived it as just another of many historical efforts by

the federal government to control them and suppress Indian rights. "The IGRA did not authorize, but limited Indian nation rights by requiring that they compact with the states" (Hill, 1994, p. 2).

Then-president Ronald Reagan signed the IGRA into law on October 7, 1988. The act defined and legitimized three separate categories of gaming.

Class I gaming: Games solely for prizes of minimal value. This class included the traditional forms of gaming that tribes had historically enjoyed and participated in as part of tribal celebrations or socialization.

Class II gaming: Included nonbanked games such as bingo (including high-stakes bingo), pull-tabs, selected card games (including poker), and tribal lotteries. These games were to be provided in conformity with and not expressly prohibited by the laws of the state in which the tribe resided.

Class III gaming: Included full casino-style gaming, such as blackjack, slots, roulette, craps, and all other forms of gaming not listed in Class I or Class II. This class included gaming where the gambler bet against the house. Parimutuel betting was also included (25 USC, 2703, Sec. 4).

In addition to defining classes of gaming, the IGRA defined the regulations regarding tribal gaming. Class I games were established and regulated entirely by local tribes. Class II games were regulated by local tribes and the National Indian Gaming Commission. Class III games would be operated on tribal lands only if they were "authorized by tribal resolution; located in a state that permits such gaming for any purpose, by any person, organization, or entity; and are conducted in conformance with a tribal state compact" approved by the chairman and National Indian Gaming Commission (25 USC, 2710, Sec. 11). Class III games are subject to conditions of regulation by both the tribe and state, established by the compact.

The nationwide explosion of Indian gaming since the establishment of the IGRA has focused much attention recently on problem-gambling behaviors unique to American Indian populations. Indian gaming in the United States produced an estimated $4 billion in revenue in 1995—representing nearly 10 percent of the $44.4 billion total gaming revenue nationwide. There are currently 130 tribes involved in 145 compacts for legalized gambling operations in 24 states throughout the United States (Christiansen, 1996). In addition, the substantial number of smaller gambling operations, such as video poker units, bingo, and pull-tabs, in reservations are difficult to enumerate.

Positive Consequences of Gaming for American Indians

Indian gaming opportunities available since the passage in 1988 of the IGRA have established previously unheard-of economic growth, employment opportunities, and purchasing power for American Indian families. Reservation casinos have become a lighthouse for displaced American Indians in search of employment, financial stability, and self-sufficiency. The value of increased personal esteem from employment, productivity, job advancement, economic stability, and relinquishment of the chains of welfare dependency is substantial and often immeasurable. Many tribal governments, once limited to merely managing federal or state programs, are now enjoying legitimate financial integrity and security.

In Michigan, for example, the unemployment rate across seven reservations was 65 percent before organized Indian gaming and the IGRA. Within five years of the introduction of formalized Indian gaming, the unemployment rate had dropped to 15 percent. Estimates of unemployment rates in the hard-to-serve rural areas of Michigan were reduced by as much as 77 percent within the same five-year period (Michigan Gaming Enterprise, 1993). Although no direct causal association has been made between the development of formalized Indian gaming and employment levels, no previous tribal economic development effort had corresponded to such a marked change in unemployment for these same reservations.

In addition, a study of eight Minnesota nonurban counties that had developed tribal gaming with various starting dates between 1987 and 1992 documented an overall 14 percent decrease in Aid to Families with Dependent Children recipients, compared with a 17 percent increase for AFDC recipients statewide within the same five-year period (Minnesota Indian Gaming Association, 1992). In 1993 combined tribal gaming in Minnesota was ranked as the seventh-largest employer within the state, just behind Honeywell Inc. and just ahead of the IBM Corporation (Minnesota Department of Trade and Economic Development, 1991).

In a study of crime problems related to casinos, 86 percent of the tribal police chiefs and 73 percent of the Indian gaming security managers surveyed felt that crime had not increased as a result of the introduction of Indian gaming. To the contrary, many felt that local tribal incidents of crime had decreased because of the positive alternative of reservation employment (Michigan Gaming Enterprise, 1993).

Negative Consequences of Gaming for American Indians

Despite the huge economic and employment windfalls for reservations, Indian gaming is not without negative consequences. For example, American Indians who were once displaced to urban settings are returning to rural reservations. These urban American Indians have been influenced by other cultures, and they return to the reservation with different and sometimes conflicting values, lifestyles, and behaviors. They appear at times to clash with the more muted pace of rural, traditional American Indian life.

In addition, the perception that American Indian tribes are self-regulatory raised concerns about a greater potential for organized crime to infiltrate tribal gaming operations. The national media carried stories denouncing alleged corruption and increases in crime that the new gaming money had brought with it. Some focused on the corruption of local tribal leaders, while others blamed Indian gaming for the dissolution of the American Indian family.

The national media turned its attention to Indian gaming in September 1994, for example, when CBS's *60 Minutes* aired a segment reporting on the tremendous financial boom experienced by selected tribes that once had been isolated and devastated by poverty. The segment also identified the potential for financial mismanagement and corruption because of an apparent lack of operations oversight and the perceived tribal inexperience with gaming (Devine, 1994).

The IGRA also addressed concerns for potential corruption of tribal gaming within its declaration of a policy "to provide a statutory basis for the regulation of gaming by an Indian tribe adequate to shield it from organized crime and other corrupting influences, to ensure that the Indian tribe is the primary beneficiary of the gaming operation, and to assure that gaming is conducted fairly and honestly" (25 USC, 2702, Sec. 3).

In addition to concerns about corruption, there were fears about the possible increase in alcohol and multisubstance abuse, relinquishment of traditional values, youth gang development, and reduced child supervision in both single- and dual-parent families.

Compulsive Gambling Research: Risk Factors

Of all the possible negative consequences caused by tribal gaming, the most serious appears to be the development of problematic or compulsive gambling among American Indians. While there are several studies in progress that are examining unique gambling issues facing American Indians, few as yet have been completed or published. Even fewer studies focus on gambling by American Indian youths. Recent research, however, leads to some preliminary conclusions regarding the impact of gambling on American Indians. For example, many recent studies on problem gambling have identified predisposers or risk factors that place both adults and adolescents at risk for developing gambling problems. Given their histories and social conditions, American Indians, especially those within reservation systems, appear to be in a unique position to be associated with most of these risk factors.

For example, Roston (1961) found that male compulsive gamblers were more likely to possess the personality characteristics of magical thinking and social alienation than control groups. American Indian tradition and long-term exposure to prejudice may predispose American Indians to these same characteristics. As Bergler (1958) noted, persons with minority status are at greater risk for compulsive gambling because they are in a more adversarial relationship with the world. American Indians, by virtue of their minority status, may be more prone to feeling alienated and powerless. They may also lack a sense of destiny control, often identified in minority populations (Jencks, 1972).

Roston also indicated a high degree of correlation between alcoholism and the potential for gambling addiction among male gamblers. High rates of problematic and dependent use of alcohol among American Indian adults and adolescents in selected tribes have been well documented (Midwest Regional Center, 1988). A general theory of addiction supports the notion that maladaptive or addictive behaviors that can exist within the family environment (for example, alcoholism, drug abuse, food addiction) may be generalized to maladaptive and addictive behaviors associated with gambling (Jacobs, 1989).

Research also shows that persons exposed to a higher prevalence of major historical trauma events may be more inclined to develop pathological gambling characteristics (Jacobs, 1989; Taber, McCormick, & Ramirez, 1987). American Indians have a documented history of multigenerational trauma (Swonomish Tribal Mental Health Project, 1991). Furthermore, research shows that persons experiencing depression may possess a predisposition to future gambling problems (Blaszczynski, Winter, & McConaghy, 1986). The statistically high rates of depression and suicide among American Indian adolescents (May & Van Winkle, 1994) appear to place them at risk for gambling problems as well.

The cultural and historical patterns experienced by many American Indians may also be associated with addictive behaviors such as compulsive gambling. The economically impoverished existence of many reservations, in which residents may have been dependent on welfare systems, may encourage American Indians to seek opportunities that provide immediate gratification, such as winning at gambling. The welfare-dependency cycle is well established for many minority families. The "feast or famine" monthly cycle of dependency allows welfare participants familiarity with and acceptance of a similar pattern found within gambling addiction.

Finally, greater length of time exposed to and availability of gambling alternatives to individuals appear to increase the addictive potential of gambling (Livingston, 1974). Many reservations have had substantial exposure to gambling opportunities—bingo, pull-tabs, and video gambling—for twenty-five years or more, long before the establishment of present-day tribal casinos. This greater length of time exposed to gambling may place American Indians at greater risk for developing problem-gambling characteristics.

Compulsive Gambling Research: Prevalence Studies

A study completed by Elia and Jacobs (1993) in a culturally mixed, adult inpatient alcohol treatment setting found a substantial prevalence of pathological gambling among American Indian male patients: 22 percent of the American Indian respondents met the South Oaks Gambling Screen (SOGS) criteria for pathological gambling, compared with 7 percent of the male Caucasian respondents. Furthermore, 19 percent of the American Indian respondents met the SOGS criteria for problematic gambling, compared with 14 percent of the Caucasian patients. The combined rate of problem and pathological gambling among American Indian males in this study was nearly double the rate among Caucasian males.

A statewide survey of Minnesota gambling in 1990 (Laundergan, Schaefer, Eckhoff, & Pirie, 1990) established higher rates of both pathological and problem gambling among adult minority populations, including American Indians. In this study, nonwhites (American Indians and blacks) were overrepresented among pathological gamblers. While they represented only 2.6 percent of the study sample, they represented 10.6 percent of the pathological gambling group.

A comparative study of gambling behaviors of American Indian and non-Indian adolescents—ages 12 to 19—was conducted by Zitzow (1996a). The results of this study revealed that American Indian adolescents were at greater risk for developing gambling problems than were non-Indian adolescents. Compared with their non-Indian counterparts, American Indian adolescents had a significantly higher lifetime prevalence of gambling (94 percent vs. 86 percent) and started gambling for money at a significantly earlier age (average 12 years vs. 13.27 years).

American Indian adolescents also reported significantly greater frequency than their non-Indian peers for gambling involvement in state scratch tabs, tribal pull-tabs, state lottery, casino blackjack, cards for money, and bingo. There were no differences between adolescent ethnic groups regarding their participation in local sports pools, track betting, sports betting, games of skill, casino roulette, or casino craps.

Furthermore, significantly more American Indian adolescents than non-Indian adolescents positively endorsed each of twenty-two other problem-gambling survey items. They believed gambling was a fast and easy way to earn money (55 percent vs. 27 percent); they believed some of their happiest memories were of winning at gambling (32 percent vs. 8 percent); they tried to stop or cut down on their gambling, but could not (9 percent vs. 1 percent); they have lied about what they won or lost gambling (21 percent vs. 9 percent); they have used money they were not supposed to in order to pay for gambling (27 percent vs. 7 percent); and they chased earlier gambling losses (47 percent vs. 24 percent).

When the SOGS was applied to this adolescent population, a statistically significant difference was found: 9.6 percent of the American Indian adolescents were classified as pathological gamblers, compared with 5.6 percent of the non-Indian adolescents. Significant differences were also evident for adolescents experiencing problem-gambling characteristics, with 14.8 percent of American Indian adolescents displaying this pattern compared with 10.5 percent of the non-Indian adolescents.

Zitzow (1996b) conducted a similar study among American Indian and non-Indian adults. This study revealed that although these two groups did not differ significantly in gambling frequency, American Indian adults revealed significantly more gambling problems. Significantly more American Indian adults than non-

Indian adults reported the following problematic gambling behaviors: hiding gambling from family and friends; failing to complete things because of gambling; borrowing money to gamble; pawning, selling, or trading possessions to pay for gambling; believing that gambling is a fast and easy way to make money; chasing gambling losses; having been criticized by family members for gambling; having gambling debts; continuing to gamble without the money to pay for it; feeling that getting lucky in gambling is the only way of getting ahead; and feeling they have a problem with gambling.

Furthermore, significant differences were found on measures of problem and pathological gambling. Of the American Indian sample 9.1 percent were classified as problematic gamblers, compared with 4 percent of the non-Indian sample, and 2.8 percent of the American Indian sample were classified as pathological gamblers, compared with 1.6 percent of the non-Indian sample. A study of American Indian gambling in North Dakota by Volberg (1993) revealed similar results. Of the American Indian sample 6.3 percent were classified as current problem gamblers and 6 percent were classified as current probable pathological gamblers, compared with a combined problem and probable pathological gambling rate of 2 percent in the general North Dakota population.

Flaws in the Current Research

The current research investigating American Indian adolescent gambling must be regarded with the utmost caution for several reasons.

1. The tools used thus far to assess American Indian adolescent gambling behaviors were designed for adults based on adult constructs and concurrent validity studies. Scales used to assess adult gambling may not accurately assess the unique developmental gambling behaviors found during adolescence.

2. A common misconception often results in the grouping of all American Indian tribes and reservation communities into one common culture. American Indian tribes are unique and extremely diverse. Risk factors for problematic adolescent gambling behavior identified within a particular Plains tribe may not apply to other tribes. For example, some tribes have alcoholism, suicide, and unemployment rates above the U.S. average, while others are well below the U.S. average (Indian Health Service, 1991). Generalizing these results to other reservations may not be appropriate, in view of the great variation in exposure to risk factors on different reservations.

3. Gambling availability among reservations also varies greatly. Some tribes have a legacy of twenty-five or more years of legalized gambling, while others have avoided gambling altogether.

4. Finally, awareness, education programs, prevention programs, and resistance

training in the area of adolescent gambling vary from reservation to reservation. The level of resources available to devote to these programs likely affects the nature and incidence of American Indian adolescent problem gambling.

Conclusion
RECOMMENDATIONS FOR FUTURE RESEARCH
Many tribes have initiated local reservation studies to monitor the consequences of their established gaming enterprises. The recent and sometimes intense exposure of persons to gambling within selected American Indian reservations provides timely and invaluable opportunities to study compulsive gambling. Much more research is needed to continue to assess the impact of American Indian adolescent exposure to and experience with all forms of gambling. I recommend that a range of studies be conducted across the nation, within various American Indian cultures, to more clearly identify (1) the short-term impact of vicarious (family) gambling exposure on the adolescent, (2) the long-term impact of adolescent gambling on eventual adult problem gambling, (3) risk factors that could emerge as more significant predictors of adolescent problem gambling, and (4) conditions or resources that appear to enhance American Indian adolescent resistance to problem gambling.

ADDITIONAL RECOMMENDATIONS
Clearly, large-stakes gambling within the American Indian community is here to stay, at least for the foreseeable future. The potential for substantial economic tribal growth, continued reduction of unemployment, increased tribal economic control, and control of destiny, as well as individual financial control and productivity, appear to coincide with successful tribal gaming operations.

In addition to the research recommendations already mentioned, tribes are encouraged to address youth and compulsive gambling as a behavioral health priority. American Indian leaders must continue to assess and remain vigilant about the very real and growing potential for gambling addiction among American Indian people. More gambling assessment and therapy resources must be developed for the reservation communities.

Education, information, and addiction-resistance programs should be developed and implemented, even as early as the grade-school years. These programs could be added to some of the excellent substance abuse curricula already available within American Indian community schools. Tribal leaders and elders could be tapped for support and direction in addressing problem gambling. Finally, early warning detection strategies need to be developed to identify problem gamblers and refer them to gambling therapy in a timely manner.

Some tribal leaders have already made the development of gaming a positive decision for tribes by addressing the concerns for gambling addiction in an effective and straightforward manner; these tribes are to be commended for their bold and sometimes controversial efforts. I recommend that all tribes take these steps to ensure that gaming remains a positive influence on American Indian culture. The development of reservation gambling holds the key to the nation's struggle with compulsive gambling.

References

Bergler, E. (1958). *The psychology of gambling.* New York: International Universities Press.

Blaszczynski, A., Winter, S. W., & McConaghy, N. (1986). Plasma endorphin levels in pathological gambling. *Journal of Gambling Behavior, 2,* 3–14.

Christiansen, E. M. (1996). The United States '95 gross annual wager. *Gaming & Wagering Business, 17* (8), 55–92.

Devine, L. F. (Producer). (1994, September 18). Wampum wonderland. *60 Minutes.* New York: CBS, Inc.

Elia, C., & Jacobs, D. F. (1993). The incidence of pathological gambling among Native Americans treated for alcohol dependence. *International Journal of the Addictions, 28,* 659–66.

Gaming & Wagering Business. (1990, July 15). *Newsletter.*

Hill, R. (1994, October). National Indian Gaming Association raps "60 Minutes" report of Mashentucket Pequots. *Pequot (NY) Times,* p. 2.

Indian Health Service. (1991). *Regional differences in Indian health.* Washington, DC: Government Printing Office.

Jacobs, D. (1989). A general theory of addictions: A new theoretical model. *Journal of Gambling Behavior, 2,* 15–31.

Jencks, C. (1972). *Inequality: A reassessment of the effect of family and schooling in America.* New York: Basic Books.

Laundergan, J., Schaefer, J., Eckhoff, K., & Pirie, P. (1990, November). *Adult survey of Minnesota gambling behavior.* St. Paul: Department of Human Services.

Livingston, J. (1974). *Compulsive gamblers: Observations on action and abstinence.* New York: Harper & Row.

May, P., & Van Winkle, N. (1994). Indian adolescent suicide: The epidemiologic picture in New Mexico. *Calling from the Rim: Suicidal Behavior among American Indian and Alaska Native Adolescents, 4,* 2–23.

Michigan Gaming Enterprise. (1993). *Economic and social effects of Indian-owned gaming enterprises in Michigan.* Lansing, Mich.: University Associates.

Midwest Regional Center. (1988). *Midwest study of ethnic differences regarding alcohol and other substance abuse.* Chicago: U.S. Office of Education.

Minnesota Department of Trade and Economic Development. (1991). *Report of Minnesota's largest corporate employers.* St. Paul: Author.

Minnesota Indian Gaming Association. (1992). *Economic benefits of tribal gaming in Minnesota.* Minneapolis: KPMG Peat Marwick.

Roston, R. (1961). Some personality characteristics of male compulsive gamblers. Unpublished doctoral dissertation, University of California, Los Angeles.

Swonomish Tribal Mental Health Project. (1991). *A gathering of wisdoms: Tribal mental health, a cultural perspective.* Mt. Vernon, Wash.: Veda Vangarde.

Taber, J. I., McCormick, R. A., & Ramirez, L. F. (1987). The prevalence and impact of major life stressors among pathological gamblers. *International Journal of the Addictions, 22,* 71–79.

Volberg, R. A., & Precision Marketing, Inc. (1993, April 23). *Gambling and problem gambling among Native Americans in North Dakota.* Albany, N.Y.: Gemini Research.

Zitzow, D. (1996a). Comparative study of problematic gambling behaviors between American Indian and Non-Indian adolescents within and near a Northern Plains reservation. *American Indian & Alaska Native Mental Health Research, 7,* 14–26.

Zitzow, D. (1996b). Comparative study of problematic gambling behaviors between American Indian and Non-Indian adults in a Northern Plains reservation. *American Indian and Alaska Native Mental Health Research, 7,* 27–41.

Legal Citations

Public Law 100-497 25 USC

25 USC, 2702, Sec. 3, 25 USC, 2702, Sec. 3

25 USC, 2703, Sec. 4

25 USC, 2710, Sec. 11

Chapter Three

Gambling in Canada
History, Economics, and Public Health

Wayne M. Yorke

Introduction: The Social Context of Gamblers and Gambling

All gamblers are not the same, and the causes of gambling are multiple. Inherited predisposition to gambling is only one etiological factor. In addition, gambling patterns vary, often in terms of broad social context, subjective states, and environmental pressures. Labeling gambling dependency a "disease" or an "impulse disorder" does not absolve the intemperate gambler from moral responsibility. Thus, by assigning to the gambler a medical debility and moral weakness, the problem is privatized. In turn, the medical professions profit by offering their professional skills, and the gambling industry is absolved from potential blame.

The outcome of labeling excessive gambling a disease is that addictionologists become absorbed in the genetic pathogenesis of gambling with all of the inherent conflicts, stresses, trauma, personality structure, and ego defenses. Thus, victims are treated and even may be changed by clinical services, but the profiteering multinational gaming complex is accepted as the normal condition of the society (Nikelly, 1994). The approach to gambling problems is similar to the historical approach to alcohol problems: Gambling is perceived as an individualized problem, as an illness or a disease, thus diverting attention from the most important issues, those related to social policy and political involvement.

An Overview of Gambling in Canada

Canadians are "hooked" on gambling. The sleeping giant has awakened. Gambling has arrived in Canada, and it is much bigger than anyone possibly could have projected. The combination of historical time, economic climate, government, policy openness, and down-and-dirty, basic human greed have all come together to produce an environment in which legal gambling has grown into a multibillion-dollar industry.

According to Moon (1992), during the 1991 fiscal year Canadians spent more than $10 billion[1] on legal wagers and bets. However, few realize the extent to which gambling is a daily part of life for millions of people and a source of crucial revenue for governments and charities. To put this expenditure in focus, $10 billion represents more than the combined 1990 revenue of five major Canadian corporations. This expenditure represents an annual per capita expenditure of nearly $370, or more than a dollar per person per day.

The History of Gambling: The Canadian Experience

In many ways, the Canadian gambling experience has paralleled that of the United States, where legalized gambling has gone through three major waves (Rose, 1995). These waves were all characterized by a transition from prohibition of gambling to widespread availability of gambling. According to the Archives at the Fortress of Louisbourg, the first real wave of gambling in Canada began on December 18, 1754. This phase of regulated gambling helped finance the colonies and contributed to the funding of American educational institutions such as Harvard and Yale.

More than 240 years ago, the French settlers' entertainment included playing various card games. Card games were so popular that during the summer, when the town's permanent population of about 5,000 increased to more than 8,000 with the arrival of more fishermen and sailors, some 7,200 decks of cards were also imported. This shipment provided almost enough for every person in Louisbourg to have his or her own deck of playing cards. Clary Croft, a folklore researcher with the Canadian Broadcasting Corporation in Halifax, Nova Scotia, noted that by the 1750s, lotteries were so popular in Louisbourg that the government stepped in to control them. On June 19, 1779, a proclamation against gambling tables read: "In spite of the law against public gambling, this practice continues whereby the fortunes of many have been ruined and the lives of many persons lost" (Croft, 1995, p. 284). Therefore, gambling tables were no longer allowed in public houses. Thirty years later, the following item appeared in a Halifax newspaper:

LOTTO RAISES FUNDS FOR HALIFAX SCHOOL
After selling the first batch of 5,000 tickets at 20 shillings each, as advertised on Sept. 25, 1781, the public school lottery has raised £750 of the £1500 needed to build a school. Prizes totaled £4250, with the biggest prize set at £2000. The House of Assembly had passed an act the previous October permitting the lottery to defray the cost of erecting "a proper and convenient building." (Abbott, 1990, p. 132)

However, because of corruption and cheating, gambling ventures were eventually regulated and prohibited.

The second wave of gambling took place in the United States between the Civil War and the end of the nineteenth century. In Canada, various forms of gambling seemed to go hand-in-hand with the development of the railway system linking the east and west, as well as with the Klondike Gold Rush during this same period. North America currently finds itself in the third wave of gambling. In the United States and Canada, Indian tribal gambling and other gambling legislation have resulted in a dramatic expansion of gambling, which is illustrated by the growth of gambling to the year 1992:

- New Hampshire started the first state lottery in 1963.
- Quebec started the first provincial lottery in 1968.
- All provinces had lotteries in 1992.
- In 1992 every province allowed charities to raise money through bingo games and raffles.
- By 1992 six out of ten provinces offered electronic slot machines, i.e., video lottery terminals.
- By 1992 five provinces had sports lotteries.
- By 1992 three provinces had offtrack horse betting.
- By 1992 all provinces had break-open tickets.
- In 1992 Canadians bet about $1.4 billion in Las Vegas and Reno alone, contributing to the $20 billion gross revenue.[2]

However, expansion of provincial and state-sponsored gambling is not confined to North America, but is now common among many countries throughout the world. A recent article in the *(Toronto) Globe and Mail* highlighted this trend:

LOTTERY FEVER STRIKES GAMBLING-HAPPY BRITONS
Record ticket sales raise concern that game of chance is too much of a good thing. Britons have gone lottery mad. Barely 4 months since Britain became the last European nation to launch a national lottery, six out of 10 adults play weekly. A billion tickets have been sold. The average punter buys two a week on the infinitesimal chance of becoming a multimillionaire. . . . Weekly sales have topped the £60 million mark ($135 million). The weekly draw is TV's biggest show. Supermarkets have to bring in extra staff to handle the crush on Fridays and Saturdays when 70 per cent of all tickets are bought. (Koring, 1995, p. A7)

The Nature of Canadian Gambling

Legalized public gambling in Canada is a recent phenomenon that has two specific components: true lotteries and other games of chance. "Prior to 1969, the Criminal

Table 3.1. *Expenditures on Gambling in Canada, 1992*

Type of Gambling	Amount of Expenditures
All legal gambling	$9,274,266,431
Lottery	2,967,729,000
Horse racing	1,921,263,000
Bingo	1,770,694,817
Other forms of gambling*	2,614,579,614

Source: Moon (1992).

*Revenue from all other legal forms of gambling went to provincial governments or to charities.

Note: According to Moon (1992), there is one dollar of illegal gambling for every dollar of legal gambling. According to this formula, the total amount spent on all forms of gambling in 1992 was over $18.5 billion.

Code of Canada prohibited such gambling activities except for parimutuel wagering on horse races, very small-scale occasional and private lottery schemes run for charitable purposes, and lottery schemes operated at an agricultural fair" (Osborne, 1992, pp. 62). In 1969 the federal government relaxed the strict criminal prohibitions on gambling to provide certain exemptions from the criminal prohibition attached to both true lotteries and quasi lotteries.

The reason for this delegation of authority to the provinces is found in the minister of justice's words: "We are assessing public opinion in this country. We feel that public opinion is not unanimous about [gambling] and that it might vary from region to region. We are, therefore, leaving it to the regions, as that public opinion may be interpreted by their provincial governments, that their provincial Attorney Generals have control over whether or not there should be lotteries permitted within provincial boundaries" (Standing Committee on Justice and Legal Affairs, 1969, p. 331). Tables 3.1 and 3.2 portray recent gambling growth and activities in Canada.

The Economics of Canadian Gambling

Turning our attention from the history of gambling in Canada to the present growing popularity of gambling, we see that lotteries have recently been far and away the most popular form of gambling. In 1992 Canadians spent $2.9 billion on provincially owned and operated lotteries. In 1994 Canadians spent $5.3 billion. Profits from this activity went to the provincial treasuries. In addition, since 1992 there has been an extremely active marketing strategy on the part of Atlantic Lotto and all lottery commissions to expand not only traditional gaming activities but also the product

Table 3.2. *Review of Gaming Activities Across Canada, Fiscal Year 1994 Annual Reports: Lottery Corporations of Canada*

Region	Sales	Net Income
Quebec	1,551,001	536,315
Ontario	1,886,080	563,546
Western	641,982	239,208
British Columbia	769,088	239,892
Eastern	530,892	178,000
Total	5,379,043	1,756,961

Sources: Atlantic Lottery Corporation (1994), British Columbia Lottery Corporation (1994), Loto-Quebec (1994), Ontario Lottery Corporation (1994), and Western Canada Lottery Corporation (1994).

line, frequency, and prize level of its payout, resulting in a rise in sales beyond imagination. For example, in the Atlantic region, the sales went from $230 million during fiscal year 1988–1989 to $530 million during the 1992–1993 fiscal year—a $300 million increase in five years.

Horse racing attracted the second-largest group of wagerers in Canada during 1992, as gamblers across the country bet $1.9 billion on thoroughbred and harness races. Taxes on racing wagers were shared by the federal and provincial governments. During 1992 bingo players (the third-largest group of wagerers) spent $1.7 billion on their game. The profits went to charities, many of which would have otherwise had to rely on the government for funds. In Nova Scotia, for instance, approximately $100 million in sales was reported (Atlantic Lottery Corporation, 1994).

It is estimated that for every dollar spent on legal gambling, an additional dollar is spent on illegal gambling (Moon, 1992). Whatever the exact figure, the amount of money Canadians spend on all forms of gambling is immense, and many experts believe that increasing the number of outlets for legal gambling would lead to decriminalization of gambling activities, even greater revenue, and painless taxes for provinces. Some argue that if people are going to gamble, it is better to let them do it within their communities and thus provide tax revenue for governments and charities (Moon).

From my perspective, it seems that Canadians fail to realize that Canada is a nation of gamblers. During fiscal year 1992, the Canadian population of 27,197,059 spent $9.2 billion on legal gambling. While most people associate American gambling with Las Vegas or Atlantic City, Canada also has a well-developed gambling industry, but it is based on a different sociological and geographical model. The charitable gaming industry in Canada is much more highly developed than it is—or per-haps ever was—in the United States. Although not all states and provinces keep records on charitable gambling, 1994 estimates indicate that the annual per capita expenditure on charitable gambling in Canada was more than 50 percent higher than that in the United States (McQueen, 1995).[3] In addition, the annual per capita ex-penditure on lotteries was over 23 percent higher in Canada than in the United States (McQueen, 1995). Gambling revenue now represents a significant portion of provincial budgets. Money from lotteries alone accounts for about 1.3 percent of provinces' revenues.

The growth of gambling is indicated by the increasing amounts of money spent on this activity. In 1974 in the United States, the national expenditure on gambling was $17.4 billion (U.S. dollars); by 1990 it had increased to $286.1 billion (Lesieur, 1992); and by 1994 it had reached $482 billion (Christiansen & Cummings, 1995). In Canada during 1993, $11 billion was spent by a population of 28 million; in Atlantic Canada the amount spent increased from $230 million to $530 million in five years. Nova Scotia, with a population of approximately 900,000, saw an increase in reve-nue from $17.4 million during fiscal year 1992 to $75.2 million during fiscal year 1993 (Atlantic Lottery Corporation, 1994).

Colin Campbell, an expert on gambling who teaches criminology at the Univer-sity of Windsor, Ontario, comments: "Unlike the United States, where several state governments have dedicated funds for research into the nature and extent of prob-lem gambling as well as for treatment programs, in Canada authorities remain aware of—or unconcerned about—the social consequences of problem gambling, particu-larly among minorities, women, and the relatively poor" (Campbell, 1991, p. 162). Political awareness of gambling in Canada, at this point in the history of gambling, has not resulted in any direct social action program responsibility. It appears that the political concern seems to be more focused on generating financial resources for the government. Gambling posturing of this type, on the part of both provincial and fed-eral governments, has become referred to by citizens as a "money grab" or as the "poor person's task."

Prevalence of Gambling Problems Among Adults in Canada

During the period between February 22 and May 3, 1993, Omnifacts Research Lim-ited conducted a provincewide survey on behalf of the Nova Scotia Drug Depen-dency Services. This survey consisted of 810 randomly selected adults 18 years of age and older and 300 randomly selected adolescents 13 to 17 years of age.

The South Oaks Gambling Screen (SOGS) was used to determine the prevalence of problem gambling among adults and adolescents in Nova Scotia. Among the 810 Nova Scotia adults in this sample, 3.1 percent were classified as problem gamblers and 1.7 percent were classified as probable pathological gamblers (Omnifacts Research Ltd., 1993). Of the 300 adolescents surveyed, 8.7 percent exhibited signs of problem gambling and 3 percent exhibited signs of pathological gambling. Although adolescents' attitudinal and behavior patterns were clearly different from those displayed by adults, no explanation has been found for why adolescents' combined level of problem and pathological gambling was so much higher than that of adults.

One possible explanation is that the SOGS is not as valid and reliable for adolescents as for adults. An examination of this point showed that the survey items associated with pathological gambling among adolescents were not the same as the items associated with pathological gambling among adults (Omnifacts Research Ltd., 1993). However, because the sample of adolescents in this study was relatively small, further research on Canadian adolescents is required to clarify this issue.

This study also investigated gamblers' preferences for different games. This analysis revealed that both adolescents and adults with gambling problems were most likely to be drawn to video gambling, though the relationship was somewhat weaker in the former category than the latter. Researchers noted that use of video games in video arcades was a weak predictor of addictive gambling among adolescents (Omnifacts Research Ltd., 1993). A study conducted among adults in New Brunswick (Baseline Market Research, 1992) reported similar findings, revealing that the general population preferred lottery tickets over other gambling activities but that pathological and potential pathological gamblers were linked most often with video gambling machines. Researchers need to explore further the association between pathological gambling and video gambling.

The profile of the adult compulsive gambler in Nova Scotia matches that generally found in the literature: young to middle-aged males, a slight majority of whom earn less than $40,000 per year and have an educational background of high school or less. In addition to the two studies reported above, at least nine other studies have investigated the prevalence of pathological gambling among Canadian adults (Bland, Newman, Orn, & Stebelsky, 1993; Criterion Research Corporation, 1995; Ferris & Stirpe, 1995; Gemini Research & Angus Reid Group, 1994; Govoni & Frisch, 1996; Insight Canada Research, 1993; Ladouceur, 1991; Volberg, 1994; Wynne Resources Ltd., 1994; Baseline Market Research, 1992, for New Brunswick; Omnifacts Research Limited, 1993, for Novia Scotia).

These eleven studies reveal estimates of the rate of current problem gambling among the adult Canadian population ranging from 1.1 percent to 9 percent (median = 2.75 percent) and estimates of the rate of current pathological gambling ranging from .2 percent to 1.7 percent (median = 1.1 percent). Similarly, these studies reveal estimates of the rate of lifetime problem gambling among the adult Canadian population ranging from 2.4 percent to 10 percent (median = 4 percent) and estimates of the rate of lifetime pathological gambling ranging from .42 percent to 2.7 percent (median = 1.25 percent). Table 3.3 lists these estimates of the rate of problem and pathological gambling among adults in Canada.

Table 3.3. *Prevalence Rates of Problem and Pathological Gambling Among Adults in Canada*

Province	Prevalence of Problem Gambling (%)		Prevalence of Probable Pathological Gambling (%)		Year of Data Collection
Alberta(a)	5.9	(lifetime rate)	2.7	(lifetime rate)	1993
	4.0	(current rate)	1.4	(current rate)	
Alberta(b)	—		.42	(lifetime rate)	1983–1990
British Columbia	6.0	(lifetime rate)	1.8	(lifetime rate)	1993
	2.4	(current rate)	1.1	(current rate)	
Manitoba(a)	2.9	(lifetime rate)*	1.3	(lifetime rate)	1993
Manitoba(b)	2.4	(lifetime rate)	1.9	(lifetime rate)	1995
New Brunswick	4.0	(lifetime rate)	2.0	(lifetime rate)	1992
	3.1	(current rate)	1.4	(current rate)	
Nova Scotia	4.5	(current rate)	1.7	(current rate)	1993
Ontario(a)	7.7	(lifetime rate)*	.9	(lifetime rate)	1993
Ontario(b)	1.5	(current rate)	.9	(current rate)	1993–94 (pre-casino)
Ontario(c)	1.1	(current rate)	1.1	(current rate)	1995 (post-casino)
Ontario(d)	10.0	(lifetime rate)	1.0	(lifetime rate)	1995
	9.0	(current rate)	.2	(current rate)	
Quebec	2.6	(lifetime rate)	1.2	(lifetime rate)	1989
Saskatchewan	2.8	(lifetime rate)	1.2	(lifetime rate)	1993
	1.9	(current rate)	.8	(current rate)	

Sources: Alberta(a): Wynne Resources Ltd. (1994); Alberta(b): Bland, Newman, Orn, & Stebelsky (1993). British Columbia: Gemini Research & Angus Reid Group (1994). Manitoba(a)(b): Criterion Research Corporation (1995). New Brunswick: Baseline Market Research (1992). Nova Scotia: Omnifacts Research Limited (1993). Ontario(a): Insight Canada Research (1993); Ontario(b)(c): Govoni & Frisch (1996); Ontario(d): Ferris & Stirpe (1995). Quebec: Ladouceur (1991). Saskatchewan: Volberg (1994).
*If studies using the SOGS do not indicate the time frame of reported rates they are listed as lifetime rates.

Gambling Problems Among Adolescents in Canada

Studies conducted among adolescents in Nova Scotia, Ontario, Quebec, and Alberta (Govoni, Rupcich, & Frisch, 1996; Insight Canada Research, 1994; Ladouceur & Mireault, 1988; Omnifacts Research Ltd., 1993; Wynne Resources Ltd., 1996) reveal rates of subclinical gambling problems, for example, "problem" or "at-risk" gambling ranging from 8.7 percent to 33 percent and rates of clinically diagnosable gambling problems (that is, pathological gambling) ranging from 3 percent to 8.1 percent. Therefore, it seems incorrect to consider expanding gambling activities without taking into consideration those who may become future casualties of gaming. Table 3.4 illustrates prevalence rates of gambling problems among adolescents.

As Nicholas Rupcich of the Canadian Foundation on Compulsive Gambling stated, "If we've got one in twenty teenagers gambling out of control, what are we going to see up the road?" (Corelli, 1994, p. 28). It is important for society to recognize that socially accepted recreational activities with potentially addictive characteristics present real potential dangers and should be addressed appropriately to minimize their negative social impact. Many individuals in society will enjoy potentially harmful experiences (for example, bungee jumping, skydiving, drinking, and gambling) with a fair margin of safety, but every effort must be made to reduce possible harmful effects through the promotion of consumer awareness, education, and prevention programs.

Advocacy for current and up-to-date research will improve the chances that youth, when faced with the choice of a variety of life experiences and potentially addictive behaviors, will have the necessary information to make such choices. Society has an obligation to impress upon our youth that potentially addictive experiences, though possibly not harmful in themselves, put them at a higher risk of harm because of their lack of experience with these activities.

Problems related to gambling activities among adolescents include disrupting school and employment, borrowing money to gamble or to pay off debts, using lunch money and diverting other financial resources to gambling, and resorting to illegal activities. Adolescent gambling behavior in the province of Nova Scotia offers some interesting characteristics, as reported by Omnifacts Research Limited (1993):

- Money gambled in one day ranged from $1 to $500, with a median amount of $3.
- Playing pool or other games for money was the gambling activity adolescents participated in most frequently.
- Lottery tickets and slot/video poker machines were the second most frequently pursued gambling activity.
- The largest amount of money was spent on slot/video poker machines.
- Playing video games surpassed all of the gambling activities among youths with possible gambling problems.

Table 3.4. *Prevalence Rates of Problem and Pathological Gambling Among Adolescents in Canada*

Province	Prevalence of Problem Gambling (%)	Prevalence of Probable Pathological Gambling (%)	Year of Data Collection
Alberta	15.0 (current rate)	8.0 (current rate)	1995
Nova Scotia	8.7 (current rate)	3.0 (current rate)	1993
Ontario(a)	9.4 (lifetime rate)	8.1 (lifetime rate)	1994
Ontario(b)	33.0 (lifetime rate)*	4.0 (lifetime rate)	1994
Quebec	—	3.6 (lifetime rate)†	1986

Sources: Alberta: Wynne Resources Ltd. (1996). Nova Scotia: Omnifacts Research Limited (1993). Ontario(a): Govoni, Rupcich & Frisch (1996); Ontario(b): Insight Canada Research (1994). Quebec: Ladouceur & Mireault (1988).
*If studies do not indicate the time frame of reported rates they are listed as lifetime rates.
†Insight Canada Research (1994). Less stringent scale based on DSM-III criteria.

- Video-game playing had the strongest connections to adolescent gamblers with potential addictions.
- Adolescents have revealed a higher prevalence rate for both problem and probable pathological gambling than adults.

The risk of adolescents' becoming problem or pathological gamblers is a real concern. Most problem gamblers started gambling in early childhood, either in their homes or in their neighborhoods (Omnifacts Research Ltd., 1993).

Commenting on the work of Erik Erickson (1972) and Anna Freud (1958) in reference to adolescent behavior, Pursley (1991) offers the following insight:

During adolescence, there is the need for acceptance, a need for outlets of expression in physical, intellectual, and emotional fields, and a need for standards with which to conform or to rebel. There is a special need to be treated as a unique individual—with the same respect that adults automatically give to one another. There is the need to be independent. It comes as no surprise, therefore, that adolescents model adult behaviors at an early age—they smoke, drink, and gamble to express their growth toward maturity. (pp. 25–27)

The adolescents researched within the province of Nova Scotia, as compared with Canadian adults, tend to demonstrate a variety of cognitive distortions concerning the realities of gambling. The adolescents:

- are more likely to argue over moneys won or lost.
- admit more readily that they have a problem controlling their gambling.
- feel less guilty about their gambling.
- feel that gambling, for the most part, is their own affair.
- are more likely to think that there are tricks to winning at gambling activities.
- are more likely to think of gambling as a harmless pastime.
- are more likely to report that one or both of their parents gambled too much.

In addition, adolescents' involvement with electronic media, computers, video games, arcades, and gambling devices promotes an alignment of self with a machine and an avoidance of socialization. This phenomenon results in a social imbalance, leaving adolescents with diminished or developmentally delayed social skills. In addition, studies have shown that excessive pinball and video game use can lead to behavior patterns similar to pathological gambling (Fisher, 1994; Griffiths, 1992). Specific studies need to determine if pinball, billiards, and video games are the adolescent forms of adult casino gambling and if one form influences the other. Pursley (1991) offers direction for future studies regarding adolescent gambling, suggesting the need for longitudinal studies that will address the influence of drug- and gambling-saturated environments and their impact upon adolescents.

Following this understanding, Shaffer (1994) sounds an alarm of caution to policy-makers and society regarding the great risk being imposed on our young people:

> As gambling became normalized during the past three decades, the moral prohibition that historically served to regulate bidding excesses diminished. With increasing economic need, moral restraint was discarded by both policymakers and the public. Social policymakers have decided that America will gamble. It seems essential that we begin to determine how that will happen. Culturally endorsed gambling has not and will not come without a price. (p. 16)

As society moves further into the twenty-first century, our ability to socialize and relate to one another in a meaningful way becomes impeded by the technological advancements designed to assist us in improving our own communication abilities. These electronically advanced systems, when matched with the ingenuity and development of gambling devices, set a stage for a colossal calamity for the next generation—an entrapment in an illusionary world of almost virtual reality wherein everything is a game and every game may be won or lost. The game and the play have a price. Are we willing to pay the price?

Conclusion and Recommendations

This chapter provided an overview of gambling activities in Canada. In addition, this discussion examined the effects of Canadian gambling on the adolescent population as a very early attempt to identify potential problem areas related to gaming. The following is a list of recommendations, from the Canadian perspective, to increase our understanding of gambling and its effects, improve public awareness of potential problems that may emerge as a consequence of gambling, and implement programs to prevent gambling-related problems. Canadians should:

- Develop a strategy to implement a program of research on Canadian gambling activities in general, and on the impact of these events on adolescent behavior in particular.
- Study the extent of problems associated with gambling, including the social impact of gambling and the efficacy of treatment programs.
- Develop consumer awareness by developing and implementing programs of gambling education and prevention.
- Develop systematic investigations of the prevalence and nature of adolescent gambling.
- Using an epidemiologic model, develop strategies based on lifestyle risk analysis to minimize the potential adverse consequences that may be faced by youthful gamblers.

Notes

The author would like to thank Howard Shaffer and Harvard Medical School for their kind invitation and the extension of the Harvard Shield of Friendship and Community Involvement. The author would also like to thank the Senior Staff of Drug Dependency Services, with special thanks to Josephine Skinner, Sheila Amos, Brenda Wylde, Jerome Aucoin, and Katherine Côté for their invaluable advice and help during the preparation of this chapter.

1. All dollar figures in this chapter refer to Canadian dollars unless otherwise noted.

2. Atlantic Lottery Corporation (1993, 1994), British Columbia Lottery Corporation (1994), Corelli (1994), Loto-Quebec (1994), Ontario Lottery Corporation (1994), Smith (1992), Western Canada Lottery Corporation (1994).

3. All comparisons of Canadian and U.S. expenditures in this chapter use an estimated 1994 exchange rate of 1$ Canadian = $.735 U.S.

References

Abbott, E. (Ed.). (1990). *Chronicle of Canada*. Montreal: Chronicle Publications.

Atlantic Lottery Corporation. (1993). *Annual report, 1992–93*. Moncton, New Brunswick: Author.

Atlantic Lottery Corporation. (1994). *Annual report, 1993–94*. Moncton, New Brunswick: Author.

Baseline Market Research. (1992). *Prevalence survey: Problem gambling*. Report to the New Brunswick Department of Finance. Fredericton, New Brunswick: N.p.

Bland, R. C., Newman, S. C., Orn, H., & Stebelsky, G. (1993). Epidemiology of pathological gambling in Edmonton. *Canadian Journal of Psychiatry, 38,* 108–12.

British Columbia Lottery Corporation. (1994). *Annual report, 1993/1994.* Victoria, British Columbia: Author.

Campbell, C. S. (1991). Gambling in Canada. In M. A. Jackson & C. T. Griffiths (Eds.), *Canadian criminology: Perspectives on crime and criminality* (pp. 153–65). Toronto: Harcourt Brace Jovanovich, Canada.

Christiansen, E. M., & Cummings, W. E. (1995, August). The United States '94 gross annual wager. *International Gaming & Wagering Business, 17,* 29–68.

Corelli, R. (1994, May 30). Betting on casinos. *MacLean's, 28.*

Criterion Research Corporation. (1995, September). *Problem gambling study: Final report.* Report prepared for the Manitoba Lotteries Corporation. Winnipeg, Manitoba: Author.

Croft, C. (1995). Mainstreet's folklore research. Canadian Broadcasting Corporation. (RGI, Vol. 170, p. 284; RGI, Vol. 329, Doc. 157). Halifax, Nova Scotia.

Ferris, J., & Stirpe, T. (1995). *Gambling in Ontario: A report from a general population survey on gambling-related problems and opinions.* Toronto: Addiction Research Foundation, Problem and Compulsive Gambling Project.

Fisher, S. (1994). Identifying video game addiction in children and adolescents. *Addictive Behaviors, 19,* 545–53.

Gemini Research & Angus Reid Group. (1994). *Social gaming and problem gambling in British Columbia.* Report to the British Columbia Lottery Corporation. Roaring Springs, PA: Gemini Research.

Govoni, R., & Frisch, G. R. (1996). *The impact of the Windsor Casino on adult gambling in the city of Windsor.* Preliminary report. Windsor, Ontario: Problem Gambling Research Group, University of Windsor Department of Psychology.

Govoni, R., Rupcich, N., & Frisch, G. R. (1996). Gambling behavior of adolescent gamblers. *Journal of Gambling Studies, 12,* 305–17.

Griffiths, M. D. (1992). Pinball wizard: The case of a pinball machine addict. *Psychological Reports, 71,* 160–62.

Insight Canada Research. (1993). *Prevalence of problem and pathological gambling in Ontario using the South Oaks Gambling Screen.* Toronto: Canadian Foundation for Compulsive Gambling.

Insight Canada Research. (1994). *An exploration of the prevalence of pathological gambling behavior among adolescents in Ontario.* Report prepared for the Canadian Foundation on Compulsive Gambling. Willowdale, Ontario: Author.

Koring, P. (1995). Lottery fever strikes gambling-happy Britons. *(Toronto) Globe and Mail,* p. A7.

Ladouceur, R. (1991, December). Prevalence estimates of pathological gambling in Quebec. *Canadian Journal of Psychiatry, 36,* 732–34.

Ladouceur, R., & Mireault, C. (1988). Gambling behaviors among high school students in the Quebec area. *Journal of Gambling Behavior, 4,* 3–12.

Lesieur, H. R. (1992). Pathological gambling, work, and employee assistance. *Journal of Employee Assistance Research, 1,* 56–74.

Loto-Quebec. (1994). *Twenty-fourth annual report (1993–94)*. Montreal: Author.

McQueen, P. A. (1995, July 1). *North American gaming report 1995*. Supplement to *International Gaming & Wagering Business*. New York: BMT Communications, Inc.

Moon, P. (1992, May 9). Canadians are hooked on gambling. *(Toronto) Globe and Mail*, pp. A1, A4.

Nikelly, A. G. (1994). Alcoholism: Social as well as psycho-medical problem: The missing "big picture." *Journal of Alcohol & Drug Education 39*, 1–12.

Omnifacts Research Limited. (1993). *An examination of the prevalence of gambling in Nova Scotia*. Research report no. 93090 for the Nova Scotia Department of Health, Drug Dependency Services. Halifax, Nova Scotia: Author.

Ontario Lottery Corporation. (1994). *Annual report, 1993–94*. Toronto: Author.

Osborne, J. A. (1992). Licensing without law: Legalized gambling in British Columbia. *Canadian Public Administration, 35*, 56–74.

Pursley, W. L. (1991). *Adolescence, chemical dependency, and pathological gambling*. New York: Haworth Press Inc.

Rose, I. N. (1995). Gambling and the law: Endless fields of dreams. *Journal of Gambling Studies, 11*, 15–33.

Shaffer, H. J. (1994). *The emergence of youthful addiction: The prevalence of underage lottery use and the impact of gambling*. Technical report no. 011394-100. Boston: Massachusetts Council on Compulsive Gambling.

Smith, G. J. (1992). *Compulsive gambling: General issues, treatments, and policy considerations*. Report prepared for Alberta Lotteries and Gaming. Edmonton, Alberta: University of Alberta.

Standing Committee on Justice and Legal Affairs. (1969). *Proceedings (1968–69)*. Ottawa: Queens Printer.

Volberg, R. A. (1994). *Gambling and problem gambling in Saskatchewan*. Report to the Minister's Advisory Committee on Social Impacts of Gaming. Regina, Saskatchewan: Author.

Western Canada Lottery Corporation. (1994). *Annual report, 1994*. Stettler, Alberta: Author.

Wynne Resources Ltd. (1994). *Gambling and problem gambling in Alberta*. Summary report prepared for Alberta Lotteries and Gaming. Edmonton, Alberta: Author.

Wynne Resources Ltd. (1996, May). *Adolescent gambling and problem gambling in Alberta*. Report prepared for the Alberta Alcohol and Drug Abuse Commission. Edmonton, Alberta: Author.

Chapter Four

What Are My Chances?

Using Probability and Number Sense to Educate Teens About the Mathematical Risks of Gambling

Terry W. Crites

The last 20 years have seen gambling explode; it now pervades our society. Andersen (1994) recounted that before 1978, the year casino gambling came to Atlantic City, "Nevada was the only place in America where one could legally go to a casino, and there were just fourteen state lotteries" (p. 45). Furthermore, "as recently as 1990, there were just three states with casinos, not counting those on Indian reservations; now there are nine. Lotteries have spread to 37 states. Indiana and five Mississippi River states have talked themselves into allowing gambling on riverboats" (p. 45).

Although Nevada and Atlantic City are considered the centers of the gambling world, casinos can be found throughout the United States, in large part because of the Indian Gaming Regulatory Act of 1988 (IGRA). Hellman (1994) identified 179 Native American casinos in 27 states; the number of casinos is now larger and continues to grow. In fact, the number of casinos in each of three states—Minnesota, Wisconsin, and Arizona—is greater than the number of casinos in Atlantic City (Hellman, 1994; Sowers, 1995). According to Fujii (1994), only Hawaii and Utah have resisted gambling's lure by "banning all forms of commercialized gambling, including lotteries" (p. 83).

Gambling is also big business. According to Hellman (1994), legalized gambling's total "handle" (the total amount of money wagered) in 1992 was $329 billion, which was greater than the gross national product of Australia and Argentina combined; the total revenue from legal gambling was $30 billion. Hellman also gave an example of the various states' interest in casino gambling when he described the arrangement between the Mashantucket tribe and the state of Connecticut. In return for being allowed to install slot machines in its casinos, the tribe annually pays the state "25 percent of the slot-machine gross, or $100 million, whichever is bigger. The tribal ante is expected to hit $113 million in fiscal 1994" (p. 84). Under the IGRA, states and tribes must negotiate such agreements. Andersen (1994) reported, "The state of Nevada now derives half its public funds from gaming-related revenues. Nevadans pay no state income or inheritance tax" (p. 45).

Because gambling is so prevalent, America's teens need to be educated about its associated risks. They need to know why this activity is called "gambling." Teens, who will later be adults, must become "informed consumers." Then, if ever faced with the decision to gamble or not, they can be strengthened by full knowledge of their chances of winning. They will know that the odds are against the gambler—that in the long run, the gambler loses money.

To help achieve this goal, school curricula must expose students to mathematics that include discussions of probability and number sense. Many professional groups (National Council of Teachers of Mathematics, 1989, 1991; National Research Council, 1989; Mathematical Sciences Educational Board, 1990; National Council of Supervisors of Mathematics, 1989; Mathematical Association of America, 1991) support the inclusion of these two topics in the mathematics curriculum. While gambling is not the sole, or even primary, reason for studying probability and number sense, gambling does give a specific context within which an examination of these two topics may take place, creating the foundation for sensible gambling.

This chapter examines how incorporating a discussion of various games of chance into a classroom unit on probability can build students' number sense while increasing their knowledge of the likelihood of random events. Specifically, this chapter will look at the mathematics of some of the most popular and easily analyzed games: lotteries, keno, roulette, and craps. Some of the fallacies and misconceptions associated with gaming will also be presented. Finally, some suggestions on how to incorporate these ideas into the classroom will be discussed.

The Lottery—America's Obsession

Lotteries have become a part of American life. As previously mentioned, at least 37 states and the District of Columbia have at least one version of a lottery game that offers to make its players "instant millionaires." Multistate lotteries, like Powerball, award millions of dollars in prizes to players who predict all the numbers drawn. Most states' weekly drawings have a guaranteed prize of at least $1 million, and prizes of $5 million are quite common.

HOW TO PLAY THE LOTTERY

Playing the lottery is probably the simplest game of chance. Most states use some variation of the following procedure. Each player picks six numbers out of a pool; in Arizona, for example, the pool consists of 42 numbers. On a given day, a lottery official randomly chooses six numbers from the same pool—usually using some type of mechanical random-number generator. Players who match all six numbers win the jackpot. Smaller prizes may be awarded for matching three, four, or five of the six numbers.

If no player matches all six numbers, the jackpot "rolls over" and is increased for the next round of playing. As the jackpot increases, so does the interest in playing. In turn, the jackpot increases, which increases the interest in playing, and so on. This cycle continues, sometimes reaching a fever pitch, until someone wins the jackpot, which, because of the "rollovers," may have grown to $30 million, $50 million, or even $100 million.

WHAT IS THE PROBABILITY OF WINNING?

Using combinatorics, the probability of winning the lottery is easily computed. In Arizona, where players pick 6 of 42 numbers, there are 5,245,786 different ways in which someone can draw the 6 numbers:

$$\binom{42}{6} = \frac{42!}{36! \ 6!} = 5,245,786.$$

To win the jackpot, however, all 6 numbers must be correctly chosen, so there is only one way to win:

$$\binom{6}{6} = \frac{6!}{0! \ 6!} = 1.$$

Therefore, the probability of winning the jackpot in the Arizona lottery is:

$$\frac{1}{5,245,786}.$$

Students and teachers alike should find it informative to note that by increasing the pool of numbers by just 6, from 42 to 48, the probability of winning the jackpot is cut by more than 57 percent:

$$\frac{\binom{6}{6}}{\binom{48}{6}} = \frac{1}{12,271,512}.$$

Increasing the pool of numbers by 12, from 42 to 54, reduces the probability of winning the jackpot by almost 80 percent. A rather important result that all students should be aware of is that the probability of winning the jackpot is not directly proportional to the quantity of numbers in the pool from which they are picked.

The lottery game Powerball is a little different: Players pick 5 numbers from a pool of 45 and then a sixth, bonus number (the "powerball") from the same pool. The jackpot is won by the player(s) who correctly pick the 5 numbers plus the power-ball. The use of combinatorics shows the probability of winning this game is:

$$\frac{\binom{5}{5}}{\binom{45}{5}} \times \frac{\binom{1}{1}}{\binom{45}{1}} = \frac{1}{1,221,759} \times \frac{1}{45} = \frac{1}{54,979,155}.$$

Even if you examine the probability of winning something less than the jackpot, the odds are not very favorable. Many lotteries award a "free play" (which is typically worth $1) or maybe a $2 cash prize to players who correctly choose 3 of the 6 numbers picked. In Arizona, where the pool consists of 42 numbers, the probability of picking 3 of the 6 numbers drawn is:

$$\frac{\binom{6}{3}\binom{36}{3}}{\binom{42}{6}} = \frac{10,200}{374,699} = 0.02722.$$

Not only is winning the jackpot highly unlikely, but the probability of picking only 3 numbers is very low as well as is the probability of correctly picking 4 of the 6 numbers:

$$\frac{\binom{6}{4}\binom{36}{2}}{\binom{42}{6}} = \frac{675}{374,699} = 0.0018.$$

And the probability of correctly picking 5 of the 6 numbers is:

$$\frac{\binom{6}{5}\binom{36}{1}}{\binom{42}{6}} = \frac{108}{2,622,893} = 0.00004.$$

The probability of winning the lottery looks especially slim when compared with other, more serious, chance events. McGervey (1986) reported that fatalities from driving a car a distance of 60 miles without wearing a seat belt, flying in a commercial plane for 10 hours, and smoking a total of 2 cigarettes occur with a probability of 1/1,000,000, which is more than 50 times as likely as winning Powerball. Paulos

(1988) gave the following fatal probabilities: being killed by a terrorist 1/1,600,000, dying in a bicycle crash 1/75,000, choking to death 1/68,000, drowning 1/20,000, and dying in a car crash 1/5,300. All of these events have probabilities that do not even come close to matching the probability of winning any state lottery. Yet for some reason—perhaps poor number sense or a misunderstanding of probability— people perceive the chance of winning the lottery to be much higher than the chance of dying while driving a car without wearing a seat belt.

CAN THE PROBABILITY OF WINNING BE INCREASED?

Despite the claims of numerous books, magazines, and video tapes that offer "secret" or "mystical" systems for winning the lottery, the probability of winning cannot be increased. Any 6 numbers are just as likely to be picked as the next, regardless of what numbers have been picked in the past. Numbers are inanimate objects that do not possess the ability to remember when they have been previously selected. It is a misunderstanding of randomness that ruins many players of games of chance, especially in games that involve dice, cards, or picking numbers.

The only sure way of winning the lottery is to buy enough tickets to cover all number combinations. Students may wonder why multimillionaires do not guarantee themselves the lottery jackpot by doing exactly this, especially if it is a large sum, like $100,000,000.[1] To guarantee a win in Powerball, you would have to buy 54,979,155 tickets. It is an interesting exercise for students to estimate and then calculate how long it would take a person to buy close to 55 million lottery tickets.

LOTTERY FACTS AND MYTHS

Numerous misconceptions surround the picking of lottery numbers. Many people believe they should select numbers that are evenly distributed throughout the range of choices. For example, the typical person on the street might think the numbers 4, 12, 18, 21, 28, and 35 would have a better chance of being selected than, say, 1, 3, 5, 7, 8, and 9, or 34, 35, 36, 37, 38, and 39. They might think to themselves, "It isn't very often that the numbers drawn are all less than 10 or are all consecutive. They are usually spread throughout the range of possible numbers." The problem with this thinking is that while it is true that the chance of nonconsecutive numbers being drawn is greater than the chance of consecutive numbers being drawn, and that the chance that all the numbers will be higher than 10 is greater than the chance that all the numbers will be less than 10, these are not bets you are allowed to make. You do not get to choose "consecutive" or "not consecutive," "all less than 25," or "uniformly distributed"; you must choose 6 numbers. On that level the numbers 1, 2, 3, 4, 5, and 6 are just as likely as 5, 10, 15, 20, 25, and 30, or 4, 12, 18, 21, 28, and 35. Any group of 6 numbers is just as likely to be chosen as another.

Others may think it is wise to pick the same 6 numbers every time. If their usual 6 numbers were chosen during a time when they did not play the lottery, however, most people would pick a different set of numbers when playing the next time. "The probability of the same 6 numbers coming up twice in a row is astronomical," they would say. But again, this is not the bet you are allowed to make. You are not betting that the next two lottery drawings will be the same; you are only betting that the next one is going to be your 6 numbers. The probability of a specific set of 6 numbers being drawn from a specific pool is always the same, regardless of what has happened before. The probability of being able to predict any two consecutive lottery picks, be it the same 6 numbers coming up twice in a row or two different sets of 6 numbers coming up on consecutive picks, is identical. Students' numbers sense and comprehension of probability will improve once they understand this notion of random selection.

The lottery agencies do nothing to help improve these notions, however. Their job is to get people to buy lottery tickets, not to promote the risks. The probability of winning the jackpot is never as highly publicized as the size of the jackpot. Lottery officials never advertise that people are much more likely to be killed in a bicycle crash than to win the jackpot. In addition, people are induced to play the lottery through promises of instant wealth with slogans like "Someone has to win" and "You can't win if you don't play." In the stories that identify the winner, the amount of money lost by lottery players is never mentioned.

Another common practice is for lottery agencies to publicize photographs and demographic information of jackpot winners. Many believe that if "common people" win—maybe people who share their hometown, line of work, or economic stratum, or people who buy their lottery tickets at the same market—their own chances of winning are somehow improved. An elderly woman who won the jackpot was heard to say on a radio commercial, "I'm living proof that even the little person can win the lottery." These advertisements are designed to capitalize on the public's tendency to personalize chance events: "If they can win, so can I!"

However, even if you beat the odds and win a $1 million jackpot, the lottery officials will not write you a check for that amount. Instead, they will typically pay a $1 million winner by purchasing an annuity (for an amount much less than $1 million) that makes 20 annual payments of $50,000, before taxes. Although most of us would be quite happy to be guaranteed $50,000 for the next 20 years, it is not quite the same as having $1 million in hand to invest today, for two reasons. First, as a result of inflation, the future value of $50,000 is considerably less 10 or 15 years from now than $50,000 today. Second, use of the compound interest formula[2]

$$A = P\left(1 + \frac{r}{n}\right)^{nt}$$

shows that $1 million invested today at 6 percent would grow to at least $3.2 million in 20 years.

Mark Number of Spots or Ways Played					Price Per Way			Price Per Game	
					Number of Games			Total Price	
1	2	3	4	5	6	7	8	9	10
11	12	13	14	15	16	17	18	19	20
21	22	23	24	25	26	27	28	29	30
31	32	33	34	35	36	37	38	39	40
41	42	43	44	45	46	47	48	49	50
51	52	53	54	55	56	57	58	59	60
61	62	63	64	65	66	67	68	69	70
71	72	73	74	75	76	77	78	79	80

Fig. 4.1. Sample Keno Card

Keno and Roulette—Cousins to the Lottery

The games keno and roulette have much in common with the lottery. All three games are based on the same principle: The players bet that they can predict what number(s) will be chosen by the game's operator. The only differences are the quantity of numbers chosen and the method by which the game's operator chooses them. Versions of many of the lottery facts and myths are also found in keno and roulette; and as with the lottery, these games can be analyzed by using combinatorics. Keno and roulette, therefore, provide an excellent context within which the concepts of probability and number sense can be developed.

HOW TO PLAY KENO
In the simplest version of the game, the player selects 1 to 15 numbers from a card marked with numbers from 1 to 80 (see figure 4.1).

At a later time, the casino draws 20 different numbers from 1 to 80. The players win, lose, or break even, depending on how many of these 20 numbers they match. The winnings are paid according to a schedule that is carefully constructed by the gaming establishment. A portion of a payoff schedule from a Laughlin, Nevada,

Table 4.1 *Schedule of Winning When Playing Keno*

PICK 10 NUMBERS

Numbers "Caught"	Payoff on a $1 Bet	Payoff on a $3 Bet	Payoff on a $5 Bet
10	$50,000	$50,000	$50,000
9	$5,000	$15,000	$25,000
8	$1,000	$3,000	$5,000
7	$160	$480	$800
6	$20	$60	$100
5	$1	$3	$5

casino (table 4.1) shows that if players chose 10 numbers, they would win or break even if they "caught" 5, 6, 7, 8, 9, or 10 of the 20 numbers drawn by the casino.

WHAT IS THE PROBABILITY OF WINNING AT KENO?

Computing the probability of winning in keno is similar to computing the probability of winning the lottery. After the casino draws its 20 numbers, the pool of 80 original numbers is effectively split into two groups: the 20 numbers that were chosen and the 60 numbers that were not. Therefore, if the player has chosen m numbers, the probability of catching n of the 20 numbers drawn is given by

$$\frac{\binom{20}{n}\binom{60}{m-n}}{\binom{80}{m}}$$

for $1 \le n \le m$. The probability distribution, along with the associated payoff, for the case described above ($m = 10$) is given in table 4.2.

An examination of the probability distribution shows that when you pick 10 numbers, the probability of losing money (catching 0, 1, 2, 3, or 4 numbers) is 93.5 percent, the probability of breaking even (catching 5 numbers) is 5.1 percent, and the probability of winning money (catching 6, 7, 8, 9, or 10 numbers) is only 1.4 percent. Computing the expected value for this distribution results in a mean winning of –29 cents. This means that when you play the game many times, you will average a loss of 29 cents for every $1 you bet—giving the house a 29 percent advantage. While this particular analysis is based on picking 10 numbers, similar outcomes would result from examining other possible choices for the quantity of numbers picked. With a house advantage of around 25 percent for all options, it is easy to see why casinos

Table 4.2 *Probability Distribution and Resulting Payoff When Playing Keno and Picking 10 Numbers*

PICK 10 NUMBERS

Numbers "Caught"	Probability	Payoff on a $1 Bet
0	0.0457907008	–$1
1	0.1795713756	–$1
2	0.2952567811	–$1
3	0.2674023678	–$1
4	0.1473188971	–$1
5	0.0514276877	$0
6	0.0114793946	$19
7	0.0016111431	$159
8	0.0001354194	$999
9	0.0000061206	$4,999
10	0.0000001122	$49,999

and other gaming establishments love the game of keno. It is also easy to understand why Ortiz (1986) advised, "the best strategy one can ever hope to fashion for keno is to stay away from the game" (p. 221).

HOW TO PLAY ROULETTE

Roulette uses a large wheel with pockets around its outer edge. These pockets are numbered from 1 to 36 and are arranged nonsequentially in alternating colors of black and red. Two green pockets—numbered "0" and "00"—complete the roulette wheel. The operator spins the wheel and drops a white ball into a small groove around the rim. Gravity eventually forces the ball to drop into one of the numbered pockets.

Players can make various bets on where they think the ball will stop, that is, in what numbered pocket the ball will land. A layout on the roulette table is used to facilitate the betting (see figure 4.2). Roulette players place chips in strategic locations of the layout to make any combination of the 11 wagers described in table 4.3.

WHAT IS THE PROBABILITY OF WINNING AT ROULETTE?

The probability of winning a particular roulette wager can be calculated by dividing the quantity of numbers covered in a particular bet by 38. For example, the probabilities of winning a "straight-up" bet, a "column" bet, or a "red" bet are 1/38, 6/19, and 9/19, respectively. However, it is important to note that these probabilities are significantly less than what the casinos pay to the winners. For example, the odds against winning a straight-up bet are 37 to 1 (that is, 37 ways to lose and 1 way to

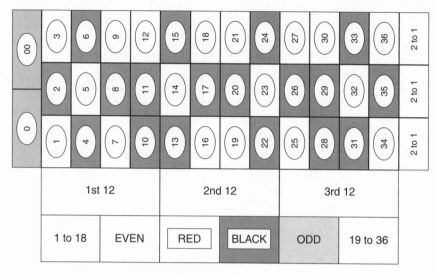

Fig. 4.2. Layout for Roulette Table

win), but the casino pays off at only 35 to 1. In other words, the casino uses the two extra pockets ("0" and "00") to its advantage in calculating the odds against a win by a gambler, but does not include these two possibilities when calculating the payout. This 2 out of 38 (5.26 percent) shortfall is the "house advantage"—how the casino owners convert your money into their money. While not as great as the roughly 25 percent advantage the casino enjoys in keno, the house advantage ensures that you will eventually run out of money if you have an average loss of 5.26¢ for every $1 you bet. This disadvantage is inescapable because of the presence of the "0" and "00" spots. Unless you have made a five-number bet or have bet these numbers straight up, you lose if either the "0" or "00" comes up. Because of these two spots, all wagers except for the five-number bet have a house advantage of 5.26 percent.

Some may think that the five-number bet, therefore, is the proper bet to make. It is not. The five-number bet is the worst roulette bet possible. By paying off at 6 to 1 odds—equivalent to 30 to 5 odds—rather than the true odds of 33 to 5, the house gives itself a 7.89 percent advantage on this wager. The salient point is that regardless of what system you use to make wagers, the casino will always have you at a disadvantage. As Royer (1994) advised, "any prolonged exposure to the game of Roulette will inevitably lead you to lose money" (158).

Craps—A Study in Conditional Probability

The game of craps can be very intimidating. It has a complex layout, there are many betting options, and the game is fast paced. However, the basic game is fairly simple

Table 4.3 *Possible Roulette Wagers*

Wager	Description	Payoff
Straight-Up Bet	This is a wager on 1 of the 38 numbers.	35 to 1
Split Bet	This is a wager on either of 2 adjoining numbers.	17 to 1
Street Bet	This is a wager on any of 3 numbers located in the same row.	11 to 1
Corner Bet	This is a wager on any of 4 numbers that are in a square formation.	8 to 1
Five-Number Bet	This is a wager on any of "0," "00," "1," "2," or "3."	6 to 1
Line Bet	This is a wager on any of 6 numbers located in 2 adjoining rows.	5 to 1
Column Bet	This is a wager on any of the 12 numbers located in a single column.	2 to 1
Dozen Bet	This is a wager on 1 of 12 consecutive numbers.	2 to 1
Red and Black Bets	This is a wager on a number of a particular color.	1 to 1
Odd and Even Bets	This is a wager on any of the odd numbers (or any of the even numbers).	1 to 1
1 to 18 and 19 to 36 Bets	This is a wager on 1 of the 18 low numbers (or 18 high numbers).	1 to 1

and easily understood. For our present purposes, craps provides a context in which to discuss the elusive concept of conditional probability. *Conditional probability* is defined as the probability of an event's occurring, given that another event has already occurred. Confusion about conditional probability leads to many of the misconceptions about the lottery (and, by extension, keno and roulette) described above.

Unlike the three games previously examined, where the various game events are independent and the probability of winning is constant and fixed from the outset, the probability of winning a particular game of craps is dependent on the first roll of the dice (the "come-out" roll). This distinction between independent and dependent events is an important piece in students' conceptual development of probability and number sense.

HOW TO PLAY CRAPS

In the basic game, one player (the "shooter") rolls a pair of dice and the sum of the two numbers that appear is observed. If the sum on the come-out roll is a 7 or 11, the shooter wins immediately. If the come-out roll results in a 2, 3, or 12, the shooter loses immediately ("craps out"). If the come-out roll is a 4, 5, 6, 8, 9, or 10, then this number becomes the shooter's "point." The dice are rolled repeatedly until the sum is either a 7 or the shooter's point number. If the point number is rolled before rolling a 7, the player "makes his point" and wins. If a 7 comes up before the point number is rolled, the player loses. Other players at the craps table participate in the game by wagering whether individual shooters win ("pass") or lose ("don't pass").

WHAT IS THE PROBABILITY OF WINNING?

The probability that a player wins immediately is the probability of rolling a 7 or an 11 on one roll of the dice. This probability is:

$$\frac{6}{36} + \frac{2}{36} = \frac{2}{9}.$$

Now assume that some other number (for example, an 8), comes up on the first roll. The conditional probability that the shooter will win, given that an 8 came up on the first roll, is equal to the probability that an 8 will come up again before a 7 is rolled. As described by DeGroot (1975), this probability is the same as the probability of rolling an 8 when the outcome is limited to either an 8 or a 7. Using the formula

$$P(A \mid B) = \frac{P(A \cap B)}{P(B)}$$

this conditional probability can be computed to be

$$\frac{\frac{5}{36}}{\frac{6}{36} + \frac{5}{36}} = \frac{5}{11}.$$

Therefore, the probability of rolling an 8 on the come-out roll and then winning the game is

$$\frac{5}{36} \times \frac{5}{11} = \frac{25}{396}.$$

Similarly, conditional probability can be used to compute the probability of winning with the other possible point numbers: 4, 5, 6, 9, and 10. These probabilities turn out to be

$$\frac{1}{36}, \frac{2}{45}, \frac{25}{396}, \frac{2}{45}, \text{ and } \frac{1}{36},$$

respectively. Finally, the total probability of winning a game of craps is the sum of all of the possible individual outcomes described above:

$$\frac{2}{9} + \frac{1}{36} + \frac{2}{45} + \frac{25}{396} + \frac{25}{396} + \frac{2}{45} + \frac{1}{36} = \frac{244}{495} = 0.4929.$$

Therefore, when playing the basic game of craps, you will lose slightly more than half of the time.

From the analysis above, it is clear that the house advantage when playing craps is about 1.42 percent. While this is not as high as the other games described, it is still significant. If you play the basic game long enough, you will have an average loss of $1.42 for every $100 bet. Once again it should be emphasized: In the long run, the odds in all casino games are against you.

Classroom Implications

Much of the previous discussion has dealt with reinforcing teachers' background knowledge about probability. It is then their responsibility to communicate the mathematical facts about gambling to their students. Teachers are quite capable of sifting through this discussion of games of chance and integrating into their lessons what they consider to be the appropriate pieces. However, as a guide, some sample classroom activities are illustrated below. It is critical to stress that the goal of these activities is not to glamorize gambling, nor is this chapter designed to teach teens how to gamble. It is illegal for any underage person to play casino or lottery games. While the mathematics and number sense that teachers can help students develop through these activities are important, the overriding social message is that gambling is a losing proposition. These activities are to be considered successful if they cause teens to think twice about starting to gamble.

ACTIVITY 1—LOTTERY SIMULATION

Using a random number generator (computer, calculator, table, etc.), simulate lottery drawings by picking 6 numbers from a pool of 42. Have each student make several six-number selections. Then pool the results for the whole class.

1. Record the frequency of each number chosen. Does each number get chosen with equal frequency? Is this to be expected? Why or why not?
2. Notice the number of times "special" results occur (consecutive numbers, all numbers less than 10, the same 6 numbers occurring twice in a row, etc.). Discuss the mathematical implications of your result. Are any of the results unexpected?

Answer: Each student should make several six-number selections and examine his or her individual results. In addition, the class should pool all the results to form one large-sample frequency distribution. Although the distribution of the pooled results may be more uniform than that of the individual results, students should not expect to see numbers chosen with equal frequency. Nor can any special significance be attached to any particular result.

ACTIVITY 2—LOTTERY NUMBER SENSE

In which of the following lotteries would you have the best chance of winning the jackpot?

A lottery where:

1. 3 numbers are chosen out of a pool of 15
2. 4 numbers are chosen out of a pool of 20
3. 5 numbers are chosen out of a pool of 25
4. 6 numbers are chosen out of a pool of 30

Answer: Students with good number sense will be able to reason that choosing 3 numbers out of 15 will have the highest probability of success. The probability of winning the jackpot in each lottery game is given below.

1. .00220
2. .000206
3. .0000188
4. .00000168
5. .000000149

ACTIVITY 3—A GUARANTEED LOTTERY WIN?

The billionaire oil tycoon J. D. Stonefeller lives in a state whose lottery game involves picking 6 numbers out of a pool of 48. The jackpot prize has reached $20 million, and Mr. Stonefeller plans on guaranteeing himself the prize by buying every possible number combination.

1. Assuming that it takes 30 seconds to buy a lottery ticket (including filling out the form), how long would it take to buy every possible lottery number combination? Do you think this scheme can work? Why or why not?
2. Assuming that Mr. Stonefeller succeeds in buying every possible number combination, is there anything that can go wrong with his plan?

Answer: There are $(48/6) = 48!/42!\,6! = 12{,}271{,}512$ different number combinations in this lottery. Therefore, assuming that it would take 30 seconds to buy a lottery ticket, it would take Mr. Stonefeller 30 seconds multiplied by 12,271,512 tickets = 368,145,360 seconds = 102,262.6 hours = 4,260.94 days = 11.67 years to buy all the possible number combinations. Obviously, Mr. Stonefeller would have to have many friends help him buy all of these tickets. Furthermore, it would cost him at least $12,271,512 to cover the numbers. With a $20,000,000 payoff, Mr. Stonefeller would be in trouble if he had to split this money with another player who also had the winning numbers.

ACTIVITY 4—CHOOSING KENO NUMBERS

In most keno games, you can select from 1 to 15 numbers. This activity leads you to answer the question: Is there an optimal quantity of numbers to pick? That is, how many numbers should you select to maximize your chances of winning a keno game? The advantage a casino holds over a keno player can be determined by computing the player's expected winnings. If this value is positive, then the game is in the player's favor; if this value is negative, then the casino has the advantage.

Fill in the missing values in the following probability distributions. Then compute the player's expected winnings and the casino's advantage.

PICK 1 NUMBER

Numbers "Caught"	Probability	Payoff on a $1 Bet
0	_____	–$1
1	_____	$2

Player's expected winnings: _____ Casino's advantage: _____ %

Answer:

PICK 1 NUMBER

Numbers "caught"	Probability	Payoff on a $1 Bet
0	0.75	–$1
1	0.25	$2

$$E = 0.75(-1) + 0.25(2) = -0.25$$

Player's expected winnings: –$0.25 Casino's advantage: 25%

PICK 2 NUMBERS

Numbers "Caught"	Probability	Payoff on a $1 Bet
0	0.5601	–$1
1	0.3798	–$1
2	_____	$11

Player's expected winnings: _____ Casino's advantage: _____ %

Answer:

PICK 2 NUMBERS

Numbers "Caught"	Probability	Payoff on a $1 Bet
0.00	0.5601	–$1
1	0.3798	–$1
2	0.0601	$11

$$E = 0.5601(-1) + 0.3798(-1) + 0.0601(11) = -0.2788$$

Player's expected winnings: –$0.28 Casino's advantage: 28%

PICK 3 NUMBERS

Numbers "Caught"	Probability	Payoff on a $1 Bet
0	0.4165	–$1
1	_____	–$1
2	0.1387	$0
3	_____	$43

Player's expected winnings: _____ Casino's advantage: _____ %

Answer:
PICK 3 NUMBERS

Numbers "Caught"	Probability	Payoff on a $1 Bet
0	0.4165	−$1
1	0.4309	−$1
2	0.1387	$0
3	0.0139	$43

$E = 0.4165(-1) + 0.4309(-1) + 0.1387(0) + 0.0139(43) = -0.2497$

Player's expected winnings: −$0.25 Casino's advantage: 25%

PICK 15 NUMBERS

Numbers "Caught"	Probability	Payoff on a $1 Bet
0, 1, 2, 3, 4, or 5	0.875	−$1
6	0.08635	$0
7	0.02989	$6
8	0.007331	$24
9	0.001267	$119
10	0.0001521	$299
11	0.00001234	$2,299
12	0.0000006496	$6,999
13	0.00000002068	$24,999
14	0.0000000003505	$49,999
15	0.000000000002336	$49,999

Player's expected winnings: _____ Casino's advantage: _____ %

Based on the computations you determined for the four games above (and the fact that similar results hold for all other keno games), do you believe there is an optimal quantity of numbers to pick when playing keno? Why or why not? Is it wise to play keno?

Once you decide how many numbers you are going to pick, is there an optimal strategy for which numbers to pick (for example, picking consecutive numbers, numbers that are spread throughout the card, numbers in the same column or row)?

Pick 15 Numbers: $E = 0.875(-1) + 0.08635(0) + 0.02989(6) + 0.007331(24) + 0.001267(119) + 0.0001521(299) + 0.00001234(2299) + 0.0000006496(6999) + 0.00000002068(24999) + 0.0000000003528(49999) = -0.2900$

Player's expected winnings: −$0.29 Casino's advantage: 29%

There is no real optimal quantity of numbers to choose. The casinos vary the payoffs in the individual games so that their advantage is always somewhere between 25 percent and 29 percent. Some students may argue that picking 3 numbers (which has a casino advantage of 25 percent) is better than picking 15 numbers (which has a casino advantage of 29 percent). The important point to stress is that anybody would be foolish even to play a game in which the player has such a great disadvantage. It really makes little difference if you lose 25¢ or 29¢ of every dollar you wager—eventually you will lose it all!

Other classroom discussion may center around ways in which casinos present the game of keno so that it appears to be attractive to the player. Some of the ways in which casinos could try to make keno more attractive include: (1) listing only the winning "catches" in payoff tables (rather than the losing ones as well), (2) having large payoffs (up to $50,000 for a $1 wager), even though the probability of winning large amounts is astronomically small, and (3) having numerous winning "catches" (in relation to losing catches), even though the probability of catching those numbers is small.

For example, if you pick 15 numbers, there are 6 "catches" on which you lose money and 10 on which you either win or break even (see probability distribution for "Pick 15 Numbers" above). To the mathematically naive, this might appear to be rather good odds. However, if you look at the probability of catching those particular quantities, you'll find that the probability of catching any one of the 6 losing quantities is .875, while the probability of winning or breaking even is only .125.

There is no optimal strategy for picking numbers. Just like the lottery, the numbers are randomly chosen and all sets of 20 numbers are equally likely.

There is also a psychological game being played here. People will normally be willing to take greater risk when they perceive the payoff to be more meaningful for them—which is why the rich are less enamored with gambling as a path to wealth. Even though the expected payoff is basically identical across all different keno games, players are more likely to pick a quantity of numbers that have a potential payoff of $50,000 than one that has a maximum payoff of $500.

ACTIVITY 5—LOTTERY NUMBER SENSE

Use reference books (*The World Almanac, Information Please,* or a set of encyclopedias) to estimate the probability of the occurrence of the following events:

1. Being audited by the Internal Revenue Service
2. Dying from a heart-related disease
3. Being a drowning victim
4. Being hurt in a fall at your home
5. Being struck by lightning

How do these probabilities compare with the probability of winning your state lottery?

Answers will vary.

ACTIVITY 6—ROULETTE: PLAYING THE THIRD COLUMN

If you look at the roulette layout, you will notice that the third column contains 8 red numbers and only 4 black numbers. A player tries to exploit this "flaw" by betting $10 on the third column and $20 on the black. Therefore, the player has 18 black numbers covered and on the column bet, twice as many red numbers as black numbers. Analyze this betting system and decide whether this player has improved his or her chances of winning.

Answer: No, the player has not improved his or her chances of winning. Assume that the player bets $30 as described above for 38 consecutive spins of the roulette wheel. Also assume that each of the 38 numbers comes up one time. By working through the payoffs, you can see that the player will have a net loss of $60 on a $1,140 bet. This is a 5.26 percent average loss, which is the expected loss when playing roulette.

ACTIVITY 7— LOTTERY FACT OR FICTION?

Break into small groups and discuss the following questions. Be prepared to defend your answers to the entire class. Situation: Your state lottery consists of a game where six numbers are drawn from a pool of 48. You always choose the same six numbers, which are a combination of relatives' birth dates: 3, 9, 12, 14, 17, and 25.

1. During a week when you were vacationing out of state and didn't play, your six numbers were picked. Do you pick another set of numbers for next week's drawing? Why or why not?
2. Someone tells you that playing birth dates is not a good idea since the lottery uses numbers through 48 and birth dates never go past 31. How do you respond?
3. Your friend wants to pick the numbers 1, 2, 3, 4, 5, and 6. He asks you if this is a wise choice, since he has never seen six consecutive numbers drawn. What do you tell him?
4. One week your next-door neighbor wins the lottery. She tells you that you should save your money and quit playing for a while. She reasons that the probability of two people who live next door to each other both winning is astronomical. How do you respond?
5. If you win the lottery, you can be paid with one of two plans. You can either collect half of the jackpot in one lump-sum payment, or you can collect the full amount in 20 annual payments. Is one method superior to the other? Are there certain factors and situations that would make one method superior to the other?

Answer:
1. It makes no difference whether you pick a new set of numbers or not. Each set of six numbers is equally likely to come up during next week's drawing. In other words, your set of six numbers is just as likely to come up as any other set of six numbers.
2. It makes no difference whether you use the entire range of numbers or not. All

the possible sets of six numbers are equally likely to come up during next week's drawing.

3. It makes no difference whether he chooses this set of six numbers or any other set. A particular set of six numbers is just as likely to come up as any of the other sets of six numbers during next week's drawing.

4. Your chances of winning are not affected. The numbers do not know that your next-door neighbor has recently won. It is a random process, so your chances are the same each time no matter what has happened the last time.

5. Generally, you would be better off if you took the lump-sum payment and invested it. This would be the case if you did not mind risking your winnings and were knowledgeable about investments. If you wanted the 20-year guarantee of financial security and were willing to settle for a lesser overall amount, then the annual payments would be a better option. For example, if you won a million dollars, you could take either a lump sum of $500,000 or $50,000 a year for 20 years. If you invested the $500,000 and received a 6 percent annual return, you would have $1,603,567.74 after 20 years, compared with the $1,000,000 you would receive if you took the annual payments. However, a 3.5 percent annual return would leave you with $994,894.43 after 20 years.

ACTIVITY 8—BETTING SYSTEMS

Critique the following betting systems. Be prepared to present your analyses to the entire class.

1. In a game of craps, the odds of a shooter "passing" is about 1 to 1, but the odds against a shooter passing three times in a row is about 7 to 1. Therefore, a player waits until the shooter has passed twice in a row and then bets against him or her.

2. We have seen that the presence of "0" and "00" on the roulette wheel is what gives the house its advantage. Therefore, a player "bets with the house" by making frequent five-number bets and "insures" all even-money bets by making a split bet on the "0" and "00."

3. A player at the craps table has a wagering system where the size of the bet is doubled after each loss. For example, if you bet $2 and lose, you bet $4 next time. If this bet loses, you bet $8 the next time. Lose—bet $16 next time. Eventually you will have to win. In this example, if you win your fourth wager of $16, you wipe out your previous losses and are left with a net profit.

4. While at a roulette table, a red number comes up 12 times in a row. Knowing about the "law of averages," a player decides that it would be smart to cover all the black numbers since they are "overdue."

5. Unlike the lottery, it is feasible to cover every number on the roulette table. Therefore, a player bets every number straight up. One of these numbers must come up, and the player is guaranteed a win.

Answer:

1. This strategy doesn't help. The outcomes of the rolls are independent. Passing twice in a row doesn't affect the probability of passing the third time.

2. This is also a losing system. As shown above, the five-number bet is the worst bet on the table. Insuring your even-money bets with a split bet on "0" and "00" doesn't help either. If you analyze this the same way you did in Activity 6, you'll see that you will have a net loss of $4 on $76 bet, for a 5.26 percent casino advantage.

3. This system has several problems. One is that the tables usually have a maximum bet. Therefore, if you have a long losing streak, you could reach a point where you might not be able to double your losing bet, and you would never be able to recoup your losses. Second, under this system, when you do win, your net profit will only equal your initial bet. You will have to wager a great deal of money to try to win a small amount. (In this example, you wager $30 to win $2). Finally, your expected winnings at true odds is $0. Since no casino offers true odds at roulette, you will lose money in the long run.

4. This decision is illogical, since the spins of the roulette wheel are independent. The wheel cannot remember that it came up red 12 times in a row.

5. This system will lose two betting units each time. It will cost $38 to bet $1 straight up on every number. The amount you bet on a number (in this case, $1) is returned to you if that number wins. Since a straight-up bet pays only 35 to 1, you will win $36 and lose $38 on each spin of the wheel.

Conclusion

Many people gamble as a form of entertainment and consider their losses as a contribution to their state's treasury or the casino owners' pockets. There are others who gamble seriously and believe they have a good chance of winning. From a mathematical viewpoint, however, gambling, cannot be viewed as anything but a losing proposition. In all games of chance, the odds are against the player. While a gambler may occasionally have some short-term success, in the long run he or she will lose money. Therefore, if you are going to gamble, you should bet only with money you can afford to lose. Furthermore, you must be prepared to lose all of the money you are betting.

By discussing these topics and incorporating these concepts into classroom lessons, teachers can give students specific insight into the workings of the lottery and the games of keno, roulette, and craps. In addition to teaching necessary concepts of probability, these lessons can promote a better awareness of the nature of random events, encourage students to think more critically about games of chance in general, and improve students' overall number sense.

Notes

1. In fact, this strategy was attempted in a recent lottery drawing in Virginia. A conglomerate of businessmen tried to buy all of the possible number combinations. They ran out of time before they could cover all the numbers, but the winning ticket was among the ones they did manage to buy.

2. In this formula, P = the original principle you invest, r = the annual percentage rate, n = the number of times per year that interest is compounded, and t = the number of years your money is invested.

References

Andersen, K. (June 10, 1994) Las Vegas, U.S.A. *Time*, 42–51.

DeGroot, M. H. (1975). *Probability and statistics*. Menlo Park, CA: Addison-Wesley.

Hellman, P. (1994, March). Casino craze. *Travel Holiday*, 80–87, 132, 134, 143–147.

Fujii, J. (1994, March). Defending Hawaii against casinos. *Travel Holiday*, 83.

Mathematical Association of America. (1991). *A call for change: Recommendations for the mathematical preparation of teachers of mathematics*. Washington, DC. Author.

Mathematical Sciences Education Board. (1990). *Reshaping school mathematics: A philosophy and framework for curriculum*. Washington, DC: National Academy Press.

McGervey, J. D. (1986). *Probabilities in everyday life*. New York: Ballantine.

National Council of Supervisors of Mathematics. (1989). Essential mathematics for the twenty-first century: The position of the National Council of Supervisors of Mathematics. *Mathematics Teacher, 82*, 388–91.

National Council of Teachers of Mathematics. (1989). *Curriculum and evaluation standards for school mathematics*. Reston, VA. Author.

National Council of Teachers of Mathematics. (1991). *Professional standards for teaching mathematics*. Reston, VA. Author.

National Research Council. (1989). *Everybody counts: A report to the nation on the future of mathematics education*. Washington, DC: National Academy Press.

Ortiz, D. (1986). *Darwin Ortiz on casino gambling*. New York: Carol Publishing Group.

Paulos, J. A. (1988). *Innumeracy: Mathematical illiteracy and its consequences*. New York: Hill and Wang.

Royer, V. H. (1994). *"Casino magazine's" play smart and win: How to beat today's most popular casino games*. New York: Fireside.

Sowers, C. (1995, May 13). Fort McDowell recalls standoff 3 years ago with FBI. *The Arizona Republic*, B1, B4.

Chapter Five

Youth-Gambling Treatment Issues

Sirgay Sanger

Introduction

Gambling touches on every aspect of personality, relationship, and impulse. Thus, the techniques used to treat adolescents who gamble may resemble the psychotherapy of all youngsters. This chapter will focus on a helpful core of essential skills and concepts that practitioners and administrators can use to influence the young personality with this addiction. It is assumed that professionals who treat this population have a foundation in the following underlying clinical skills and standards: interviewing techniques, motivating family support of therapy, structuring and limit setting within the therapeutic relationship, confidentiality, gathering information from school and camp, insisting on abstinence, and recommending groups and Gamblers Anonymous attendance (see Gupta & Derevensky, 2000).

Professionals should be familiar with such developmental issues of adolescence and pre-adolescence as consolidation of morality and ethics, resolution of ambivalent thinking, relinquishment of magical thinking, and mastery of oppositional (contrarian) posturing. Other global achievements to be considered are the ability to grieve for real and imagined childhood pleasures, to set realistic goals, to balance personal and social demands, to transcend shame, and to have a sufficiently firm identity allowing empathy and love. A full discussion of developmental issues is available in standard texts on adolescence (Bird, 1995; Caplan & Lebovici, 1969; Holmes, 1964; Pearson, 1992).

Obviously, adolescents have a lot on their plates. However, what is often left out of the picture is that their protection by family and society enables them to take risks in searching out, experimenting with, and experiencing the sensations and pleasures of life. Given the influence of the media, advertising, and group fashion, as well as the "worship" of idealized young bodies and sports, adolescents often feel impelled and entitled to have as much fun and freedom as possible. Measuring themselves against such aspirations, they may suffer from feelings of loneliness, inadequacy, and desperation. They may feel bored or may wish to challenge themselves to determine what levels of excitement are suitable. How far can one go before it gets scary? When does the bright side of danger darken? Nearly all adolescents think they know more than they do. Furthermore, they want to make their own mistakes and do not welcome correction. They pretend they can defy the laws of chance and influence any risk they encounter. This is a temporary attitude, but it is one that persists in those who go on to gamble (Derevensky, Gupta, & Cioppa, 1996).

The Attraction of Quick Solutions and the Path to Gambling

Adolescents are primed for immediate impulse gratification and to perpetuate positive arousal and thrill (Apter, 1992). They cannot bear the experience of anhedonia (lack of pleasure in acts that are usually pleasurable). Privileged youngsters from intact families are susceptible to these motives. Marginalized teenagers—dysfunctionally parented, poor, undereducated, and abused (with nutritional and neurophysiological early life stress)—are even more vulnerable; their intolerance of frustration is even greater.

Immediate gratification is seen in alcohol and drug use, fast driving, promiscuity, pranks, stealing, and gambling. It can also be a motivator for turning toward the productive pursuits of art and music, the history of ideas, athletics, dramatics, explorations, and physical challenges. Which avenues youngsters may take are determined by their own characters, as well as their teachers, coaches, and friends. Are healthy opportunities or unhealthy gratifications available? Often when there is urgency to the unpleasure, the path of gratification is to toy with one's own thinking patterns, to unlink cause and effect, idea and its felt component. In general, adolescents poorly identify the boundary between playing and serious life issues, ignoring consequences in order to pursue instant relief and positive gratifications.

The therapy of gambling youths must address this conscious dismantling of maturity. Clarification and interpretation such as, "I needn't tell you what you already know, do I?" are needed. Developmentally, adolescence is the era when the mind "comes together," knits an identity, solidifies life purposes, and learns how to maintain states of calm and consistency. What experiment could be more sensational (and wanton) than to mishandle the mind, to play with one's contemplative self, and to allow dissociation (uncoupling) to flourish? One comes to avoid relating present rational, logical experiences with their relevant patterns of past history. In essence, it is a process that allows one to suspend effective intelligence, to be negligent, to unthink, to allow irrationality and unmodulated impulses to prevail. This is a process that makes the adolescent appear to be stupid.

Pseudostupidity and Treatment

From the perspective of what is reasonable, this misuse of the emerging organization of personality, this fragmentation, is mental gambling.[1] Internal chaos and anarchy of mind precede actual gambling. From any consideration of psychotherapy, there can be no effective remediation of the behavior of problem gambling without first addressing the prior mental components. Once exposed and thoroughly understood in all its self-destructive forms, pseudostupidity can release its grip on the youth's natural intelligence. Then youths can stop derailing their developing mental prowess, and the arrested intellect can begin to grow again.

If the developmental arrest began in early childhood, the therapist may note the onset of refreshing curiosity in an otherwise childish and inept youngster. Successful therapy should yield young people who are smarter, make better use of their time, and have calm, deeper characters. When the process of therapy fails to address pseudostupidity, adolescents often amplify the process of mind-wasting with other compulsive activities. It is striking how much mindless busyness problem gamblers can generate as they age.

Intelligence and Dissociation

In the structured setting of my office with its nonhumiliating one-on-one conversation, youths rarely claim they can beat the odds. Elsewhere, however, when placing a bet, they think they can and will win. They report a sense of being lucky, being smarter than the odds, or wanting to get into some "action" and be like everyone gambling around them (even if it is a totally blind wager). What allowed them to yield to the impulse to gamble was the prior suspension of rational and logical memory connections. They do this neutering intelligence through dissociation of their thinking, that is, to deny, ignore, or split off memories of their parents' influence and their own remembered experiences of reality. This deconstructive dynamic of mind is prevalent among much of the gambling population I have encountered.

The Developmentally Delayed

A second group of young gamblers comprised individuals who never formed an integrated self, and present as lost, odd, spacy, chronically angry, anxious, and/or suspicious. Dysfunctional parenting can have caused meager structuring of thought, logic, and rationality. These individuals feel alive only with intense projects, sensations, or crises. These serve to unify the internal chaos and make them "feel real." Otherwise, they suffer from chronic boredom, feelings of deadness, and confusion.

Whereas those who use dissociation wish to feel less aware, in this second cluster, the young people use gambling to feel more alive. Such individuals can be included in diagnostic categories as varied as pervasive developmental disorders, posttraumatic stress disorder, low borderline personality disorder, inadequate personality, and attention deficit disorder with or without hyperactivity. For members of this population, who lack both self-discipline and the ability to organize themselves for experiences of normal life challenges and pleasures, any preoccupation is welcome. Gambling in particular offers a comprehensive "solution" to the tedium and deadness.

Related to this category are youngsters whose immature thinking has a magical characteristic.[2] They persist in the belief that wishing can make something happen, that seemingly unrelated events are connected and influenced by mysterious forces. These unrealistic fictions offer inner excitement and intensity.

Memory and Identity Deficits

Dissociation and developmental delay affect structured memory and identity. Unexamined and obscured life experience cripples a viable memory. How can a comparison of poor versus useful outcomes be made? Adolescents who have memory and identity deficits rely on chance, lacking alternative options. In some teenagers who have a modicum of a work ethic, there is a façade of actively trying to handicap or creating pseudoschemes of magical formulas that give a veneer of having "worked" at some point in the gambling cycle. To deal with this primitive and distorted thinking I will sometimes say, "I wish you could succeed using your methods. Nice try— what you are doing is quite clever. However, there may be some missing pieces to your method. Can you think of what they are?"

To understand and offer therapy for pathologically wagering teenagers, experience with adolescent group process can bring peer dynamics to help channel their risk behavior. In-patient and out-patient experience is highly useful, as these young gamblers are seriously mentally compromised. For some, ironically, the activity of gambling may be a "step up" from even more deteriorated and irrational behavior. For others, gambling may serve as a protective device, helping to prevent regression to even more primitive states. Gambling needs to be slowly and delicately examined for its benefits before an attempt is made to implicate its costs and to substitute more productive activities. As professionals, we have to contain our opinion that all wagering is costly, dubious, and must stop.

"Addiction" to Anticipation

Universal in childhood and adolescence is the experience of looking forward to something happening: birthdays, holidays, competition, exams. However, when these years are wretched, filled with disappointments, a youth may present a fantasy of what-is-yet-to-come. Gambling, as an activity that involves much anticipation, is more satisfying in this regard than speeding in a car, stealing from stores, or getting drunk. It has the added advantage that the expectation of a win can be engaged in secretly. Any interpersonal therapy removes the secrecy part of gambling and substitutes the comfort of being heard and sharing.

Acting Out: From Thoughts to Action

Young people have a propensity for putting thought into action. It is their primary way to learn about their relationship to the animate and inanimate world. It is a way to test, to try out. Therefore, when a youth has been indulging in dissociated thinking (as a coping mechanism to alleviate misery), he or she, in the larger context of risk issues, may have an impulse to wager, and then they go right into action. Gambling provides a particularly tempting arena. The notion of pushing the limits, trying anything new and different is confirmed by the evidence that where gambling is available, youths will gravitate to it.[3] The treating professional must question young gamblers about the risk/gain relationship in gambling; therapy can focus on how, using reason, they can set up actions so that no one gets hurt and much is learned. The enjoyment of acting out risky magical thinking is the dynamic to be analyzed.

Psychotherapy for Problem-Gambling Youth

The thrust of therapy is to ensure that dissociation as a mental mechanism is kept within productive limits. Artists and writers, for inspiration, supposedly "dip" into dissociative thinking. Similarly, teenagers can make effective use of disjointed thinking to have flights of fantasy and playful ideas. Treatment should address and bolster the part of the mind that monitors thinking, that leads to discernment (the observing ego). The youngster needs assistance to differentiate the realistic from the fanciful, to determine when to put thoughts into action, and to determine when to limit experiments from going too far. For example, in a theater, one can smell smoke and imagine a disaster in the making. This scenario calls for some action. One can desperately need money, and there may be a casino nearby. This scenario calls for inaction.

Therapists need to help young people ask themselves useful questions that require them to pause and take time to consider alternative choices. The following are useful phrases: "You know many of the sensible answers, so how do you manage to undo that and pretend ignorance?" "Have you taken enough time to examine carefully all the alternatives you can think of?" "You seem to rush to decision. Is speed an essential part of being in power? Is it because you prefer to focus on the rash, risky, and problematic?" "You must have thought a lot about this issue, and as you are intelligent, you probably have a range of possibilities. How can you narrow down this field?" "By now you have a good idea of what I'd say." "I'll back your drift of thinking if it's genuinely your thought, then we'll learn from it." Developmentally, the professional is encouraging the adolescent to hold onto the benefits of wariness, watchfulness, and second thoughts before plunging into most actions.

Therapeutic Concerns and Crises: Strategies and Tactics for Developing and Maintaining a Safe Haven

Character evolves during childhood and adolescence. Changing it is difficult. So long as a youngster continues to dissociate and wager, he consolidates an immature identity. Lacking adultlike, mature, reasonable thought patterns, he solidifies a dys-functioning and defective mind. Even when not actively gambling, such an adolescent remains dysphoric and at risk of engaging in rash experiments that offer immediate reactions. This atmosphere of urgency permeates the diagnostic inter-views and the start of therapy. Therapists are pressured to "do something" immedi-ately to satisfy the wagering teenagers' habitual action orientation. When added to the pent-up demands of family, school, and law enforcement officials, the relation-ship experiences pressures that may work against therapy.

Everyone needs to slow down, to resist the pressure to act, to develop wariness. Therapists can establish the necessary room be emphasizing that treatment is not magic or instantaneous. For therapy to be effective, it has to be, in addition, intense and diverting, a counterpoint to the distraction and action sought in wagering. Therapy liberated from unreasonable expectations must be a process that intrigues. It also must offer a safe emotional "container" for the youth's thoughts to be heard and verbalized. If the therapist is stampeded by the current crisis into action, for ex-ample, rescuing the youngster from school obligations or allowing stealing to go on, objectivity within that relationship is lost, and the adolescent will have found an ac-complice for his pathology.

Most adolescents are mildly suspicious of "helping" adults and of violation of their privacy. They will have, in addition, discomfort about trusting older profes-sionals. Thus, clinicians should examine excessive wariness just as much as excessive risk. All the while exploration of this youngster's mind continues, there is estab-lished a warm, understanding atmosphere, nonhumiliating and nonthreatening, that lets him get emotional support.

The next therapeutic tactic is for clinicians to impress the adolescent with their ability to capture in words or to epitomize the young person's current emotional state. This technique bridges the generation gap and demonstrates skill to describe human behavioral patterns. This tactic serves as a model for having a conversation. After all, psychotherapy is a talking experience, and most adolescents have under-developed verbal communication skills. Clinicians should continue to recognize that conversation is the matrix of any beginning relationship and that gambling would have headed the adolescents into increasingly lonely and secretive byways. In time, youthful patients may be able to ask for the personal support they have avoided so studiously.

During early sessions, clinicians will find it helpful to present a developmental point of view: that we embody our early experiences and any dysfunctional behavior results from multiple causes. Parents and significant others share responsibility with youngsters for some of their symptoms and woes. Therapeutic exploration need not hurt; it is meant to achieve a fulfilled life rather than to label the youngsters as sick.

All topics are useful to discuss insofar as they provide the occasion for ideas and words. For some youngsters, the therapist's ability to make sense and meaning from the facts of their lives may seem like mind reading. It may be the first time that someone has become a nonthreatening mirror to their situation and made a verbal version of themselves. Nonetheless, adolescents may not be pleased by what they hear. The professional runs the risk of being too quiet, boring, and unimpressive or too dazzling, energetic, and overpowering. Adolescents' unfamiliarity with the diagnostic/therapeutic situation itself is challenging or strange. Therapists should address this issue right away and emphasize that therapy can be a productive, new experience. This unfamiliarity should be welcomed. It may not be comfortable and may not eliminate young gamblers' woes, but a clinician might characterize it as a primer or a "class in yourself."

A sociable atmosphere is established so long as labels are avoided. Children and young adults cannot bear to be characterized by terms such as *nervous, afraid, underachieving,* or *misbehaving.* Such labels are confining and remind the teen of parents who blame or criticize. In addition, therapists should avoid medical language such as *ill, patients, getting therapy,* and *having appointments for treatment.*

The next task of therapy is to explore the "healthy" aspects of gambling. Is the gambling activity a way of belonging to a group? Does it offer brief but predictable pleasures—relaxation, excitement, hope, new opportunity, a way to feel trashy or brave? Is it a way of getting close to family or distant? Behavior has meaning. Is it a way to earn money or trick and triumph over certain "unfair" rules? Adolescents will be intrigued by such an approach. They may suspect, correctly, that in time, any clinician will be exploring the negatives of gambling such as losing, covering debts, being wrong about "lady luck," dropping out of the mainstream. Therefore, it is both honest and correct in therapy for clinicians to admit that they first want to acknowledge the good in every situation, saying for example: "You've caught me being upbeat, trying to be optimistic and pleasant—is that so terrible? We're not here to attack you but to think together, to discuss the pros and then the cons."

Motivation for Therapy: Clinical Responses

The vast majority of youngsters are brought to a professional's office. Thus, motivation for a talking therapy comes at first from parents or other responsible adults. Therapists must not assume that the adolescent chose therapy. It is part of therapists' "mind reading" to bring this issue out into the open. Therapists may be stuck unless they know how to expose the unpleasantness of being "dragged" somewhere. In many cases, part of the young person will resist, while another part will welcome a professional entering the family system. This contradiction is like the ambivalent, dissociative thinking that underlies adolescent gambling: one side of them enjoys the experience, another experiences invasive threat.

It helps to revisit those efforts parents make that succeeded and those that misfired. While most parents try not to humiliate, most still manage to hurt their children's feelings. This situation can then lead the professional to a discussion of the differences between acrimonious power struggles and "lovers' quarrels." All families get into battles between the generations and need to learn how to avoid becoming bitter. The therapist can compliment the family for airing its interpersonal issues in the presence of a professional and giving problems the respect they merit. At the same time, the therapist can criticize the family where there has been procrastination in addressing chronic disturbances.

Delinquent Gambling

If the youth has little respect for authority and carries a grudge against society, the mental health professional may be trying to treat a delinquent who just happens to be gambling. This is a very different undertaking and is much less promising than treating a dissociating youngster who is gambling and who at times may have defied authority or broken some rules in order to keep gambling. With the delinquent who gambles, the therapist will uncover a long history of moral difficulties and angry entitlements, along with school and family reports of truancy, petty theft, aggressive behavior, and lack of personal control. Therapy with this population has not been very effective outside of residential placement.

In fostering a therapeutic alliance, clinicians can try to highlight in themselves those qualities the youth respects in others. If young gamblers suspect clinicians of trying to gain influence by being agreeable, they will dislike the clinician immediately. Therefore, psychotherapists should wisely volunteer at the outset that they are trying to hear about all of their young patient's experiences. In time, however, the therapist will want to explore—when the adolescent is sufficiently comfortable—those memories of interactions with parents and the adult world that were abrasive, less useful, or simply wrong. Clinicians can explain how little benefit there is to being confrontational. It is helpful to explain that a comfortable atmosphere—

which all therapists try to establish—is most conducive to helping people think their best thoughts and elicit new solutions.

Psychotherapists can also explain their need to be in contact with all sources of information, favorable and not, so as to better know the other points of view that the young gambler is experiencing. This tactic, added to tempering any urgency, will help establish a less crisis-driven situation. The therapist may appear to be the youth's tool or champion. We can explain that no one can learn under pressure and that to slow everything down is to better find and understand solutions.

Treatment and Resistance: Integrating Strategies and Tactics for a Strong Therapeutic Alliance

After several weeks, therapists may find their reaching out is met with battling and objections. Nonetheless, at the same time these are signs of a growing sense of relatedness—a hopeful sign of a developing therapeutic alliance. The goal of this alliance is to be able to look together, and with some objectivity, at how the adolescent handles the stresses, disappointments, and pleasures of dating, infatuations, feelings of loneliness, defeats, and triumphs, and at how those experiences can cause risk-taking impulses, some leading to gambling.

The adolescent's punctuality for sessions, the wish to extend the length of sessions, richer conversation, and the curiosity about the therapist all serve to indicate an emerging therapeutic alliance. With its further development clinicians are enabled to ask about how it feels to have an irresistible impulse, how the youth breaches all rational and logical guidelines, how magical thinking (with its disregard for the law of averages, its wish-come-true expectations, its counting on being lucky or ingenious) takes over. Only then can a therapist inquire about feelings of being diminished, needy, or desperate. This is a propitious moment in therapy, as adolescents will feel strange and surprised to be communicating such thoughts for the first time. To protect the therapeutic alliance, the therapist can show how such new, exciting, scary revelations signify progress in discovering the sources of the unbearable feelings that in turn provoke dangerous dissociating avoidances. In this conversation a youngster may discover that thinking out loud is the precursor of rethinking and reexamining one's self and one's world, that when thinking serves only to splinter and fragment one's thought, it induces risks that can be dangerous. In other words, playful thought is welcome at all times, but "playing with thought" is less safe.

Developing a Sense of Self

Parallel to dialogue, therapists need to listen for those hardly audible personal interests, talents, and preferences that can form the basis of a realistic sense of self. Emphasizing these interests tells adolescent gamblers who they truly are. Teenagers who gain the pleasure of positive self-discovery may begin to contrast these natural qualities with the less substantial ones of gambling. At this stage (usually several months), gambling activities may be seen as originating from impulses that were acted out because of a personality weakened by dissociation.

Clinical Caveats

Once the patient and therapist uncover these newly found interests and talents, the impulse to wager may become only one of many possible choices. In conversation, there is room for healthy silliness, grossness, linking one concept to another, gossip, and candid mockery of family and friends. There is intellectual scope for searching out those themes that link diverse topics, even themes that are macabre, grotesque, or tangential. At the same time, the adolescent needs to be reminded of two important points: (1) the flow of ideas, however bizarre, is an integral and essential part of therapy, and (2) this free conversation needs to be adapted for talk on the outside.

For both practical reasons and reasons of politeness, therapists have to make a stand for tact, consideration, and privacy. Also, teenagers need to learn that therapists are trained individuals who have a breadth of acceptance and personal security that lets them be joked with and at. Therapists must be able to weather the buffeting while continuing to be trustworthy, confidential, and good-natured—this type of personal relationship is special. Adolescents in therapy need to be forewarned that if they try some of the riffs or linkages made in therapy on others, they run the risk of appearing strange, outrageous, insulting, or dismissable.

Responding to Resistance

There may come a phase of therapy when the adolescent wants to cancel or arbitrarily change appointments. This situation is tricky for any therapist to handle because allowing absences may be too indulgent and insisting on attendance may be too parental. The only path is to interpret what is going on and to be flexible. The therapist's puzzlement can help the youth empathize with the complex nature of a treatment process.

Sometimes in the middle phase of therapy, the adolescent gambler will express an interest in attending medical or graduate school. Often a pipe dream that has no seeming logic, incorporating the identity of the therapist, may be a subtle way to continue the therapeutic process of making connections. This is a "trial balloon," and the therapist should greet it with mild encouragement. It is part of the healthy adolescent process of trying on the different hats of adult life. This process represents the restarting of developmental rehearsing that was stifled and paralyzed by the dissociating and gambling. It is decidedly better to dream about being a veterinarian than to dream of gambling riches. The examination of math and science, curiosity about biology, and learning how people behave individually and in groups, for example, will form a paradigm for how the adolescent examines ideas and impulses to eventuate in considering future goals.

Ambivalent Thinking and Its Effect on Therapy

The highly ambivalent thinking that marks the experience of both early adolescents and addicts of all ages may present in therapy in a variety of ways (Shaffer, 1994). This sort of thinking can be described as either/or, win/lose swings, extremes of attitude, and lack of a middle ground. The therapist will see a person thinking without compromise. Flexibility and reasonableness, on the other hand, which result from continual resolution of ambivalence, are rare. For example, therapists can make this point by saying, "All in all, I can see this point in shades of gray; it doesn't have to be all black or all white." Problem gamblers tend to exhibit this type of ambivalent thinking pattern. Child and adolescent psychiatrists should be skillful at exposing the inefficiency and pitfalls that can result.

A failing therapy is self-evident: The adolescent may not show up for the scheduled appointments or may remain awkwardly silent. Similarly, therapy may "oversucceed," crossing an invisible line and failing because adolescents are so in need of the therapist's good opinion that they are afraid to reveal thoughts or actions that they are ashamed of. Extremes of attitude toward therapy ("It was good; now it isn't") may be obvious. The technique for handling these issues is part of general training in mental health.

Guilt and Shame: Emotional Engines for Dissociation

Unless therapy addresses the guilt and shame aspects of the adolescent's conscience, treatment may only partially succeed. Guilt has much to do with the opinion of others; social atonement and "I'm sorry" are accepted mechanisms for handling it. However, shame—an underlying issue for gamblers—concerns one's opinion of oneself and is harder to handle. Shame, usually associated with dirtiness and humiliation, is deeply uncomfortable and gives immediate rise to a need to banish it. A first impulse is to hide, wish the ground would open up. A second impulse is to gain respect by being favored by lady luck, to be brave in a big wager, and/or to become a winner.[4]

If shaming is overused by parents in communication or as a disciplinary tactic, children will incorporate it as part of themselves. They cope with internalized shame by using the primitive defense mechanisms of denial, isolation, projection, and, as is common in the case of youthful gamblers, dissociation (Gupta & Derevensky, 2000). Children cannot tolerate being made to feel ashamed for long. Forced to cope with humiliation, they will protect themselves with some of the following coping mechanisms: "It isn't me" (dissociation); "It doesn't hurt" (psychic numbing, dissociation of feelings from the events); "You do it too" (imitation); "You made me do it" (projection); "Since I can't ever get your respect, I might as well be as bad as I can be" (negative identity, fatalism); and "I'll be just like you, give you a taste of your own medicine, and show you just how rotten I am" (identification with the aggressor).

These ways of coping can be characterized as disconnections. In therapy, teenagers need to realize that their parents misused a powerful negative method, that authoritativeness and firmness should have been used in place of shaming. Rarely, however, is a child below age 12 able to sort this out, and often the therapist will note that dissociation has become a habitual and ingrained defense. An advantage in having adolescents in treatment is that they can be helped to develop a perspective on how their parents behaved and to imagine more respectful, endurable alternatives.

A number of factors can contribute to the use of this parenting style. Low-income, socially precarious, and marginalized communities have been found to use overstrict, arbitrary child discipline too frequently and too early. Teenage parents use language with their babies and toddlers that is shaming and ridiculing. They often see their children as playthings—little toys that will forget being overpowered, capriciously mocked, or physically abused. For some teenage mothers, the fun is over once labor begins, and the new mother may soon resent the child for causing pain and having needs. Getting a baby to cry is a predictable and controllable activity that serves immature parents with a push-pull amusement.

Children may sense that they were an "accident" or unwanted, or that the next baby was brought into the family to make up for their parents' disappointment in them. For such children, dissociation can be the predominant shield against shame. Dissociation can protect them from feelings attached to unbearable ideas. The parents themselves may use dissociation, too. They will disavow behavior that signals their lack of commitment. Their children will sense that the "giants" on whom they depend do not make sense (as they are deeply afraid of being honest). Once shame and its concomitant dissociation entrench, therapy must include the entire family, in order to be successful. Adolescents will come to see that with this pattern of dissociation, every aspect of character and motivation aims not to find fulfillment in love but to find a hiding place that avoids humiliation or being caught.

In treatment, adolescents may be so relieved to have found an environment where there is pride and safety from shame that they just want to bask, dutifully keeping appointments but not necessarily being productive. This pattern becomes evident when the quantity and quality of the material the adolescent brings to the session becomes stale and repetitious.

Dissociation and Language

For adolescents whose dissociation of life experiences began in the preverbal era, the ability to describe their thoughts and emotions in words is severely impeded. Therefore, these alexithymic young people (unable to identify/articulate feelings, which are often described as physical symptoms) and their therapists have to create a new language to describe and attempt to explain and integrate bodily states and sensations that are fragmented. For example, the early treatment sessions may need to focus on the sudden fast pounding of the heart, clammy hands, sensations of being closed in, or inexplicable sleepiness. Physiological experiences need to be connected to verbal labels. This is a difficult process to accomplish with adolescents, who resent labels of any kind and make a cult of the inarticulate ("Yuh know," "I want," "No hassle," "Cool," "Whatever"). Nonetheless, it is the path to improvement.

Self-Knowledge, Identity, Arousal, and Calming: Architecture for Self-Regulation

There has to be a self before there can be self-knowledge. Once clinicians sense that the teenager has a modicum of self, then there can be an exploration of what sorts of activities, mental and physical, keep it aroused, stimulated, and challenged, and whether, in experiencing and activating a self, one crosses the line into overly risky behaviors. The goal at this stage is to identify those special abilities and talents that are safe to develop further. Individual standards for arousal or calm can have deep roots in the earliest months of life.

For example, certain patterns can be seen among those who were premature as infants and had to depend so much more on the environment for calming. As adults, these people may have a habit of wiggling their leg or playing with their hair, or they may need a steadying friend. They may be overly wary or may throw themselves into situations too quickly. These people may act irritable and "wired."

By not being helped to self-modulate during the early years, young people can develop certain misconnections. They may come to associate curiosity with frustration, exploration with disappointment. Pessimistic that wishes come true, they are sometimes categorized as "pain dependent." They may have a history of colic or other painful physical conditions. This population of youth is difficult to treat. Their faces often reflect unhappiness even when they are most calm. They do not feel real when they do something that is pleasurable. During treatment, it is useful for therapists to identify this "miswiring" and instruct young gamblers that they consciously have to tell themselves, when they are away from wagering, that they are fine. Their standards of a comfortable zone have bypassed the healthy range and are self-destructive. Numbing and security achieved through dissociation always need direct therapeutic intervention.

Another impediment to self-development occurs when oppositional attitudes persist into adolescence. In this case, the individual gives responses that block or are contrary to whatever is being suggested. This is a misnamed syndrome. Instead of oppositional behavior, this pattern should be called the "Need for Assertion of Initiative" syndrome. For those with this syndrome, no one else's suggestions are acceptable. Only self-generated ideas are valuable. These adolescents need to take initiative but do not quite know how. Suggestions threaten this group of teenagers with feelings of unreality (for example, being a toady, a follower, or invisible). This thinking, hypersensitive to anyone else's, forces the young person to reject expected norms and behave with dramatic impulsiveness.

Identifications throughout adolescence are like hats tried on or partially worn. They try to imitate, incorporate different personalities. Some are quite convincing; it takes a wise parent to know what to pass off as a temporary fancy and what to take seriously. This process of parent mirroring and validating resembles the care giving of infants and requires patience and humor. The parental function of monitoring should be turned over gradually to the adolescent.

In the case of teenagers whose parents themselves lack self-integration, have impaired self-monitoring, and frequently dissociate (for example, parents who abuse alcohol or drugs or rely on denial when facing challenges), therapy provides the first opportunity for adolescents to experience an adult capable of reflecting their integrative needs. In time, the monitoring and self-observing functions can be taken on by the adolescents themselves. Gradually they act to discriminate, assign red, green, and yellow lights, and determine which boundaries and options they want to test.

Young people can also encounter social situations that call for bending the rules, overriding certain strictures. These circumstances may arise when the hyperalert or chronically fearful young person turns to rigidity and narrowness of vision, resulting in shyness, withdrawal, and constriction. Many adolescents who give the appearance of limit testing, trying activities such as intoxications, near arrest, and close physical danger, are setting out to have a "past" so as to say that they do not need to do that again and that they have learned from experience.

In the frequently missed case of the under-stimulated, very bright adolescent, math, science calculations, and intellectually challenging games can play a role. These individuals may be treated through educational methods. Extra readings, one-on-one tutorials, after-school clubs, theater workshops, and the like can provide extra maturational stimuli.

Summary and Conclusion

In summary, gambling can perniciously lead adolescents into addiction because it acts synergistically with dissociative thinking. The intensity and seductions of the wagering behavior in all its forms help to contain the loosely organized or fragmented mental state so typical of adolescence. Gambling helps to protect youngsters from the emotional pain that can result from their characteristically inadequate relationships and needy selves. Adolescents avoid the anguish of feeling lost, lonely, and helpless through the use of a number of postures, alterations of consciousness, trances, internal struggles, self-deceptions, impulsivities, and reckless behaviors. Furthermore, young people who have had too much shaming in their background will conceal hurts. This energizes compulsive escaping behavior. However, these methods of coping come at a considerable cost and cannot lead to a wholesome outcome. Inevitably these young people become desperate due to the insidious money needs and deteriorating relationships.

The greatest obstacle to therapy is confronting young gamblers with what they have been trying to avoid all along: integrated thinking. These adolescents usually are not grateful to professionals who eagerly offer answers and explanations, as their minds do not automatically revert to cohesiveness when mildly jogged. Although their compulsive self-remedy of gambling has not worked, their avoidance of mature thought remains. Once forced into therapy, their only protection is to set up barriers that allow the fragmentation of self to continue. They cannot allow themselves to listen to any one adult, for they are certain this person will bring them humiliation.

These youths need to carefully control and regulate their clear thinking so that this new experience will not cause intolerable personal distress. Maturity is often signaled by a willingness to grant that the therapist has something of value to offer.

The feelings of warm security that accompany a therapeutic alliance can displace the brief pleasures of winning at gambling. These feelings can be contrasted with episodes of dysphoria and panic. The anticipation of a win or a loss mimics the persistent hope of the shamed child in a dysfunctional family that something, anything, will soon give relief. It will take quite a while in therapy for the teenager to come to enjoy realistic expectation of mastery in academics and socializing. These pursuits require continuity of self-observing skills and the relinquishment of illusion. Gambling is dangerously soothing for those youths who have the prior "addiction" of avoiding linked-up thinking. In therapy, their contrived illusory anticipations and linkages can be replaced by real satisfactions and associations.

Notes

1. Readers interested in more information on the concept of dissociation are referred to Jacobs, 1988.

2. For a discussion of the magical thinking normally present in children up to 6 years of age, see Fraiberg, 1959.

3. This evidence is reviewed in chap. 12, "Adolescent Gambling Research: The Next Wave," by Henry Lesieur.

4. For more information on guilt and shame as these concepts relate to therapy for pathological gamblers, see Rosenthal & Rugle, 1994.

References

Apter, M. J. (1992). *The dangerous edge: The psychology of excitement.* New York: Free Press.

Bird, H. R. (1995). Psychiatric treatment of adolescents. In H. I. Kaplan & B. J. Sadock (Eds.), *Comprehensive textbook of psychiatry,* vol. 6 (pp. 2439–46). Baltimore: Williams & Wilkins.

Caplan, G., & Lebovici, S. (Eds.) (1969). *Adolescence.* New York: Basic Books, Inc.

Derevensky, J. L., Gupta, R., & Cioppa, G. D. (1996). A developmental perspective of gambling behavior in children and adolescents. *Journal of Gambling Studies, 12,* 49–66.

Fraiberg, S. H. (1959). *The magic years.* New York: Charles Scribner's Sons.

Gupta, R., & Derevenksy, J. L. (2000). Adolescents with gambling problems: From research to treatment. *Journal of Gambling Studies, 16,* 315–42.

Holmes, D. J. (1964). *The adolescent in psychotherapy.* Boston: Little, Brown and Company.

Jacobs, D. F. (1988). Evidence for a common dissociative-like reaction among addicts. *Journal of Gambling Behavior, 4,* 27–37.

Pearson, G. S. (1992). Nursing interventions with children and adolescents experiencing thought disorders. In P. West & C. L. S. Evans (Eds.), *Psychiatric and mental health nursing with children and adolescents* (pp. 329–43). Gaithersburg, MD: Aspen Publishers, Inc.

Rosenthal, R. J., & Rugle, L. J. (1994). A psychodynamic approach to the treatment of pathological gambling: Part I. Achieving abstinence. *Journal of Gambling Studies, 10,* 21–42.

Shaffer, H. J. (1994). Denial, ambivalence, and countertransference hate. In J. D. Levin & R. Weiss (Eds.), *Alcoholism: Dynamics and treatment* (pp. 421–37). Northdale, NJ: Jason Aronson, Inc.

Chapter Six

Gambling in a Familial Context

Joni Vander Bilt and Joanna Franklin

Introduction

Familial and friendship frameworks pose the context in which compulsive gambling lives. Although a compulsive gambler can be isolated from a family of origin or a family of choice, the more usual situation is that of a compulsive gambler acting and interacting with related others. Specifically, compulsive gambling by an adult has been shown to have significant consequences for a partner/spouse (Darvas, 1981; Heineman, 1987; Lorenz, 1987; Lorenz & Shuttlesworth, 1983; Lorenz & Yaffee, 1988), for children (Jacobs et al., 1989; Lesieur & Klein, 1987; Lesieur & Rothschild, 1989; Lorenz, 1987), for siblings (Lorenz, 1987), and for parent(s) (Heineman, 1987; Heineman, 1989; Lorenz, 1987). Similarly, adolescent compulsive gambling also adversely affects parent(s) (Moody, 1989) and other family members. Domestic/family violence is just one potential consequence of compulsive gambling, and it is an area that has generally been neglected in gambling research. This chapter will first explore some of the ramifications for family relationships that result from a family member (or members) with a compulsive gambling problem. The chapter specifically focuses on domestic violence in this context. It then looks at treatment, discussing interventions specific to the needs of various family members as well as of the family system. Several examples from clinical experience are used to illustrate and support concepts and hypotheses.

Today every American experiences the effects of the proliferation of gambling. Adolescents, however, are confronted with the advent of legalized and condoned gambling at a stage in their lives when the formation of individual values, habits, judgments, and behaviors is most easily influenced. Depending on the state and on the gambling activity, institutionalized or government-sanctioned gambling (for example, lottery, casinos, and racetracks), is not legally accessible to those under 18 or 21 years of age (Rose, 2002). However, gambling is not a rare event for most adolescents. Research indicates that lottery agents sell lottery tickets to adolescents as young as 9 years of age (Lesieur, 2002). One study reported 47.1 percent of seventh-grade students purchased lottery tickets at some point in their lifetimes; by twelfth grade, the number increased to 74.6 percent (Shaffer, 1994). In addition, 64 percent of underage students at one Atlantic City high school reported they had gambled at casinos (Arcuri, Lester, & Smith, 1985).

Parents and grandparents alike have children line up to buy "their tickets" as a way of rewarding or entertaining the child. It is not uncommon for these parents and grandparents to deny that the child is in fact gambling, rationalizing, "It's only a lottery ticket; that's not gambling." In response to this situation, some states, such as Massachusetts, have passed laws mandating the posting of age limits in outlets selling lottery tickets, and a few casinos have proactively instituted an educational campaign citing the risks of underage gambling, such as Harrah's Project 21 (Satre, 2002).

The lack of stigma associated with gambling and the increased opportunity for gambling have resulted in a generation of young people who gamble more than the previous generation did at the same age. In fact, the prevalence of compulsive gambling is currently higher among adolescents than among adults (Addiction Research Foundation, 1995; Jacobs et al., 1989). High school and college students also exhibit higher prevalence rates for probable pathological gambling than adults (Lesieur & Klein, 1987; Lesieur et al., 1991). Some adolescents will gamble occasionally, some regularly, but approximately 4.4 percent to 7.4 percent are considered pathological gamblers (Shaffer & Hall, 1996).

Two recent studies examined the levels of involvement of Massachusetts adolescents in various illicit activities, including the lottery (Shaffer, 1994; Shaffer et al., 1995). Of six illicit activities (for example, substance use or lottery participation) that researchers investigated among students in grades seven through twelve, lifetime prevalence of involvement with the lottery is exceeded only by lifetime prevalence of alcohol use. One such teenager had been increasingly involved with peers in a sports book system; when unable to pay his debts, he was threatened by his peers, then taken forcibly from his home, driven to a distant location, and released to find his way home alone. Although his peers intended just to frighten the teen, they were sought out by authorities and subject to kidnapping charges.

Likewise several teens have been introduced to treatment services following drug charges (possession of a controlled and dangerous substance with intent to distribute) just to have the treatment team discover the drug charges were not related to a drug-use problem but rather to drug selling as a means to fund their gambling activities. The parents of one such youth expressed great relief at finding out their teenage son had, not a drug problem, but rather a gambling problem. "Thank God," the mother said, "it's only a gambling problem. We were afraid he had a serious addiction."

Some adolescents who gamble but do not meet diagnostic criteria for compulsive gambling also experience negative consequences. For example, young people who experience subclinical gambling problems, that is, they are not identified by a diagnostic screen, are distracted from their homework, family chores, and social activities because of their gambling. They are not fully engaged in the kinds of activities that would ultimately lead them to make professional, academic, scientific, athletic, or other contributions to society (Shaffer, Hall, Walsh, & Vander Bilt, 1995).

The proliferation of gambling during the 1980s and 1990s and the increased prevalence of adult gambling behavior have resulted in a generation of children growing up in households and families where gambling is increasingly common. Although research has much to say about children raised in homes with an alcoholic parent (Juliana & Goodman, 1992), little research apart from clinical observation has been done to ascertain the impact of adult compulsive gambling on a child. The extant research reports that children of pathological gamblers are more likely than children of nonpathological gamblers to develop gambling problems themselves (Lesieur & Klein, 1987; Lesieur et al., 1991).

Not only are more children being raised in an atmosphere where one or both parents engage in gambling behavior, but also societal approval of gambling behavior translates into a lack of stigma and criticism of gambling behavior. Parents are aware of their children's gambling activity but do not disapprove of it (Derevensky, Gupta, & Cioppa, 1996; Ladouceur & Mireault, 1988). Some casinos have constructed elaborate amusement centers around the casino to promote the idea of gambling as a family activity. In addition, the increasingly popular use of the term *gaming,* as opposed to *gambling,* encourages families to consider a trip to a casino complex fun and games. "The family that gambles together stays together," however, is an image constructed by marketing strategists and does not reflect the reality of the impact of compulsive gambling on a family. Moderate gambling or compulsive gambling, like substance abuse, is more than an individual problem and must be viewed in the context of family and social systems (Juliana & Goodman, 1992).

Consequences of Youth Gambling

Adolescents who gamble compulsively are often facing other obstacles in their lives. Although it is unclear which behavior precedes the other, research demonstrates that a higher proportion of adolescent compulsive gamblers abuse substances than do adolescents who do not gamble (Jacobs, 1987). They are also more likely to be depressed, attempt suicide, and have lower grades (Ladouceur & Mireault, 1988; Lesieur & Klein, 1987). Problem gambling can result in a disruption of friendship that cannot withstand the burden of the friend's covering up for or repeatedly loaning money to the gambler. Two studies found that 9 percent to 10 percent of high school students admitted to supporting their gambling behavior by engaging in illegal activities (Ladouceur & Mireault, 1988; Lesieur & Klein, 1987).

For some adolescents, gambling serves as an escape from the challenges they face. Winning the lottery, doubling their money at a casino, or betting their allowance on a baseball game could reestablish some footing in the world and improve self-esteem. Unfortunately, it is much easier to lose in gambling than it is to win; adolescents counting on a win to improve their situation are usually thrown into an increasingly frustrating cycle of loss.

Consequences of Gambling on Youth Who Reside in Gambling Households

Youth experience the effects of their parents' addictive behaviors. Adolescents growing up in a household with one or more compulsive gamblers not only are more likely to have a gambling (Lesieur & Klein, 1987) or substance abuse (Lorenz & Shuttlesworth, 1983) problem themselves, but also experience the instability of the gambler's financial and emotional swings (Franklin & Thoms, 1989). Other adverse effects of parental compulsive gambling include significant behavioral or adjustment problems such as running away from home and being arrested on charges of theft (Jacobs, 1989; Lesieur & Rothschild, 1989; Lorenz & Shuttlesworth, 1983; Shaffer, Hall, Walsh, & Vander Bilt, 1995). Although these behaviors can be seen as ways the adolescent copes with the household conflict, they nonetheless have the potential of introducing adverse consequences for the adolescent's future.

Family Violence

Although little research has examined the association between compulsive gambling and domestic violence, this chapter will lay the groundwork for the hypothesis that this association not only is feasible but is one that treatment providers, policymakers, and the gambling industry should be aware of. The implications of violence for youth—both as recipients of family violence and as witnesses of family violence—are important to consider. The definition of family violence includes the following:

1. action or omission of behavior that produces damage to members of the family group
2. intentionality
3. negative incidence on an individual's physical or psychic development
4. negative incidence on the subject's perception about himself/herself
5. negative incidence on subject's physical and/or psychic health (Kornblit, 1994).

First, we will briefly review the epidemiology of violence against women, adolescents, and children.

VIOLENCE AGAINST WOMEN

A major cause of morbidity and mortality for women is physical abuse, often perpetrated by husbands or male intimates. Research from a wide range of countries reveals that between 20 percent and 50 percent of women interviewed have been beaten by a male partner (Heise, 1994). Women in the United States are more likely to be assaulted and injured, raped, or killed by their former or current male partner than by all other types of assailants combined (Council on Scientific Affairs, 1992). Statistics from the 1982–1984 National Crime Survey reveal that for violent crimes in which the victim and the offender are related, 77 percent of all victims are women (Klein, Martin, & Kaufman, 1988).

The National Committee for Injury Prevention and Control estimates that each year in the United States, one million women receive emergency medical services for injuries related to battering (Dannenberg, Baker, & Li, 1994); 22 percent to 35 percent of women treated in hospital emergency departments evidence injuries or symptoms of physical abuse (Horton, 1995). Although motor vehicle crashes are responsible for more than one-third of all female unintentional injuries (34 percent), women make almost three times as many medical visits for treatment of injuries related to physical abuse as they do for injuries related to motor vehicle crashes (Dannenberg, Baker, & Li, 1994). Women are 2.4 times more likely than men to be strangled or beaten to death (Sorenson & Saftlas, 1994). Furthermore, of all battered women presenting in an emergency department, 30 percent were injured as a result of domestic violence (Sugg & Inui, 1992). Estimates of violence against women often originate from emergency room studies or medical records. Given the nature of domestic violence and the disincentive for women to report violence or even seek direct help for fear of retaliation and other factors (Frieze & Browne, 1989), it can be expected that these estimates are conservative.

Women living in violent and abusive situations have limited resources, both emotionally and physically, to attend to themselves and to their children. In addition, research shows that children's development and behavior is affected by witnessing domestic violence. Even when the violent incident is not directly observed by children, they are nonetheless aware of and affected by parental conflict and violence (Wolfe & Korsch, 1994). In a review of the behavioral and emotional problems suffered by children who witness domestic violence, Wolfe and Korsch describe high levels of distress and adjustment problems among preschool and early school-age children. School-age children suffer significant emotional difficulties, including undermined self-esteem and confidence in their future. Some children experience guilt as a result of believing that somehow they could stop the violence.

VIOLENCE AGAINST CHILDREN

Children and adolescents are also the victims of direct violence and abuse. Two million cases of child abuse and two thousand deaths from child abuse are reported each year in the United States (Marwick, 1994). Adolescents (ages 12 to 17) represented one-quarter of all of the cases reported to child protective services in 1990 (Council on Scientific Affairs, 1993). In one study, adolescent-onset abuse (as differentiated from childhood-onset abuse) was associated with periods of high stress in families. Risk factors for adolescent maltreatment include high levels of interparental conflict. Health consequences associated with a history of sexual abuse among adolescents include delinquency, alcohol and other drug abuse, and increased attempts of suicide (Council on Scientific Affairs, 1993).

Recognizing the Problem

Pathological gambling, like other addictive behavior, is not an isolated activity. The formation in 1960 of Gam-Anon, an organization designed to provide support for the pathological gambler's family and friends, represents one of the first indications that the family of the compulsive gambler is as affected by gambling as the gambler. In fact, 58 percent of one sample of males attending Gamblers Anonymous (GA) cited "his wife's threatening to leave" as a precipitating factor to entering GA (Livingston, 1974). Gamblers Anonymous is the oldest and largest treatment group available for problem gamblers. Based on Alcoholics Anonymous' twelve steps of recovery, GA is a self-help program for those who desire to stop gambling.

One of the consequences of excessive gambling is the deception gamblers use to create the illusion of control—both for themselves and for the sake of others who may be involved with them. In a study of spouses of compulsive gamblers, 25 percent of the respondents did not recognize that a problem existed until nine or more years after the start of the marriage (Lorenz & Shuttlesworth, 1983). High percentages of these spouses characterized their gambling partners as liars (93 percent), dishonest (89 percent), and emotionally ill (100 percent) (Lorenz & Shuttlesworth, 1983).

In another example, 81 percent of a sample of GA conference attendees reported hiding their gambling from their spouse (Lorenz & Yaffee, 1986). However, the response rate of this study was only 30 percent. Furthermore, 97 percent of the respondents were male, so this study cannot be considered representative of the gambling population. However, the high prevalence of deceptive behavior reported by this sample confirms the high levels of marital discord for pathological gamblers and their spouses reported by Lorenz and Shuttlesworth (1983). Clinical evidence from gamblers and their families who enter treatment also supports this interpretation (Steinberg, 1993).

Gambling and Family Violence

Adding the tensions generated by problem gambling to the existing interactions among family members may increase the possibility of violence, particularly if the relationships are already unsteady. Money tends to be a highly charged issue for any family; in fact, money can be the primary cause of marital disagreements ("Speaking of money," *Boston Globe*, December 26, 1994). Adding addiction and the often-associated patterns of secrecy and betrayal to the money component could escalate problems into violence. Children who witness violent arguments about money may be attracted to gambling as a way to relieve their guilt at potentially being responsible for the arguments by winning enough money to "fix it."

In one of the few studies assessing the extent of violence among pathological gamblers, 43 percent of the Gam-Anon members surveyed reported that they had been emotionally, verbally, and physically abused by their gambling spouse or partner (Lorenz & Shuttlesworth, 1983). Ninety-eight percent of the respondents were women. Approximately 10 percent of the Gam-Anon members surveyed also reported that the gambler had abused the children, and 12 percent of the respondents had attempted suicide (Lorenz & Shuttlesworth, 1983). Of the 12 percent who attempted suicide, 50 percent reported being physically or verbally abused by their spouse (Lorenz & Shuttlesworth, 1983). In an earlier, British study, 45.8 percent of physically battered wives reported that their spouses gambled heavily: 19.8 percent had gambled heavily occasionally and 26 percent had gambled heavily frequently (Gayford, 1975). A Canadian study determined that 23.3 percent of the respondents who were pathological gamblers had abused their spouses and 16.7 percent had abused their children (Bland, Newman, Orn, & Stebelsky, 1993). Neither of these studies collected data from a control group, so the relative severity of the prevalence rates cannot be determined.

Female spouses of male pathological gamblers are more likely than their general population counterparts to attempt suicide (Lorenz & Shuttlesworth, 1983). There is also evidence that being in a relationship with a problem gambler negatively affects a spouse's physical health. Medical complaints made by wives of gamblers attending a Gam-Anon conference include chronic or severe headaches, gastrointestinal problems, and depression (Lorenz & Yaffee, 1988). The levels at which these women manifested these symptoms were higher than in a comparison sample of hospital patients. Alternative explanations for these differences, apart from involvement with a compulsive gambler, were not explored in this study.

Children of pathological gamblers also are victimized by their parents' gambling behavior and are often abused physically and verbally (Lorenz, 1987). One of the few existing studies investigating this area revealed that children of pathological gamblers were more likely to have experienced physical violence and abusive violence than nationally normed samples of children (Lesieur & Rothschild, 1989). Children of pathological gamblers also attempt suicide twice as often as their classmates (Jacobs et al., 1989; Lesieur & Rothschild, 1989).

A significant positive association has been found between adult pathological gambling and the gambling behavior of both parents (Lesieur, Blume, & Zoppa, 1986). However, despite evidence for increased prevalence of adolescent gambling (Jacobs, 2002), little research has been done to determine the relationship between parental pathological gambling and the gambling behavior of their adolescent children.

Several problems are inherent in the sparse data investigating the incidence of violence among pathological gamblers and their families. The samples are almost entirely nonrepresentative and very small, lessening the precision of the estimates. Respondent groups are rarely compared with control groups, which would help isolate the incidence of the violence associated with gambling. In addition, the methods used to measure "violence"—verbal abuse or physical abuse—are not consistent across studies. Methodologists are just beginning to examine the differences among the scales and instruments designed to measure violence. For example, the questions researchers asked to elicit percentages of respondents experiencing abuse are not always specifically elaborated in the articles and reports.

Family-Related Items in Gambling Screening Instruments

The general impact of pathological gambling on the family has been recognized by specific items included on a variety of screening instruments used to measure the severity of pathological gambling patterns. The Massachusetts Gambling Screen (MAGS) has three questions that specifically relate to family:

1. Does any member of your family ever worry or complain about your gambling?
2. Has your gambling ever created problems between you and any member of your family or friends?
3. Have you ever neglected your obligations (for example, family, work, or school) for two or more days in a row because you were gambling? (Shaffer, LaBrie, Scanlan, & Cummings, 1994)

An earlier version of the South Oaks Gambling Screen (SOGS) included "disrupted family or spouse relationship due to gambling" as one of seven possible criteria used in classifying an individual as a pathological gambler (Lesieur, Blume, & Zoppa, 1986). However, in later versions the language became more direct:

1. Have you ever hidden betting slips, lottery tickets . . . from your spouse, children, or other important people in your life?
2. Have you ever argued with people you live with over how you handle money?
3. If you borrowed money to gamble or to pay gambling debts, who or where did you borrow from? . . . from your spouse? (Lesieur & Blume, 1987; Wallisch, 1993)

The fourth edition of the American Psychiatric Association's *Diagnostic and Statistical Manual of Mental Disorders* (DSM-IV) also changed the criterion associated with the effects of gambling on the family. In the third edition of the manual, the criterion referred to "disrupted family or spouse relationship"; in the fourth edition, the criterion was changed to (1) "lies to family members or others to conceal the extent of involvement with gambling" and (2) "has jeopardized or lost a significant relationship, job, educational, or career opportunity because of gambling" (Shaffer et al., 1994; American Psychiatric Association, 1994).

Finally, the Gamblers Anonymous twenty questions, developed by GA to help pathological gamblers identify their problem, has two questions relating to family:

1. Is gambling making your home life unhappy?
2. Does gambling make you careless of the welfare of your family? (Alcoholics Anonymous Central Service Committee, 1995)

A Void in the Existing Research: Gambling and Domestic Violence

Despite the recognition of gambling-related family problems on the various gambling problem screens, there has been a dearth of research specifically investigating gambling and domestic violence. There are various reasons for this gap, including lack of funding sources, perception of gambling as a socially accepted activity, and a slow response by treatment providers to meet the demands of problem gamblers. Professional treatment for pathological gamblers is relatively new: The first treatment program opened in 1972. At the time this book went to press, there were approximately 139 treatment programs for pathological gamblers and their families existing in the United States, clearly an insufficient number to meet the needs of those seeking treatment.

Treatment options for compulsive gambling include individual, group, couples, family treatment, and self-help. Treatment programs established for family members of pathological gamblers address the ways in which pathological gambling has affected and disrupted the family. For example, group therapy for female spouses of male gamblers participating in long-term outpatient therapy has focused on the spouse's therapeutic needs. Franklin and Thoms (1989) mention some of the issues confronting the spouse of the gambler: depression, isolation, marital discord, poor parenting, and poor communication skills.

Lorenz enumerates similar difficulties facing the family of a pathological gambler: poor communication, unsatisfactory sexual relations, ineffective parenting, and poor conflict resolution (Lorenz, 1987, p. 72). In addition, families that include a compulsive gambler commonly experience financial and legal difficulties (Darvas, 1981; Heineman, 1994; Lorenz, 1989; Lorenz & Shuttlesworth, 1983; Wildman, 1989). In a study of a sample of 144 spouses of compulsive gamblers, 99 percent of the respondents reported financial problems directly related to gambling (Lorenz & Shuttleworth, 1983).

Although some of these family problems could be related to domestic violence (for example, marital discord or poor conflict resolution), domestic violence as a specific consequence of gambling is conspicuously absent from these problem lists. Similarly, much of the treatment research examining issues aggravated by compulsive gambling has failed to consider domestic violence as a potential consequence of excessive gambling. Common characteristics of families in which violence occurs include "social isolation and certain particularly stressful situations such as unemployment or financial problems" (Bergman, Larsson, Brismar, & Klang, 1988)—a profile that fits many situations in which one or more family members are having a problem with gambling.

Supporting the likelihood of pathological gamblers' violence toward their family is a study of female spouses of pathological gamblers that found "almost half of the women had experienced abuse, either physical or verbal, from the gambler" (Wildman, 1989, p. 295). Similarly, a higher percentage of parents, one or both of whom were compulsive gamblers, used a violent tactic in resolving conflict with their children than did parents in a nationally normed sample (Lesieur & Rothschild, 1989).

Violence can be a way of acting out when the pathological gambler reaches a certain stage in the disorder. In the four-phase course of gambling progression constructed by Rosenthal and Lorenz (1992), the pathological gambler is said to become "irritable, quick-tempered, and sometimes abusive to family members" in the third or "desperation phase." According to this model, some gamblers progress to the fourth phase, the "giving-up phase," in which they no longer care that they are losing but gamble for the sake of action or excitement alone (Rosenthal & Lorenz, 1992). Although research confirms that most violence that causes injury is perpetrated by men against women (Council on Scientific Affairs, 1992; Heise, 1994, p. 15), no studies to our knowledge have been conducted specifically to investigate the causal role that gambling plays in stimulating domestic violence.

Male gamblers can also become targets of attacks from their female spouses. In one study, 61 percent of the female spouses physically struck or threw something at the gambler. These episodes were related to the gambler's physical or verbal abuse of his partner or his children, or to financial problems. This study failed to make a comparison with national norms (Lorenz, 1981). These statistics need to be confirmed by further research.

Other studies on gamblers' violence suggest that pathological gamblers rarely resort to violent acts against strangers (Brown, 1987). Although several studies have found it common for pathological gamblers to admit to illegal activities that support their gambling, these crimes are most often of a financial, nonviolent nature (Rosenthal & Lorenz, 1992). "Violence is only threatened by the gambler as part of a more desperate property crime, such as armed robbery, and is rare even then" (Brown, 1987, p. 107).

Violence and Pathological Gambling as Impulse Disorders

Compulsive gambling is defined as an impulse disorder by the American Psychiatric Association. Individuals who act impulsively in one domain might be expected to have difficulty regulating their impulses in other areas. For example, individuals who have difficulty regulating their impulses with respect to gambling might be more apt to act out in other areas of daily living, such as eating and substance use. Currently, the relationship among these areas is unclear. A study of 61 prisoners in a special protection wing did not support the hypothesis of a "multi-impulsive personality disorder"; in fact, pathological gambling was not related to substance abuse, aggression, or self-harm (Kennedy & Grubin, 1990). Further research is necessary to explore these relationships.

Although violence is a manifestation of societal structures of differential power and economics, a violent incident by an individual can also be a manifestation of a lack of control. An improved understanding of the underlying impulse control mechanisms and the influence of this regulatory mechanism on violence and gambling is fundamental to the prevention and treatment of violence in general and gambling-related violence in particular. In both cases, a more comprehensive study of gambling will provide the forum for exploring the dynamics of domestic violence.

Relationship Among Violence, Pathological Gambling, and Substance Abuse

Any inquiry into gambling and domestic violence remains incomplete without a consideration of substance use and abuse. Several studies examining various populations agree that approximately 50 percent of pathological gamblers has or has had problems with substance abuse and dependence (Linden, Pope, & Jonas, 1986; Ramirez, McCormick, Russo, & Taber, 1983; Rosenthal & Lorenz, 1992). In a Canadian study, pathological gamblers were significantly more likely to have substance use disorders than nongamblers (Bland et al., 1993). Conversely, approximately 10 percent to 20 percent of substance abusers qualify as pathological gamblers (Elia & Jacobs, 1993; Lesieur, Blume, & Zoppa, 1986; Spunt, Lesieur, Hunt, & Cahill, 1995).

A study of children of compulsive gamblers discovered that children of "multiple-problem families" (defined as children who, in addition to having a compulsive gambling parent, also had an alcoholic, drug-abusing, and/or an overeating parent) were different from children of "pure gamblers." Children of multiple-problem families were more likely to smoke, drink, and overeat than a control group, while children of pure gamblers were less likely to gamble more than they could afford and only slightly more likely than the control group to smoke, overeat, or drink (Lesieur & Rothschild, 1989). These findings underscore the importance of considering the role of substance abuse in the consequences of compulsive gambling problems.

Research has established an association between substance abuse and family violence (Frieze & Browne, 1989; Leonard & Jacob, 1988). An estimated 50 percent of all domestic abuse cases involve alcohol or drug abuse, while alcohol is a factor in 55 percent of all home assaults (Substance Abuse Project Task Force, 1995). For example, a study released by the Quincy District Court in Massachusetts revealed that 71 percent of batterers appearing before the court system had an alcohol problem (Harshbarger & Winsten, 1993, p. 20). Other states have comparable rates of substance abuse among batterers (Adams, 1989).

Although substance abuse is not always present in domestic violence, when it is present the violence tends to be more severe (Frieze & Browne, 1989). A study examining whether parental physical abuse is present when parents exhibit both gambling and substance abuse problems found that multiple-problem parents were more abusive than parents who gambled but did not abuse substances (Lesieur & Rothschild, 1989). Since a high percentage of pathological gamblers engage in substance abuse (Murray, 1993; Ramirez et al., 1993), research is needed to isolate the effect that each behavior has on domestic violence and to determine how the two addictive behaviors might act synergistically as a component of domestic violence.

Research Questions

There are many questions that emerge when we consider the expanding impact of gambling in the contemporary United States. What is the prevalence of domestic violence among pathological gamblers—of either gender? In what direction does the identified violence manifest itself? For example, how is female-to-male violence among one or more pathological gamblers contextually different than male-to-female violence and how prevalent is violence directed at children? Does violent behavior change depending on whether the gambler enters a treatment program? Is gambling-related domestic violence associated with family and household structure, for example, nuclear families, one-parent families, same-sex relationships, or extended households? What are the coping mechanisms adopted by family members of a problem gambler? In what way is violence in the family related to who is doing the gambling?

No longer can we assume the traditional scenario of a male gambler married to a female nongambler with two nongambling children. It is time to reconsider conventional patterns, particularly if we want to refine previous research that relied on samples of gamblers that were not representative of the full range of problem or pathological gamblers. Opportunities for gambling have increased dramatically in recent years, especially for children; family compositions now take many forms. Determining the risk factors associated with gambling-related domestic violence is instrumental to developing primary and secondary prevention measures that can decrease the incidence of gambling-related violence within the family.

Violent behavior can be antecedent or consequent to excessive gambling. In situations where gambling and violence coexist, it is difficult to determine which behavior came first. Is violence a way of releasing the stress of financial loss, deception, and other consequences of gambling, or is gambling a way of escaping from the cycle of violence and the frustrations of family conflict? Or are both related to a third factor, such as impulse control? New research must identify the different patterns of violence/gambling relationships.

Treatment

Given the extent to which gambling and abusive behavior may coexist, it is crucial that therapists be aware of as many of the unique issues involved in working with compulsive gamblers and their families as possible. As research continues into family treatment, clinicians are finding that problem gambling shares much in common with other addictions. The late Dr. Robert Custer has been quoted as saying that gambling addiction is 90 percent similar to substance addictions. Although the remaining 10 percent is small, it is a critical difference to consider when seeking a successful treatment outcome.

For example, gamblers do not overdose. Given an unlimited supply of money the gambling behavior can continue without the body reaching a "maximum point" and slipping into an unconscious state or vomiting. Likewise, without a blood or urine test the counselor is forced to examine outward signs of gambling or relapse to monitor progress such as budget or financial management. And as has been noted by Joseph Ciarrocchi, there have been cases reported of alcoholics who regain their physical strength and whose bodies can recover from the ravages of alcoholism, but there is not one case of a spontaneously regenerated bank account on record for any gamblers in recovery.

A remarkably important fact to note for the family in recovery with the gambler is the long sentence they also sign onto when a restitution plan reaches into ten, fifteen, or twenty years of the gambler's life. Many of these families who have chosen to remain together have also chosen to forfeit their homes, retirement accounts, vacations, and entire lifestyles in order to support the gambler in recovery. Gamblers are heavily in debt and trying to work a restitution plan, perhaps stay out of jail, and repay the victims of their gambling disorder while making amends to their families. As months and years pass sometimes the initial sincere support of a spouse or parents gives way to a growing sense of resentment and bitterness. This critical area of recovery for the family must be anticipated by the counselor and appropriate strategies prepared to empower and help the family redefine their life in recovery, complete with all its choices.

In an attempt to meet this need for integration of research with therapeutic intervention, we now focus on the applied science of gambling treatment. Here the sharing of constructs and intervention strategies that effectively meet the needs of compulsive gamblers and their family members can best be examined in the laboratory of the family in treatment. The courage and hope of these families who have presented for treatment services have allowed the counselors and therapists to translate and evolve treatment strategies to meet the needs of these children, their parents and family members.

FAMILY THERAPY FOR CHILDREN OF COMPULSIVE GAMBLERS

Many parents caught in the chaos of a gambling crisis find themselves resorting to "secret keeping" as the easiest way to deal with the children in the family. Conflicting feelings of shame, hurt, anger, love, and concern often leave parents hiding the truth about the crisis and trying desperately to minimize the effects of the trauma on the children. Such protective feelings are sometimes more in the interest of the parents than the children. The easier thing to do is make up excuses for the gambler's behavior—behavior that is difficult for both the gambler and the spouse or partner to understand (Heineman, 1994; Steinberg, 1993). It can be even more difficult for parents to explain to young children the many absences from home, arguments, lack of money, strange phone calls, or even the sudden need to move. Consequently, the unspoken conspiracy begins as the parents join forces to "protect" the children from the truth of the family's circumstances, an approach that can have some serious short- and long-term consequences.

Some of the excuses for a gambling parent's whereabouts include "working late"; an inpatient treatment stay or extended gambling absence is often explained away as a "business trip." Some parents go to elaborate means to convince young teens or adult children that these lies are in fact the truth. This deceptive behavior destroys the basis of trust, making it even more difficult for children and parents once the truth becomes known.

One example of secret keeping involves a young couple who were pleased they had been able to keep the truth about their gambling crisis from their three young daughters. The parents hid the reason for Dad's job change, Mom's return to work, and the need to sell their home. They went to court for the gambler's sentencing hearing without saying a word about the possibility of Dad not coming home for three to seven years. In fact, after the sentencing the defense attorney had to plead with the judge to give the gambler some time to explain his prison sentence to his three unsuspecting daughters. Such a disclosure so late in the game made the two older children feel betrayed and untrusted (the youngest was not yet 3 years old).

AGE-APPROPRIATE HONESTY WITH CHILDREN: PERCEPTIONS AND INTERPRETATIONS

Parents in a gambling household are encouraged to share with children the reality of the family situation in a language that is simple, honest, and age-appropriate for the children. Much of the work in such disclosures actually focuses on preparing the parents to tell the truth and think long-term about the impact on the family. Conversely, when asked whether they would want their children to protect parents from the truth or trouble they may be experiencing, parents do not agree with secret keeping. Typically, parents feel very strongly about "being there" for their children no matter what. Once the discussion on the power of role modeling and double standards has concluded, parents are ready to have the "tough conversation" and begin searching for the language to use during their disclosure.

A counselor or therapist can be instructive and supportive in helping parents choose the right words. The age of the children is only one variable to consider. The counselor should also assess the communication styles of the parents and children, as well as review the "functional age" of the children, because many children are old or young for their age. Deciding how to approach the issue should be based on what all parties believe the children are able to understand. For children from 4 years of age to 6 or 7, an introduction to the specifics could include analogies about "play." For example,

Q: When might you get in trouble for playing?

A: If it is time to go inside and eat dinner or get ready for bed.

Q: Do you get punished for not listening when your parents ask you to stop playing?

These simple questions introduce the concepts of "in control" and "out of control" to even very young children. This same age group already has an awareness of what illness or "being sick" is all about, so with patience and simple explanations, a meaningful dialogue about problems, responsibility, and support can be concluded with everyone winning. Adolescents and late-latency-age children are often able to understand far more than parents give them credit for. These older children have a sense of the tension and stress in the home whether or not they are told the reasons for it. They frequently know of money problems, even if they do not know the full extent of the gambling problems. Likewise, they have a sense of what human service agencies and self-help groups are all about. It is often easy to draw parallels between drug and alcohol treatment and Alcoholics Anonymous and gambling treatment and Gamblers Anonymous.

An important element for parents to consider should be the child's perceptions and interpretations of the truth. As many divorced couples have experienced, children decide for themselves what the reality of the divorce is, based on available information and on their perceptions and interpretations. At this time children often decide that they are to blame for the divorce in spite of the denials voiced by the parents. Parents should be prepared to reassure their children and reaffirm that they are not responsible for the consequences of the gambling problem, such as their father going to jail.

THE SECURITY OF STRUCTURE AND THE POWER OF ROLE MODELING

Adolescents and young children alike have a need for structure. Their sense of security comes largely from consistent structure in the home (Satir, 1967). The children of pathological gamblers complain about the lack of such structure; consequently, as adolescents they demonstrate some of the more typical ways of acting out insecurities by drinking, smoking, using drugs, and eating more than their peers from non-problem-gambling homes (Jacobs et al., 1989). When asked about role modeling, many parents with gambling problems find themselves from the "Do as I say, not as I do" school. Negative role modeling for these families includes teaching children not to face the painful truths in their lives, admit to a problem, or reach out for help. They also learn to lie to protect those they are closest to and care most about. Once presented with the way children perceive these messages, parents realize how different the messages are that they truly want to convey. This ensuing motivation and reasoning allow the parents to know that though honesty may be difficult, it teaches children to own their problems, take responsibility and not blame, admit a need, and reach out for help.

Parents should thoroughly discuss factors such as the timing and content of any disclosures. Both parties (if there is a gambler and a spouse/partner) should agree to any negotiations or compromises before making any disclosures. It is important for the children to see parents working in a united front toward the resolution of problems. This also limits children's ability to split the parents by siding first with one parent and then the other. For many children and adolescents, age-appropriate pursuit of mastery over their own lives often includes manipulating their parents' lives. At such times a history of open, honest, and consistently structured communication can minimize trauma and maximize growth opportunities. Timing should not be left to "I can't hide this from them anymore," nor should poor timing allow the nongambling spouse (if there is one) to punish the gambler by informing on them.

THERAPEUTIC ISSUES AND STRATEGIES

Parents will often find children and young adolescents to be primarily nonverbal regarding trauma and conflicts. At these times it is helpful to have available to the child a counselor familiar with play therapy, art therapy, and physically expressive therapies. Such work should always include age-appropriate education on problem gambling for the children. Education materials on this subject can be found through the National Council on Problem Gambling, local state affiliates, local gambling treatment programs, GA, and Gam-Anon, as well as Gama-Teen literature.

In relationships consisting of a gambler and a nongambler, the role of the nongambler in therapy is critical (Berman & Siegel, 1993; Heineman, 1994). In many treatment programs the spouse or partner is not considered a primary client, yet partners or spouses of problem gamblers are at times in greater need of therapeutic services than the gambler (Ciarrocchi & Reinert, 1993). Unfortunately, as de facto crisis managers for the family, partners are under great stress and struggle to maintain the stability of the home.

Similar to families struggling with substance abuse problems, all members of the family will continue to be affected by the financial and emotional consequences of the gambler's behavior long after the gambling has stopped, and in many cases for the duration of the restitution period. Such circumstances frequently breed resentment and bitterness if left untreated (Darvas, 1981). Typically, the nongambler has assumed the parenting responsibilities abdicated by the gambler. Under these conditions the nongambling partner, without appropriate support and education, is understandably tempted to take the path of least resistance in resolving conflicts with the children.

The gambler's role in the family during recovery cannot be limited to abstinence and restitution. Rather, it must include a reassessment of the primary relationship with the partner or spouse. With this improved foundation, parenting skills can be further developed to meet the needs of the nongambler, the children, and the gambler in recovery. Such skills include appropriate limit setting, clear marking of boundaries, modeling of good communication skill, and investing the care and support that nurture the child (Steinberg, 1993). Gamblers' partners are often told in Gam-Anon that the program is for them, with or without the gambler. Recovery resources are available to the family members who seek them.

TREATMENT SERVICES FOR ADOLESCENT COMPULSIVE GAMBLERS

Typically, the family of an adolescent seeking treatment services for a mental or behavioral health concern would turn first to the school counselor, nurse, or perhaps mental health professional specializing in adolescent psychiatry or psychology. Unfortunately, it is rare for most of these professionals to be aware of or experienced with problem or pathological gambling. So, like their adult counterparts, adolescent gamblers are frequently left with one of three options: (1) continue to see the care provider regardless of the lack of specialized knowledge or training, (2) go to Gamblers Anonymous, or (3) follow the recommendation of the treatment professional and contact an agency, program, or treatment professional specializing in pathological gambling. Of course, there is also the not uncommon fourth option of one or more members of the family believing in the transient nature of the problem and forgoing treatment altogether.

The drawbacks for each of these approaches to adolescent treatment needs are readily apparent. Usually parents of a teen gambler seek the help of a health care professional just after they have found out about the extent of their child's gambling. As a result, this search often occurs in a state of shock, disbelief, hurt, and anger. Counselors rarely see self-motivated adolescents early on in the progression of their gambling problems, eager to find some way to stop the gambling and restore manageability to their lives. Instead, adolescents often have reality issues forcing them to seek help, such as the threat of being expelled from school, losing a job, being threatened for nonpayment of gambling-related debts, or prosecution for a gambling-related crime. Sometimes increased depression and thoughts of self-destruction have frightened teens into seeking help.

However, some adolescents enter treatment in denial, presenting a formidable challenge for the professional therapist. Parents are eager for the counselor to fix or cure the problem and are often all too eager to hear and believe in a promise of "I will never do it again" and then forego the pursuit of treatment services. The need for specialized knowledge and training in gambling treatment can make the difference between engaging the client in the therapeutic process and losing the client to a control battle no one can win.

School counselors may be the first health professionals parents call on for help. Sometimes they are aware of the warning signs of gambling and know where local referrals can be made, yet most times they are not. One family brought their 15-year-old son to the school counselor for help with a gambling problem that included several thousand dollars owed to bookies, stolen items from the parents' home, and plummeting grades. The well-intentioned counselor was unfamiliar with gambling problems and recommended that the teen limit his gambling to ten-dollar bets only on weekends. This adolescent was encouraged to attend the after-prom party with the Las Vegas night theme, at which students were encouraged to gamble "play" money as an alternative to drinking and driving. Yet this counselor was trying to help this student learn to control his gambling.

Counselors are cautioned that treating gambling problems is a subspecialty area within the specialty area of adolescent treatment. Sometimes, however, a counselor who specializes in adult services and gambling problems is unavoidably asked to counsel an adolescent with a gambling problem. This is a concern if the counselor is not an experienced adolescent counselor with specialized knowledge and experience in counseling youth. The developmental milestones, upheaval of hormones, identity crises, separation and individuation conflicts, need to rebel, natural impulsiveness, and family dynamics all must be understood and grounded in solid intervention techniques and age-appropriate educational information (e.g., Sanger, 2002). Few adolescent gamblers have access to such expertise.

Many adolescent gamblers find themselves pursuing help through Gamblers Anonymous, the oldest and largest treatment group available for problem gamblers. Based on AA's twelve steps of recovery, GA offers an anonymous self-help program for those with a desire to stop gambling. Historically, GA has been unable to attract and keep adolescents in its fellowship, because many adolescents find themselves quite uncomfortable in a typical GA meeting. They are often the only teens attending the meeting; most GA meetings in the United States and Canada are attended by white, middle-aged men who are offering advice and sharing their own experiences with gambling.

This is usually a difficult group for adolescents (and women and minorities) to feel comfortable in; it also, more often than not, triggers the negative transference and countertransference feelings that will send a teen running from the group. The adolescent has heard ten or fifteen "fathers" telling him or her what to do and how to do it. The harder the group tries to help the teen, the harder the teen tries to distance from the group. When unable to leave the group because of a court order or parental insistence, the teen distances instead from the message "stop gambling." Such an approach, poorly timed, rarely keeps the teen engaged (Haubrich-Casperson & Van Nispen, 1993). Feeling immortal as many teens do, they find it even more difficult than their adult counterparts to admit to the unmanageability of their lives and almost impossible to surrender to the higher power, as they are encouraged to do within the GA fellowship.

However, age-appropriate use of support groups has met with some encouraging success. In these cases, the counselor or GA group has gone to some effort to connect one recovering teen with another and then another. Enough adolescents at about the same stage in the recovery process can support each other and have a greater chance of being able to relate to each other. For this approach to work, it is in the best interest of the school counselors, local GA members, and mental health professionals to cooperate and refer the adolescents to a common source of help. GA, like all twelve-step groups, is meant to function as a peer group. No matter where adolescents enter the health care delivery system, it is important that they be directed to whatever specialized services exist in the local community.

TREATMENT OF THE FAMILY SYSTEM: SOME COMMON MISTAKES

It was Todd's fifth birthday. The party had just ended, the guests had gone home, and Todd was full of joy and excitement from his big day. He approached his father to say good-night and show him his favorite new toys. Todd's father was busy watching a football playoff game. Todd did not know that his father had a month's pay riding on the game and was making a desperate attempt to double up and get out of debt to his bookie. When Todd touched his father's knee and said, "Look what I have, Dad," his father grabbed him by the arm and sent him sprawling across the room. Todd hit his head and was unconscious for a minute or so, and was left with a broken arm. Todd's father was horrified at what he had done. He stated over and over again, "I only shoved him away. I didn't mean to hurt him."

Todd's father was telling the truth: He did not mean to hurt his son, and he had no idea how hard he threw the child. But Todd never forgot the incident. Ten years later when Todd came to the attention of the staff at the local mental health center, he discussed with defiance and pride his current gambling binge, related thefts, and recent school suspension for gambling as the only thing he had in common with his father. The dynamics involved in Todd's family were complicated and demanded the attention of an experienced family therapist familiar with gambling problems. The therapist, however, treated only the family dynamic issues, then waited for the "symptom" of gambling to disappear—a common mistake. Todd's relationship with his parents improved, his grades stabilized, but his gambling continued, leading to yet another crisis a few months later.

It is just as important for the counselor not to overlook the importance of the family system and the need for the family to be involved in the counseling process. Gambling speaks loudly to an adolescent, and it sometimes becomes the preferred form of communication in the family and the focus of control battles. Stopping the gambling is only one part of the recovery process. The entire family often needs to find more productive ways to communicate and to cope with stress. Distances between adolescent gamblers and their parents can sometimes be unintentionally increased if the teen commits to a recovery program without family involvement. Once the family is involved, continued support and encouragement is necessary to maintain that involvement.

EDUCATION FOR THE PROBLEM-GAMBLING ADOLESCENT

Since developmental stages dictate that adolescents feel immortal, omnipotent, and all-knowing, it is sometimes difficult to engage them in the learning process regarding problem gambling. It can be most helpful to apply the principles of stages of change as outlined by James Prochaska and his colleagues (Prochaska, DiClemente, & Norcross, 1992). Many control battles can be avoided if counselors set appropriate priorities based on the client's readiness to change. The importance of providing adolescents with accurate, understandable gambling information to better prepare and eventually motivate them to engage in the therapeutic process, and not just attend counseling sessions, cannot be overlooked.

Detailed information on adolescent gambling is beginning to accumulate in the gambling treatment and research fields and is a small part of available Gamblers Anonymous literature. When presented within the stage-change model, such resources can be used by the adolescent counselor to effectively educate and inform adolescent gamblers. To present too much too soon can distance rather than engage adolescents as they prepare to ignore the latest lecture. Motivational work, giving adolescents choices, and simple contracting can combine to help effect lasting change. The "when" to engage adolescents gamblers becomes equally important as the "how" to engage them. Adding the necessary gambling treatment information to the already existing skills of the experienced adolescent counselor would be an efficient use of limited treatment dollars and scarce training funds. This approach allows those adolescent treatment programs and professionals already established in a community to offer a new service built on their existing skills. This is especially appropriate for those clinicians who already provide substance abuse services for teens.

Counselors who have experience with gamblers but have not been trained in family therapy can find themselves trying to do individual counseling with each member of the family instead of applying family therapy techniques and strategies to the entire system. Relapse prevention can be increased when lasting changes to the gambler's entire family system are the focus of treatment (Darvas, 1981).

Referral of the adolescent gambler demands even more effort on the part of the counselor. Client matching is the single most important element in the referral process. The adolescent should be assessed, and the counselor should know if the local GA groups have any young members, if there is a local gambling treatment program with an adolescent specialist on staff, and if the staff of the local adolescent service programs know anything about gambling treatment. If the answer to many of these questions is no, the next task for the counselor or family member is to begin building a network of support and services. Perhaps the local GA group members can share the philosophy and principles of the program with local clinicians. The local affiliate of the National Council on Problem Gambling (there are 34 state affiliates) could be contacted for information on training and education programs available for clinicians, PTAs, Student Assistance Programs, and so forth. Although establishing a treatment and support network is labor intensive, it will be available for as long as there are families in need of the services.

Directions for Future Research on Youth and Family

Patterns of behavior and activity often remain undocumented until new questions are asked. Child abuse, for example, remained relatively unexplored until research protocols, clinician guidelines, and a shift in societal expectations enabled more discussion and documentation of maltreatment of children. Similarly, as substance abuse counselors, school counselors, and practitioners in other fields begin asking questions and screening for gambling-related problems, a broad and diverse group can be identified and can then receive treatment and guidance. If questions about domestic violence are included in the intake and screening procedures at gambling treatment centers, new patterns may emerge that will have far-reaching treatment implications.

Although this chapter has focused on domestic violence, other gambling-related violence also affects the family. Many gamblers who fall into debt from gambling losses become familiar with a network of individuals whose priority is to recoup their money. As the gambler finds it more and more difficult to repay, a continuum of potentially violent experiences emerge, including threatening phone calls and physical assaults. Much of gambling-related violence involves illegal gambling ventures, making research into this area challenging. However, the disruptive events that occur as a result of gambling contribute to an emotional climate within the family that deserves further investigation.

One aspect of child maltreatment not discussed in this chapter is child neglect. Neglect is a caretaker's failure, either deliberately or through inability or negligence, to take the necessary actions to provide a child with shelter, minimally adequate food, clothing, supervision, medical care, emotional growth and stability, or other essential care (Felix, Berman, & Carlisle, 1995). No research has been done to determine whether pathological gamblers are at risk of neglecting their children. However, a preoccupation with gambling and chasing losses could correlate with having less time to provide children with adequate care. Financial recklessness on account of gambling might also be considered neglect, if it deprives children of the resources necessary to feed and shelter them. Further investigation into the impacts of adult gambling on their children will result in more understanding and prevention of these potentially negative sequelae.

In addition, as women and children begin gambling as frequently or even more often than men, and with similar adverse consequences, family dynamics are likely to change accordingly. Research must stay attuned to demographic trends in gambling to provide policy and treatment recommendations as well as to offer a deeper understanding of the manner in which pathological gambling affects in meaningful ways not only the individual but also those around the gambler.

References

Adams, D. (1989, July/August). Identifying the assaultive husband in court: You be the judge. *Boston Bar Journal, 33* (4), 23–25.

Addiction Research Foundation. (1995). Review of the literature on problem and compulsive gambling.

Alcoholics Anonymous Central Service Committee. (1995). *Beginner's pamphlet.* Boston: Author.

American Psychiatric Association. (1994). *Diagnostic and statistical manual of mental disorders: Fourth edition.* Washington, DC: Author.

Arcuri, A. F., Lester, D., & Smith, R. O. (1985). Shaping adolescent behavior. *Adolescence, 20,* 935–38.

Bergman, B., Larsson, G., Brismar B., & Klang, M. (1988). Aetiological and precipitating factors in wife battering: A psychosocial study of battered wives. *Acta Psychiatrica Scandinavica, 77,* 338–45.

Berman, L., & Siegel, M. (1993). *Behind the eight ball: A guide for families of gamblers.* New York: Simon & Schuster.

Bland, R. C., Newman, S. C., Orn, H., & Stebelsky, G. (1993). Epidemiology of pathological gambling in Edmonton. *Canadian Journal of Psychiatry, 38,* 108–12.

Brown, R. I. F. (1987). Pathological gambling and associated patterns of crime: Comparisons with alcohol and other drug addictions. *Journal of Gambling Behavior, 3*, 98–114.

Ciarrocchi, J. (1993). Rates of pathological gambling in publicly funded outpatient substance abuse treatment. *Journal of Gambling Studies, 9*, 289–94.

Ciarrocchi, J., & Reinert, D. F. (1993). Family environment and length of recovery for married male members of Gamblers Anonymous and female members of Gam-Anon. *Journal of Gambling Studies, 9*, 341–52.

Council on Scientific Affairs, American Medical Association. (1992). Violence against women: Relevance for medical practitioners. *Journal of the American Medical Association, 267*, 3184–89.

Council on Scientific Affairs, American Medical Association. (1993). Adolescents as victims of family violence. *Journal of the American Medical Association, 270*, 1850–56.

Dannenberg, A. L., Baker, S. P., & Li, G. (1994). Intentional and unintentional injuries in women: An overview. *Annals of Epidemiology, 4*, 133–39.

Darvas, S. F. (1981, October). The spouse in treatment: Or, there is a woman (or women) behind every pathological gambler. Paper presented at Fifth National Conference on Gambling and Risk-Taking, Lake Tahoe, NV.

Derevensky, J. L., Gupta, R., & Cioppa, G. D. (1996). A developmental perspective of gambling behavior in children and adolescents. *Journal of Gambling Studies, 12*, 49–66.

Elia, C., & Jacobs, D. F. (1993). The incidence of pathological gambling among Native Americans treated for alcohol dependence. *International Journal of the Addictions, 28*, 659–66.

Felix, A. C., Berman, R. A., & Carlisle, L. K. (1995). *1994 child maltreatment statistics.* Boston: Massachusetts Department of Social Services.

Franklin, J., & Thoms, D. R. (1989). Clinical observations of family members of compulsive gamblers. In H. J. Shaffer, S. A. Stein, B. Gambino, & T. N. Cummings (Eds.), *Compulsive gambling.* Lexington, MA: Lexington Books.

Frieze, I. H., & Browne, A. (1989). Violence in marriage. In L. Ohlin & M. Tonry (Eds.), *Family violence. Crime and justice: A review of research* (Vol. 11), pp. 163–18. Chicago: University of Chicago Press.

Gayford, J. J. (1975). Wife battering: A preliminary survey of 100 cases. *British Medical Journal, 1*, 194–97.

Harshbarger, S., & Winsten, J. A. (1993). *Report on domestic violence: A commitment to action.* Boston: Authors.

Haubrich-Casperson, J., & Van Nispen, D. (1993). *Coping with teen gambling.* New York: Rosen Publishing Group, Inc.

Heineman, M. (1987). A comparison: The treatment of wives of alcoholics with the treatment of wives of pathological gamblers. *Journal of Gambling Behavior, 3*, 27–40.

Heineman, M. (1989). Parents of male compulsive gamblers: Clinical issues/treatment approaches. *Journal of Gambling Behavior, 5*, 321–33.

Heineman, M. (1994). Compulsive gambling: Structured family intervention. *Journal of Gambling Studies, 10,* 67–76.

Heise, L. L. (1994). *Violence against women: The hidden health burden.* Washington, DC: World Bank.

Horton, J. A. (1995). *The women's health data book: A profile of women's health in the United States.* Washington, DC: Jacobs Institute of Women's Health.

Jacobs, D. F. (1987, August). Effects on children of parental excess in gambling. Paper presented at the Seventh International Conference on Gambling and Risk-Taking, Reno, NV.

Jacobs, D. F. (1989). Illegal and undocumented: A review of teenage gamblers in America. In H. J. Shaffer, S. A. Stein, B. Gambino, & T. N. Cummings (Eds.), *Compulsive gambling: Theory, research, and practice* (pp. 249–92). Lexington, MA.: Lexington Books.

Jacobs, D. F., Marston, A. R., Singer, R. D., Widaman, K., Little, T., & Veizades, J. (1989). Children of problem gamblers. *Journal of Gambling Behavior, 5,* 261–68.

Jacobs, D. F. (2003). Juvenile gambling in North America: Considering past trends and future prospects. In H. J. Shaffer, M. N. Hall, J. Vander Bilt, & E. George (Eds.), *Futures at stake: Youth, gambling, and society* (epilogue). Reno: University of Nevada Press.

Juliana, P., & Goodman, C. (1992). Children of substance abusing parents. In J. H. Lowinson, P. Ruiz, R. B. Millman, & J. G. Langrod (Eds.), *Substance abuse: A comprehensive textbook* (pp. 808–15). Baltimore: Williams & Wilkins.

Kennedy, H. G., & Grubin, D. H. (1990). Hot-headed or impulsive? *British Journal of Addiction, 85,* 639–43.

Klein, D., Martin, S., & Kaufman, K. (1988). The most commonly asked questions about domestic violence. In *Domestic violence: A training curriculum for law enforcement.* San Francisco: Family Violence Project, District Attorney's Office.

Kornblit, A. L. (1994). Domestic violence: An emerging health issue. *Social Science & Medicine, 39,* 1181–88.

Ladouceur, R., & Mireault, C. (1988). Gambling behaviors among high school students in the Quebec area. *Journal of Gambling Behavior, 4,* 3–12.

Leonard, K. E., & Jacob, T. (1988). Alcohol, alcoholism, and family violence. In V. B. VanHasselt, R. L. Morrison, A. S. Bellack, & M. Hersen (Eds.), *Handbook of family violence* (pp. 383–406). New York: Plenum Press.

Lesieur, H. R. (2003). Adolescent gambling research: The next wave. In H. J. Shaffer, M. N. Hall, J. Vander Bilt, & E. George (Eds.), *Futures at stake: Youth, gambling, and society* (chap. 12). Reno: University of Nevada Press.

Lesieur, H. R., & Blume, S. B. (1987). The South Oaks Gambling Screen (SOGS): A new instrument for the identification of pathological gamblers. *American Journal of Psychiatry, 144,* 1184–88.

Lesieur, H. R., Blume, S. B., & Zoppa, R. M. (1986). Alcoholism, drug abuse, and gambling. *Alcoholism: Clinical & Experimental Research, 10,* 33–38.

Lesieur, H. R., Cross, J., Frank, M., Welch, M., White, C. M., Rubenstein, G., Moseley,

K., & Mark, M. (1991). Gambling and pathological gambling among university students. *Addictive Behaviors, 16,* 517–27.

Lesieur, H. R., & Klein, R. (1987). Pathological gambling among high school students. *Addictive Behaviors, 12,* 129–35.

Lesieur, H. R., & Rothschild, J. (1989). Children of Gamblers Anonymous members. *Journal of Gambling Behavior, 5,* 269–81.

Linden, R. D., Pope Jr., H. G., Jonas, J. M. (1986). Pathological gambling and major affective disorder: Preliminary findings. *Journal of Clinical Psychiatry, 47,* 201–3.

Lorenz, V. C. (1981, October). Differences found among Catholic, Protestant, and Jewish families of pathological gamblers. Paper presented at the Fifth National Conference on Gambling and Risk-Taking, Lake Tahoe, NV.

Lorenz, V. C. (1987). Family dynamics of pathological gamblers. In T. Galski (Ed.), *The handbook of pathological gambling* (pp. 71–88). Springfield, IL: Charles C. Thomas.

Lorenz, V. C. (1989). Some treatment approaches for family members who jeopardize the compulsive gambler's recovery. *Journal of Gambling Behavior, 5,* 303–12.

Lorenz, V. C., & Shuttlesworth, D. E. (1983). The impact of pathological gambling on the spouse of the gambler. *Journal of Community Psychology, 11,* 67–76.

Lorenz, V. C., & Yaffee, R. A. (1986). Pathological gambling: Psychosomatic, emotional, and marital difficulties as reported by the gambler. *Journal of Gambling Behavior, 2,* 40–49.

Lorenz, V. C., & Yaffee, R. A. (1988). Pathological gambling: Psychosomatic, emotional, and marital difficulties as reported by the spouse. *Journal of Gambling Behavior, 4,* 13–26.

Marwick, C. (1994). Health and justice professionals set goals to lessen domestic violence. *Journal of the American Medical Association, 271,* 1147–48.

Moody, G. (1989). Parents of young gamblers. (Special issue: Gambling and the family.) *Journal of Gambling Behavior, 5,* 313–20.

Murray, J. B. (1993). Review of research on pathological gambling. *Psychological Reports, 72,* 791–810.

Prochaska, J. O., DiClemente, C. C., & Norcross, J. C. (1992). In search of how people change: Applications to addictive behaviors. *American Psychologist, 47,* 1102–14.

Ramirez, L. F., McCormick, R. A., Russo, A. M., & Taber, J. I. (1983). Patterns of substance abuse in pathological gamblers undergoing treatment. *Addictive Behaviors, 8,* 425–28.

Rose, I. N. (2003). Underage gambling and the law. In H. J. Shaffer, M. N. Hall, J. Vander Bilt, & E. George (Eds.), *Futures at stake: Youth, gambling, and society* (chap. 7). Reno: University of Nevada Press.

Rosenthal, R. J., & Lorenz, V. C. (1992). The pathological gambler as criminal offender. *Clinical Forensic Psychiatry, 15,* 647–61.

Sanger, S. (2003). Youth-gambling treatment issues. In H. J. Shaffer, M. N. Hall, J. Vander Bilt, & E. George (Eds.), *Futures at stake: Youth, gambling, and society* (chap. 5). Reno: University of Nevada Press.

Satir, V. (1967). *Conjoint family therapy: A guide to theory and technique.* Palo Alto, CA: Science and Behavior Books.

Satre, P. (2003). Youth gambling: The casino industry's responsibility. In H. J. Shaffer, M. N. Hall, J. Vander Bilt, & E. George (Eds.), *Futures at stake: Youth, gambling, and society* (chap. 9). Reno: University of Nevada Press.

Shaffer, H. J. (1994). *The emergence of youthful addiction: The prevalence of underage lottery use and the impact of gambling.* (Technical Report No. 011394-100). Boston: Massachusetts Council on Compulsive Gambling.

Shaffer, H. J., & Hall, M. N. (1996). Estimating the prevalence of adolescent gambling disorders: A quantitative synthesis and guide toward standard gambling nomenclature. *Journal of Gambling Studies, 12,* 193–214.

Shaffer, H. J., Hall, M. N., Walsh, J. S., & Vander Bilt, J. (1995). *The psychosocial consequences of gambling.* Boston: Federal Reserve Bank.

Shaffer, H. J., LaBrie, R., Scanlan, K. M., & Cummings, T. N. (1994). Pathological gambling among adolescents: Massachusetts Gambling Screen (MAGS). *Journal of Gambling Studies, 10,* 339–62.

Shaffer, H. J., Walsh, J. S., Howard, C. M., Hall, M. N., Wellington, C. A., & Vander Bilt, J. (1995). *Science and substance abuse education: A needs assessment for curriculum design* (SEDAP Technical Report No. 082595-300). Cambridge: Harvard Medical School Division on Addictions.

Sorenson, S. B., & Saftlas, A. F. (1994). Violence and women's health: The role of epidemiology. *Annals of Epidemiology, 4,* 140–45.

Speaking of money: For many couples, that's not so easy. (1994, December 26). *Boston Globe,* sec. A., pp. 1, 10.

Spunt, B., Lesieur, H., Hunt, D., & Cahill, L. (1995). Gambling among methadone patients. *International Journal of the Addictions, 30,* 929–62.

Steinberg, M. A. (1993). Pathological gambling and couple relationship issues. In W. R. Eadington & J. A. Cornelius (Eds.), *Gambling behavior and problem gambling* (pp. 197–214). Reno, NV.: Institute for the Study of Gambling and Commercial Gaming.

Substance Abuse Project Task Force. (1995, March). *A matter of just treatment: Substance abuse and the courts.* Boston: Author.

Sugg, N. K., & Inui, T. (1992). Primary care physicians' response to domestic violence: Opening Pandora's box. *Journal of the American Medical Association, 267,* 3157–60.

Wallisch, L. S. (1993, September). *Gambling in Texas: 1992 Texas survey of adolescent gambling behavior.* Austin: Texas Commission on Alcohol and Drug Abuse.

Wildman II, R. W. (1989). Pathological gambling: Marital-familial factors, implications, and treatments. *Journal of Gambling Behavior, 5,* 293–301.

Wolfe, D. A., & Korsch, B. (1994). Witnessing domestic violence during childhood and adolescence: Implication for pediatric practice. *Pediatrics, 94,* 594–99.

Chapter Seven

Underage Gambling and the Law®

I. Nelson Rose

Finally 21, and Legally Able To Do Everything I've Been Doing Since I Was 15
  Bumper Sticker

Introduction: Age Limits for Gambling

How old should a child be before he or she is allowed to gamble?

This question is not merely rhetorical. Every government has both the power and the obligation to set the minimum age to gamble once it has legalized that activity. Not establishing an age limit is itself a decision, a legal declaration that anyone, even a small child, can legally wager.

The regulation and control of gambling comes under a government's police power, the power and obligation of a government to protect the health, safety, and welfare of its citizens. In the United States, as in most parts of the world, the police power has almost always been reserved to local governments, primarily the states, but also to cities, counties, and Indian tribes.

Federal governments, on the other hand, do not normally have police power over local issues, such as gambling. The powers of a federal government are usually limited to those explicitly listed in a constitution. Congress and other branches of the federal government of the United States, for example, probably do not have the power to set a minimum age for gambling, unless authority can be found in the U.S. Constitution, such as Congress's power over interstate commerce and Indian tribes.

The police power of a state is virtually unlimited—even constitutional rights are put aside. Historically, situations calling for police power actions often have been emergencies, like fires and plagues, when there was no time for considerations such as the due process right to a trial.

The Nevada Supreme Court has gone so far as to declare that when it comes to legal gambling, there are no federal civil rights.

We view gaming as a matter reserved to the states within the meaning of the Tenth Amendment to the United States Constitution. Within this context we find no room for federally protected constitutional rights. This distinctively state problem is to be governed, controlled and regulated by the state legislature and, to the extent the legislature decrees, by the Nevada Constitution. It is apparent that if we were to recognize federal protections of this wholly privileged-state enterprise, necessary state control would be substantially diminished and federal intrusion invited.[1]

Taking the Nevada Supreme Court at its word: To control gaming a state may discriminate on the basis of race; federal constitutional prohibitions on discrimination would not apply. Even state constitutional rights do not apply, unless the state legislature gives its blessing. If a state can discriminate on the basis of race, it certainly can draw reasonable categories on the basis of age.

Other courts have said the Rosenthal opinion goes too far.[2] But the Nevada Supreme Court's basic approach still holds true. In cases involving legal gaming, the burden is on the individual to prove that his or her rights outweigh the important government policies behind restrictions and prohibitions.

The most striking example of how a state's police power trumps constitutional rights was decided in 2001, when the Louisiana Supreme Court ruled that some adults could be barred from gambling, purely on the basis of their age.

In 1998 the Louisiana State Legislature raised the minimum age to gamble on both the state lottery and privately owned video poker machines.[3] The state is saturated with these privately owned gaming devices, since they may be put into every truck stop, racetrack, and any other business holding an easily obtained liquor license. Other forms of gaming, including slot machines and identical video poker machines at the state's many casinos, on riverboats, Indian land, and in the heart of New Orleans, had always been limited to players over 21. A 19-year-old resident, William B. Norton, and David Melius, the owner of Bruno's Bar in New Orleans, filed suit in January 1999, claiming the new law violated the state constitutional provision against age discrimination.[4]

The argument had some merit, because 18-year-olds are legally adults in Louisiana, and the state has the strongest provision found in any state constitution against age discrimination. But on January 29, 2001, a majority of the Supreme Court of Louisiana held it was not unconstitutional to prohibit 18-, 19-, and 20-year-old adults from participating in some forms of legal gambling.[5]

Although the justices may have been thinking they were dealing with children, Louisiana law prevented them from using that word. Louisiana law is very clear that the age of majority, the year when a person stops being a child and becomes an adult, is 18; the age was lowered from 21 to 18 in 1972. The Louisiana constitution also has an unusual Individual Dignity Clause. Justice Catherine D. "Kitty" Kimball wrote a separate opinion in the recent case to emphasize that Louisiana has a "unique constitutional provision which gives greater protection against age discrimination than either the United States Constitution or any other State Constitution."

Both the trial judge, Preston Aucoin, and Justice Harry Thomas Lemmon of the state supreme court felt the state had not proved that preventing 18- to 21-year-olds from gambling would have any greater benefit to society than if any other group of adults was chosen to be barred from gambling.

The majority, however, looked to its precedent from 1996, where it upheld laws raising the minimum drinking age from 18 to 21 to protect both the young adults and society.[6] In that case the court laid down a unique, new standard: In Louisiana, a law may discriminate against 18-, 19-, and 20-year-old adults only if the state can prove the law substantially furthers "appropriate government purposes."[7] These purposes must involve a benefit to members of the public other than the 18- to 20-year-olds. The state showed that raising the drinking age improved highway safety for all. In that case, the court looked at the evidence, experience, other states, and common sense in concluding that keeping the group most likely to become involved in drunk-driving accidents off the road protected not only those young adults but society in general.

But while there is extensive evidence of the dangers of letting young people drink and drive, the United States, and in fact the entire world, has little experience with widespread legal gambling for any age group. Dr. Rachel Volberg, the leading expert on the prevalence of compulsive gambling, has found, in the relatively few studies that have been done, that 18- to 21-year-olds are three times as likely as adults 21 years of age and older to have problems with gambling. At trial, the state's expert, Dr. James Westphal, testified that "although the 18- to 20-year-old age group only comprises 8.2 percent of the total adult population, that age group makes up 22.5 percent of total adults with gambling disorders."

The problem for the law is how to deal with the fact that we treat 18-year-olds as competent for some activities and not for others. Louisiana, for example, now prohibits anyone under 21 from buying a lottery ticket or playing a video poker machine. But an 18-year-old can place a parimutuel wager at a Louisiana racetrack and bet at charity bingo, including bingo machines.

In theory, it might be difficult to show that raising the gambling age protects other members of society. Perhaps the argument can be made that, in general, 18- to 20-year-olds do not have the financial resources to lose large amounts, are more likely to bet beyond their limits, and thus would be more likely to turn to crime to support their habits. Anecdotal evidence indicates that younger gamblers are more likely to become compulsive. But the Louisiana Legislature, and virtually every other lawmaking body in the country, had already made the determination that society as a whole benefits by restricting casino gaming to specified places with controlled access and to adults over 21.

In the past, a state's police power included an element of morality. Even today, courts have no problem upholding actions by state legislatures designed to protect individuals and society from moral harms. Victimless crimes are the classic example. All parties directly involved in an illegal transaction involving gambling, drugs, or prostitution want the transaction to proceed, but the law forbids it. Illegal gambling obviously falls under police power, but police power has continued to extend to these morally suspect activities even after they have been made legal. What would be a victimless crime becomes a morally suspect industry, still subject to state controls. Examples include legalized prostitution in Nevada, decriminalized "recreational" drugs, such as marijuana, and legal gambling. All forms of gambling continue to fall under the state's police power, even if the legal gaming operation has existed for years and been established by state law or run by the state itself. As recently as 1993, the U.S Supreme Court had this to say about state lotteries:

> While lotteries have existed in this country since its founding, States have long viewed them as a hazard to their citizens and to the public interest. . . . Gambling implicates no constitutionally protected right; rather, it falls into a category of "vice" activity that could be, and frequently has been, banned altogether.[8]

How should a government decide how to use its police power in setting the minimum age to place a wager? The too-easily-given answer is to do "what is best for children."[9]

The first question, then, should properly be, "Who should decide what is best?" and not "What is best for this class of children?" Put differently, when confronted with a problem concerning the well-being of children, the policymaker should initially ask, "Is this a problem I should try to solve by legislating the best answer for every child, or is the identification of the 'best' policy something that I should leave or delegate to someone else to determine?"

State legislatures usually decide whether an existing prohibition on a form of gambling will be lifted. They thus have to decide who will determine what the standard will be, including the fundamental question of whether there should be an unwavering minimum age for participating in the activity, or whether exceptions should be made in rare cases, or whether each child should be evaluated individually.

The makers of broad public policies most often decide that their appropriate function is to allocate power and responsibility among others to determine what is best.[10] Curfews and television viewing are examples of activities where decision making is shared among governments, private industry, parents, and the children themselves. The current controversy over children's access to the Internet is a dramatic example of how society struggles with the issues of how much power each party should have.

With legal gambling coming under the state's police power, the government has always been the sole official decision maker. A mother and her 20-year-old son may agree that he is mature enough to gamble, but the minor and his mother cannot legally overrule a minimum age limit of 21 for gambling. When it comes to activities that fall within the state's police power, government almost always has the ultimate decision-making power, even if it chooses not to exercise that power. This is especially true with public policies affecting the health, safety, welfare, and morality of children. In fact, this sovereign power is sometimes called parens patriae, derived from the king's role as guardian of those of his citizens, especially children, who are legally incompetent.

Constitutional and statutory bans on virtually every form of gambling have traditionally been in place in each state of the United States. Although legalization swept through the United States two times, the complete prohibition of gambling has been the norm. As recently as 1963 there were no state lotteries and the only state with casinos was Nevada.[11] Legal gambling is a limited, explicit, governmentally created exception: a morally suspect industry created, but regulated, by state law.

Problems with Age Limits

Should there be any age limits at all? Most, if not all, jurisdictions throughout the world agree that some people simply are not competent to make certain decisions. Legal limitations based on age alone encompass and restrict every part of life, including the right to work, marry, vote, serve on juries, drive, buy alcoholic beverages and tobacco, read certain books and magazines, view certain films, make enforceable contracts and wills, sue or be sued, make decisions about jobs, schools, and medical treatments, and handle one's own finances.

In some cases, the finding of legal incompetence can be used as a shield. All states, for example, would say that a 4-year-old child who kills her baby brother simply cannot commit the crime of murder. She may be physically capable of killing, but the law states, as a presumption not subject to rebuttal, that she cannot form the requisite mental specific intent to kill, because she does not understand the consequences of her actions. The court will not allow a prosecutor to put on evidence to prove that she actually does understand the meaning and consequences of her act. In other cases, legal incompetence can be used as a sword. In some states, a 17-year-old girl cannot legally consent to sexual intercourse. A man who knowingly has sex with the underage girl commits the crime of statutory rape, even if the act is voluntary and even if the girl is an experienced prostitute.

Of course, many adults are ruled legally incompetent each year as well. A 40-

year-old man with the intelligence of a 2-year-old may be institutionalized permanently. Even though he is chronologically an adult, he has become, in the eyes of the law, like an infant: He cannot be trusted to make decisions for himself. But for anyone who has reached the age of majority, a finding of legal incompetence occurs only after a full hearing, focusing on the individual.[12] For minors being born after a designated year is enough to prove legal incompetence.

The law almost always declares that a minor is automatically legally transformed from being an incompetent child into a competent adult on the day the minor reaches a certain age. Yet we all know that 100 percent of all minors do not become instantly wiser the day they turn 18 or 21. So why is the law enforcing a legal fiction?

The answer can be seen in the examples of the 17-year-old prostitute and the 40-year-old institutionalized patient given above. The legal system has only two ways of dealing with these individuals. It can either take each and every person as he or she is at any moment and conduct extensive hearings to determine that person's actual competence. Sometimes the law starts with broad, generalized presumptions; for example, a 17-year-old is presumed to not have the capacity to commit adult crimes and is normally subject to the less harsh juvenile justice system. But these legal presumptions are rebuttable; prosecutors can put on evidence and a judge can rule at a hearing that this particular minor should be tried as an adult. In the other cases the presumptions are irrebuttable, and there is thus no need for a hearing, because no evidence of actual competence may be introduced.

It thus becomes obvious why societies impose irrebuttable presumptions in the case of the minimum age to gamble, even if the presumptions are rebuttable for other activities. If a presumption of competence is rebuttable, a tribunal, such as a court, would be required to decide whether specific individuals may engage in certain specified activities. In the case of gambling, the presumption is irrebuttable: The lawmakers simply declare that no one under a certain age, such as 21, can legally engage in the specified activity and everyone 21 years of age and older can.

As America's experiment with Prohibition demonstrated, creating laws that are not enforced can lead to, at the very least, public disrespect for the legal process. On the other, it cannot be disputed that increased availability leads to increased use: Making something like alcoholic beverages legal for adults increases forbidden use by minors. Every study on underage gambling has found that wherever any form of legal gambling is easily available to adults, a large percentage of teenagers will also participate in that form of gambling, no matter what the legal age limit. Age restrictions not only are arbitrary, they are obviously arbitrary.[13] Strict enforcement is difficult, if not impossible, and can lead to unwanted side effects. Casinos throughout the world have been subjected to stories of children locked up for hours in parked cars while their parents gambled.[14]

Both solutions for determining when a person can make certain independent decisions create real-world problems. A case-by-case analysis of each individual would burden the court system beyond its breaking point. Yet whenever the law saves judicial resources by making broad generalizations, some individuals outside the norm will be harmed.

The first solution, calling for individual hearings in all cases, would be especially unworkable for minors. A particular child of 12 may not be able to understand all the consequences of buying a lottery ticket one month but may grow in understanding the next.

There is not even a general acceptance of what it means to be "competent" to make a particular decision—for example, what is required for a person to be competent to gamble? Does competence merely involve a working knowledge of the rules of the game? Knowledge of the odds? Understanding the meaning of money? Having a moral sense of right and wrong? Valuing the work ethic? Understanding the risk of becoming a compulsive gambler? Being able to evaluate and compare the entertainment value of gambling against the risks inherent in the games?

We know there are skilled 20-year-old card-counters who know exactly what they are doing when they play blackjack and 60-year-olds who should not be trusted with their own or anyone else's money in a casino. When the law imposes a minimum age limit of 21, it prevents the 20-year-old card-counter from gambling and probably winning, while it allows the 60-year-old to gamble and probably lose.

Not only the individuals face potential harm; society also pays whenever generalities cannot be disputed. Legal gambling can have pervasive and often unrecognized impacts on nongaming individuals and institutions, including a gambler's family and job. Economic theory alone would call for barring only the truly incompetent, not individuals who have been so classified merely due to the accident of their year of birth.

Drawing the Line: A Legislative Balancing Act

Where the law draws the line is also subject to society's shifting feelings about what it means to be an adult. In setting an age into law, a state legislature is undertaking a rough balancing act. It is also recognized that raising a minimum age for any activity, such as drinking or gambling, from 18 to 21, not only affects that age group but also makes it more difficult for even younger children to participate.

One unspoken hope is that raising the legal age will lead to reduced rates of early use, with the additional expectation that this will translate into lower rates of heavy use when the child grows up. Although this proposition may be true, there is little in the way of empirical support for it for any product or activity: Raising the age at which individuals may legally buy alcoholic beverages to 21 has not been shown to decrease the incidence of adult alcoholism. Similarly, raising the gambling age from 18 to 21 certainly will provide additional protection to 18-, 19-, and 20-year-olds, by making commercialized gambling much less available to them and their younger friends and siblings. But it seems clear that most compulsive gamblers begin betting when they are very young. In his 1995 book, *Adolescent Gambling*, Mark Griffiths discusses the empirical studies conducted up to that date, showing that significant percentages of adolescents are already problem gamblers by the time they are in high school.[15]

Another unstated goal is to ensure that minimal injustice results from the legal system's inability to judge each person individually. Exactly how much injustice is acceptable? When setting a minimum age for legal gambling, the legislature is attempting to minimize the number of individuals who will be harmed by being judged, in effect, by a stereotype. The standard is never stated explicitly; where the line is drawn is always more of a political decision than a scientific one.

Blatant use of the minimum age to gamble as a public relations ploy abounds. For example, even though Indian casinos in California have the right to allow gambling by 18-year-olds, the Lytton Band of Pomo Indians announced that it would keep the minimum age at 21, if its controversial proposal to turn the San Pablo card club into an urban casino near San Francisco is approved.[16] In late 1999, the Cherokee Tribe and North Carolina renegotiated their 1994 compact, raising the minimum age for gambling at the tribe's casino from 18 to 21. The new compact will also allow the tribe to enlarge its video gaming casino and raise the limit on its jackpots. The Associated Press reported that "tribal leaders said they suggested that the gambling age be raised because they were worried that students from nearby Western Carolina University in Cullowhee could become reckless with their college money and lose it at the casino," despite the fact the university reported "they haven't had many problems with students losing large amounts of money at the casino."[17]

State legislatures and Indian tribes do not conduct studies to determine at what ages and with what percentages individuals become competent to gamble, drink, smoke, marry, have sex, make contracts, drive cars, or vote.

What percentage of 5-year-olds are competent, under any standard, to gamble for money? Personally, I would say zero. But not every state legislator agrees, since a few have voted to put no minimum age limit on bingo, at least when the children are accompanied by an adult.[18] Ask yourself what percentage of 10-year-olds are competent to gamble by your own standards. What about 15-year-olds, 18-year-olds, 21-year-olds, 25-year-olds?

The competence percentages should grow over time but will not necessarily peak at age 21. If 21 were the peak, the percentage of 22-year-olds who are competent to gamble would have to be equal to or less than the percentage of 21-year-olds. Is it true that there are as many or more 21-year-olds than 22-year-olds who are competent? Are more 21-year-olds competent than 30-year-olds? Probably not. Of course, whatever the number, whatever the age, it will never be 100 percent. By putting the minimum age at 21, lawmakers are declaring that some unknown percentage of 21-

year-olds are competent and that a smaller percentage of 20-year-olds are competent. More importantly, because the decision is political and not scientific, legislators have decided that the percentage of 20-year-olds who are incompetent and would be hurt if they were allowed to participate in this legal activity is unacceptable to society, and that the percentage of 21-year-olds who are incompetent and will be hurt is acceptable to society, even if a smaller percent of the population would be incompetent if the minimum age were raised to 22.

The law is attempting to do rough justice by drawing a bright line at a certain age. Yes, there will be exceptions. However, the "right" result—allowing truly competent individuals and barring the truly incompetent—will occur for the overwhelming majority, in numbers ranging into the tens of millions, or political pressure will force the lawmakers to raise the minimum age.

The Politics and History of Age Limits

Individual legislators, of course, have differing standards. It does not appear that they are trying to decide when a mere majority of a given age cohort is competent. For example, no legislator would put the limit at 18 if he or she believed that only 51 percent of 18-year-olds were capable of making decisions for themselves. Still, lawmakers are not drawing the line at its optimum point. Undoubtedly, more than one legislator would agree that a larger percentage of 21-year-olds are capable of understanding the consequences of gambling than 18-year-olds, but even more 22-year-olds are competent than 21-year-olds, and even more 30-year-olds than 22-year-olds.

Politics thus plays a decisive role. It appears that the highest minimum age in the American legal system for when a person is deemed competent is found in the United States Constitution: "No person . . . shall be eligible to the Office of President . . . who shall not have attained to the Age of thirty-five Years."[19] Ohio has a humorous age limit of 60 years for bingo players, but this is limited to games played at senior centers.

On the other end, there are a few state laws that put the minimum age at 12, 13, or 14 for various activities, including marriage.[20] This is not as unusual as it seems. After all, for more than two thousand years it has been at age 13 that boys become Bar Mitzvah, while girls become obligated to fulfill Jewish laws at age 12. A 13-year-old is counted in making up the ten adult men required for a minyan, the quorum for prayer.[21] Delaying full adulthood to age 21 would have been regarded as absurd in an era when life spans were much shorter than they are now. It is modern society that is unique in promoting long childhoods.[22]

Until the mid-1960s, American society conventionally viewed 21 as the most appropriate age for full adult status, as reflected in most state and federal laws. It was not an issue of great controversy. The Vietnam War brought the age of majority status into the spotlight. Eighteen-year-olds were sent off to kill or be killed, but they could not vote. The result was the 26th Amendment to the U.S. Constitution, which lowered the voting age to 18 for all elected positions, federal and state. After the 26th Amendment was ratified in 1971, it seemed logical to change all minimum age limits to 18. If a person is competent at 18 to make decisions as to who should be elected to every office in the land, that person must also be competent to serve on juries. If a person is competent to make those types of decisions that vitally affect the lives of others, that person must be able to make similar choices for himself or herself, such as deciding to enter into legally enforceable contracts. Because the law set 18 years as the legal floor for every other activity, there seemed little reason to keep the age at 21 for drinking and smoking.

The 26th Amendment did not require the states to make any of these changes—it only required that states not discriminate against anyone 18 or over solely on the basis of age when determining who has the right to vote. The states were also free to set even lower age limits for every activity, including voting; none, however, has put the voting age at 17 or 16. The age of adulthood thus was changed throughout the United States, from 21 to 18. Today, it would be extremely difficult, politically, for an American lawmaking body to establish an age limit much below 18 for any dangerous or morally suspect activity, despite lower age limits existing in other countries. The fact that residents of the United Kingdom may buy lottery tickets at age 16 with seemingly little or no harm carries no weight with a U.S. state legislature. Furthermore, experience with the lowered age of majority has led legislators to conclude that some activities are just too dangerous for too many individuals who are only 18 years old and too dangerous for society.

In other countries, the trend is exactly the opposite. In 1969 the Bahamas set the minimum age for gambling at 21, but the minimum is now 18.[23] Similarly, in France the minimum age was 21 until 1987, when it was lowered to 18.[24]

Danger and Age Limits

The law has always recognized that some activities are more dangerous than others. Selling alcohol to a minor might result in a fine. Selling cocaine or heroin to the same minor, however, may result in years in prison.[25] In the rush to make 18 the official start of adulthood, legislatures often forgot those differences. Lawmakers chose one standard, the age a person is considered qualified to vote, and applied it to all others, including gambling. While linking age limits is common, this practice only complicates fundamental questions of fairness. Legislatures have to decide not only what the age limit should be for the baseline activity—in this case, voting—but whether the secondary, linked activity—in this case, gambling—is more like the first than some other already existing age limit, for example, the drinking age.

New Jersey's restrictions on gambling illustrate the confusion that the linking of age limits often creates. Mostly as historic accidents, New Jersey has chosen a different standard for each type of gambling permitted by law. Parimutuel betting, legalized in 1940, is prohibited to "minors."[26] Bingo, made legal in 1954, has a strict limit of age 18.[27] State lottery tickets, first sold in 1970, may not be sold or bought by anyone under 18, but a person under 18 may receive one as a gift from an adult.[28] Casino gambling in Atlantic City is limited to "the age at which a person is authorized to purchase and consume alcoholic beverages," which is currently 21.[29] Prior to 1982, the minimum ages for drinking and for casino gambling were set independently at 18. The legislature raised the drinking age to 19 in 1982. In 1983 it raised both the drinking age and the casino gambling age to 21, and tied the age for casino gambling to the age for alcoholic beverages. Each standard, on its own, makes some sense. For example, alcoholic beverages are always present in Atlantic City casinos. However, putting all these standards together in one package shows the inconsistencies inherent in such a statutory scheme. Why is a 20-year-old competent to gamble in a bingo hall, at a state lottery terminal, and at a racetrack, but not in a casino?

In the last 25 years state legislatures have moved to raise the age limits for more "dangerous" activities back to 21. The argument about young men fighting and dying without the right to vote disappeared from the American consciousness with the passage of the 26th Amendment and the end of the Vietnam War and the draft. The dangers created by minors' drinking and driving were then pushed to the forefront when legislators heard about the tens of thousands of people killed by drunk drivers each year. The major political push came from well-organized advocacy groups such as Mothers Against Drunk Driving (MADD). Their success can be seen in the states' drinking ages. Although almost every state lowered the drinking age to 18 during the early 1970s, the 1980s saw a nationwide movement to return it to 21. In 1984, Congress required a drinking age of 21 for states to be eligible for federal highway funds.[30] By 1993 the National Transportation Safety Board reported that "no state allows the sale of alcohol to persons under the age of 21."[31]

Because the proliferation of legal gambling began prior to the war in Vietnam and has continued up to the present, virtually all gambling age limits range from 18 to 21, with the ages differing according to the perceived danger of the particular form of gambling involved. As table 7.1 shows, legislatures view bingo as the most innocuous form of gambling; sometimes it is not even regarded as gambling. The law does a disservice to both parents and children when it pretends that gambling games, such as bingo, are merely another form of entertainment. Marijuana and other intoxicants are sometimes described as "recreational drugs." However, even advocates of decriminalization do not ask for the bans against use by children to be lifted.

Many states statutorily define the low-limit games of chance that proliferate at county fairs and amusement halls as nongambling. Even devices identical to slot machines are tolerated, so long as the devices accept tokens rather than coins and the prizes are merchandise. Because these are viewed as amusement games, the law places no age limits on their play. In fact, the games are often specifically designed for children. Anyone who has ever been with a child who is playing games that would be illegal if they paid out in cash, however, knows how quickly money disappears into these devices, and how mesmerizing they are to children.

The age limits for true social gambling, taking place in a private home with no house operator making a profit, present less of a problem. The statutory prohibitions were lifted in most states in the 1940s, 1950s, and 1960s, even in Hawaii, which bans every other form of gambling. Governments do not try to regulate social gambling; they simply draw a bright line in the law for the activity as a whole: It is either legal or a crime. Usually, no special attention is given to the question of the minimum age for social gambling. But every state does have general statutes dealing with corrupting minors, often specifically mentioning gambling. Technically, then, true social gambling with a person under the age of majority, which is 18 virtually everywhere, is a misdemeanor—although these laws are rarely enforced.

A larger problem arises when commercial games are opened under the disguise of "social gambling." Pennsylvania and Arizona were inundated with casino gambling when those legislatures introduced poorly written legislation. The legislatures had defined social gambling as any game in which only participants, but not bar owners, can make a profit. So, shrewd operators opened blackjack tables and roulette wheels in bars. Sometimes, to be in compliance with the new laws, the operators had to make a show of offering the bank to other players. These commercialized social games, like the regularly scheduled charity "Las Vegas Nights," are clearly a form of public gambling, even if only played for low stakes. Because social, amusement arcade, carnival, and charity casino games themselves are not thought of as being of any particular danger, or even of any importance, age limits are rarely considered.

Age limits for lotteries and racetracks, which are still viewed by lawmakers as occasional, limited, and fairly benign wagers, are usually set at age 18. Casinos, on the other hand, raise warning flags: There are nearly as many minimum ages set at 21 as at 18, and the trend is definitely in favor of the higher age limit. Iowa raised the age limit from 18 to 21 on all its riverboat casinos in 1989, five years before raising the age for the state lottery, parimutuel wagers, and low-stakes social card games.[32] Then-governor Tommy Thompson insisted that tribes in Wisconsin agree to raise the age limit from 18 to 21 when their casino compacts began expiring in 1997. All but two of the state's fifteen tribes agreed.[33] Only one tribe, the Red Cliff Chippewas, resisted and threatened to file a federal lawsuit. "The tribe contends their casino, the state's smallest, needs as many gamblers as it can get."[34] Because the tribe did eventually agree to the higher minimum gambling age, it is possible that their stance was merely a negotiation posture. In Arizona, the state legislature passed a bill requiring that the state's tribes agree to raise their casino gambling age from 18 to 21 when the tribal-state compacts came up for renegotiation. The tribes responded by agreeing to the higher minimum age, but only if the state raised the age to 21 for its legal gambling, including the state lottery and parimutuel betting. The state legislature agreed.

Lawmakers correctly view slot machines as one of the most dangerous forms of gambling, so age limits generally are 21. Lawsuits have been fought over the state lotteries' rights to operate video lottery terminals (VLTs).[35] When a state lottery is allowed to operate these devices, the age limit is usually set at 21, acknowledging that VLTs are more similar to slot machines than they are to traditional lotteries. For example, Delaware's state lottery is open to 18-year-olds, but when the legislature approved VLTs, the age limit for these slot machines was set at 21.[36]

ENFORCEMENT OF AGE LIMITS

After setting a minimum age to gamble, drink, or engage in any other activity, the legislators and regulators have to decide how to enforce that law. By definition, the law is designed to protect individuals and children who are incapable of taking care of themselves. As stated by the U.S. Supreme Court in *Thompson v. Oklahoma* (1988):

> it does not make sense to put the burden on the minor to make the right decision. In fact, the law usually deals much more harshly with the adult purveyor than the child buyer. Thus, the United States Supreme Court has already endorsed the proposition that less culpability should attach to a crime committed by a juvenile than to a comparable crime committed by an adult. The basis for this conclusion is too obvious to require extended explanation. Inexperience, less education, and less knowledge make minors less able to evaluate the consequences of their conduct while at the same time making them much more apt to be motivated by mere emotion or peer pressure than adults. The reasons why juveniles are not trusted with the privileges and responsibilities of adults also explain why their irresponsible conduct is not as morally reprehensible as that of adults.[37]

To enforce a minimum gambling age, the state has only a limited number of weapons and targets. It can mandate, or at least fund, education programs directed at minors and at selected adults, parents, teachers, gaming operators, etc. But the law usually takes a less subtle approach to a problem: Laws are designed to apply direct punishments and rewards. So, a gaming operator who violates a rule against underage gambling may be criminally punished by a court or an administrative body. The punishment is usually the imposition of a fine or the suspension or loss of the license to operate. The child can also be criminally punished, by a fine or imprisonment, either in the adult or juvenile justice systems. Because gambling involves one party winning money at the expense of the other party, either the operator or minor or both can be deprived of their winnings.

The efficacy of any of these remedies can be questioned, and no scientific studies have been done on whether they work at all. Especially suspect are criminal punishments imposed on minors who gamble. By definition, these are children who are legally incapable of making decisions for themselves, specifically, in this case, the decision of whether to gamble or not. It is possible that adults may take potential punishments into account when contemplating crimes, but even adult offenders do not think they will be caught. A child who gambles illegally is normally a risk taker, although some succumb to peer pressure. Probably the most effective deterrent for children who at least understand what gambling is would be to make it clear that they cannot collect if they win. This will work with table games and other face-to-face encounters, but it is impractical for winnings that are automatically paid by slot machines.

Applying pressure to operators is a different situation. Gambling operators and other for-profit businesses, on the other hand, are rational decision makers. If the punishment is severe and the chances of being caught great enough, safeguards will be put into place. Of course, if the punishments are small or nonexistent, then the opposite is true.

From the time Nevada casinos were legalized in 1931 until the early 1990s, no licensed operator paid as much as a penny in fines for gambling with children. Worse, if a minor lost, the casino could keep the money. If the minor won, the casino could check the winner's identification and refuse to pay—again, keeping the money. And, if Nevada state government regulators caught the casino with underage players, the casino risked no fine, let alone the suspension or revocation of its license. Under conditions such as these, a casino operator would be economically irrational not to exploit children.

It appears that most casino operators in Nevada during this era did make efforts to keep children off their floors, perhaps because of a desire to obey the law, individual ethical standards, or an attempt to create an adult-only atmosphere. When Steve Winn first opened the Mirage, there were complaints from patrons because minors could not even sit at bars to drink nonalcoholic beverages or cross the casino floor to enter restaurants.

Caesars Palace, on the other hand, seemed to take a different approach. Lawsuits were filed against this Las Vegas casino after it refused to pay a $1 million jackpot to a 19-year-old, Kirk Erickson.[38] The Nevada regulators allowed the casino to decide for itself whether it would pay the minor; not surprisingly, Caesars decided to keep the money. The author was retained by the parents of the boy approximately one year after the boy's attorney began attempts to collect, and was involved in some of the legal proceedings. During formal discovery, Caesars was required to turn over all of its internal reports of minors gambling during a two-year period. Caesars turned over less than two dozen incident reports, and most of these involved prostitution or disruptive behavior. During that same two-year period, the dozen casinos in Atlantic City reported turning away or evicting almost 400,000 minors. Unlike the casinos in Nevada during this period, operators in Atlantic City were fined if minors were discovered in their gaming areas. To this day Caesars has not paid anything to Erickson, nor has it been fined.

Even if a casino is fined for allowing minors to gamble, the casino can make an economic decision to enforce the legal age restriction less than vigorously if the fine is small enough. The New Jersey Casino Control Commission used to impose fines of about $3,000, which Caesars' casino in Atlantic City apparently considered merely a cost of doing business. But the situation changed when the commission required Caesars Atlantic City to pay more than $100,000 to treatment programs after the casino allowed Debra Kim Cohen to gamble and drink, even though it had received written notice that she was a compulsive gambler and only 15 years old.

Regulators have enormous power in this area. A recent example from Canada shows how the system is supposed to work. In June 2001 Casino Niagara was fined $112,500 for allowing a 13-year-old boy to play at its slot machines. The casino's management company pleaded guilty in Niagara Falls provincial offenses court to violating the Gaming Control Act, which imposed a minimum age of 19. The justice of the peace imposed a $90,000 fine with a 25 percent "victim surcharge." In May, the company paid a fine of $106,250 for allowing a 14-year-old boy to play blackjack and slot machines. Although there were only two fines, the size of the penalties forced the casino to stiffen its already tight safeguards. "Ab Campion, a spokesman for the Alcohol and Gaming Commission, said the casino would have been fined more if it hadn't improved security."[39]

Government regulators also chose to make examples of the offending minors and their companions. In the May hearing, the 14-year-old was fined $70 and his 17-year-old brother was fined $130 for showing false identification at the door. In the June hearing, the 13-year-old was charged under the Liquor Licensing Act and barred from all casinos in Ontario until he turns 21. His 30-year-old uncle will not be allowed into any casino in Ontario for two years.[40]

Lawmakers have to decide the degree of culpability required before an operator can be fined and whether any defenses will be allowed. Culpability can range from strict liability, through a requirement that the operator be at least negligent or reckless or that the operator is only liable if it knows it is violating the law. Strict liability is imposed under the police power even where an operator has made every effort to prevent underage gambling. Strict vicarious liability imposes punishment on an operator when one of its employees gambles with a minor, even if both the operator and the employee have taken all possible precautions. Negligence requires a finding that the operator has not taken reasonable steps to prevent minors from gambling. A tougher standard to prove is reckless, where the operator not only has to act unreasonably but has to have recognized the risk that minors might gamble.

The easiest standard for the operator is one that states it is not liable unless it has actual knowledge that a minor is gambling.

If a jurisdiction imposes strict liability in the name of protecting society, the operator is still liable, even if the minor uses a false identification. The burden can be so strict that even the truly innocent adult can be criminally liable. This is often the standard applied to liquor licensees. As a legal encyclopedia puts it, "it is an offense to sell, furnish, give, serve, or dispense intoxicating liquor to a minor, regardless of the intent or knowledge of the seller, unless, by the terms of the statute, knowledge is made an essential element of the offense."[41] Some states, such as Nevada, do allow a bartender to argue that a minor looked like he or she was of drinking age.[42] The worry here is not only of tying up the courts but also of collusion and fraud. After all, neither bartenders nor their underage customers are likely to complain.

As with the enforcement of the legal age limit for alcohol, gambling jurisdictions differ,[43] even internally, on whether an operator is strictly liable for allowing a minor to gamble or whether it can raise defenses such as lack of knowledge. For example, New Jersey's Casino Control Act provides:

> Any licensee or employee of a casino who allows a person under the age at which a person is authorized to purchase and consume alcoholic beverages to remain in or wager in a casino or simulcasting facility is guilty of a disorderly persons offense; except that the establishment of all of the following facts by a licensee or employee allowing any such underage person to remain shall constitute a defense to any prosecution therefore:
>
> 1. That the underage person falsely represented in writing that he or she was at or over the age at which a person is authorized to purchase and consume alcoholic beverages;
> 2. That the appearance of the underage person was such that an ordinary prudent person would believe him or her to be at or over the age at which a person is authorized to purchase and consume alcoholic beverages; and
> 3. That the admission was made in good faith, relying upon such written representation and appearance, and in the reasonable belief that the underage person was actually at or over the age at which a person is authorized to purchase and consume alcoholic beverages.[44]

This language has been interpreted to mean that casino operators can claim they did not know that the minor was underage, but this defense is valid only in a criminal proceeding. However, the courts of New Jersey upheld a decision by an administrative agency that a casino had to pay a fine, even though it had no way of knowing the minors were using phony identifications. The court reasoned that administrative proceedings, including hearings held by the Casino Control Commission to decide whether to levy a fine, were not criminal proceedings and thus casino licensees in Atlantic City were allowed no excuses when a minor was found in the gaming area.[45] Similarly, Mississippi has two statutes. An adult casino operator who unwittingly allows a minor to bet commits a misdemeanor.[46] If the adult knows the minor is under 21, however, the crime becomes a felony, with punishment up to two years in prison.[47]

Questions of the responsibility and role of parents or other guardians arise whenever a minor violates the law or causes damage. But under the common law of the English-speaking world, imposing civil liability or criminal punishments on parents for the wrongdoing of their children is extremely rare, unless the parent knowingly participated in the minor's deed. An interesting case developed in Louisiana,[48] illustrating how strict liability works and answering the question whether parents have a duty to keep their children out of casinos.

Although the facts of the case are somewhat in dispute, the basic legal issues are clear. On January 11, 1994, Sandi and Toni Dixon, guardians of 4-year-old Candace, brought the girl with them into the Chelsea Street Pub in the Pecanland Mall in Ouachita Parish, Louisiana. The restaurant had a separate section for its video poker machines. Signs warned that minors were not allowed to enter this gaming room. Two state troopers were also in the pub, having lunch. One testified that he saw Toni take Candace into the video poker room. Toni put coins into the machine, then showed the child, sitting on her lap, how to touch the screen to play the game.

The Video Gaming Division of the Office of State Police issued a citation to the pub owner, Carver, Inc., and petitioned to revoke its gaming license. Pulling a license worth hundreds of thousands of dollars because one 4-year-old touched a video poker screen may seem a bit extreme. But the Louisiana Legislature's Video Draw Poker Devices Control Law stated, at the time:

A. No person licensed . . . or any agent or employee thereof, shall allow a person under the age of eighteen to play or operate a video draw poker device at a licensed establishment.

B. The Division shall revoke the license of any person . . . who is found by the Division to have committed or allowed a violation of Subsection A.[49]

The division had the power to issue fines when other violations occurred. But it could impose only one penalty, license revocation, when it came to minors gambling.

Having lost the battle, and its license, the pub's owner tried to salvage some of its business by finding someone else to take the blame. It probably realized that it could not sue its own employees for letting the child into the gaming area. It did try to sue the State Police Video Gaming Division, but that, naturally, went nowhere, because the State Police have immunity from suits such as this. Carver, Inc., hired a new lawyer, George E. Lucas Jr., who decided to sue Sandi and Toni Dixon, the pair responsible for bringing in the girl. Lucas knew that most individuals do not have enough money to make a lawsuit like this worthwhile. But he also knew that homeowners' insurance often covers claims having nothing to do with houses. So, he added Louisiana Farm Bureau Casualty Insurance Company as a defendant. The lawsuit sought damages for the loss of the gaming license "and the substantial revenue generated thereby."

Both the trial court and Court of Appeal took the claim seriously, though they both agreed the lawsuit had to be dismissed. It may seem farfetched that these adults might have to pay for all of the pub's lost profits, but they did cause the pub to lose its valuable video poker license. Fortunately for the Dixons, causation alone is not enough. The pub alleged that the Dixons were negligent in letting a child play video poker.

Legally, a claim of negligence can only be brought if the defendant owed a duty to the injured plaintiff. The Court of Appeal analyzed the "moral, social and economic factors, including the fairness of imposing liability." Looking at the history and purpose of the statute and regulations, it came to the inevitable conclusion: The duty to keep children out of the gaming area rests ultimately with the licensee. Parents may have a moral duty to keep their young ones away from gambling, but they owe no legal duty to gaming operators. In the end, it all came down to money: It is the operator who would make more money if it allowed minors to gamble, so it is the operator who bears the risk.

Federally recognized Indian tribes are usually allowed to set their own age limits, with a minimum of 18. Potential conflicts can arise between a tribe, which might want to maximize its profit, and its non-Indian management company, which often worries about its image. The situation can be exacerbated in a state that imposes a minimum age of 21 on all other forms of gambling. For example, Harrah's Entertainment, Inc., one of Nevada's largest gaming companies with casinos around the world, is building a $110 million casino for the Rincon Band of Mission Indians in San Diego County. Although the tribe's compact with the state allows it to offer casino gaming, slot machines, and banking card games to 18-year-olds, the Harrah's-managed casino will have a minimum gambling age of 21.[50] This is consistent with Harrah's international corporate policy, as one of the leading proponents and sponsors of programs to prevent underage gambling.

The most recent controversy surrounding minors and gambling involves slot machines with cartoon themes. At least one Nevada casino voluntarily pulled some devices, even before regulators began questioning whether some slot machines might be unduly attractive to children.

The issue became news in October 1999, when the Nevada Gaming Commission (NGC) made public its growing unhappiness over gaming devices with cartoon themes, labeled by anti-gaming activists as "slots for tots."[51] In December 1999 the NGC circulated proposed regulations. On January 27, 2000, the commission met and adopted amendments to NGC Regulation 14, prohibiting slot machines with themes derived from products marketed to children.

The controversy gained national attention because it involved interesting subjects: children, gambling, and well-known brand names. In addition, television news shows want action and color: One slot machine is worth a thousand talking heads. Even radio could get in on this story, capturing audience attention by mentioning familiar names, such as South Park. Gambling stories are inherently newsworthy, because the very topic gives rise to strong emotional reactions, especially from its opponents.

The idea of branded slots is only a few years old. The enormous success of the "Wheel of Fortune" slot machine led manufacturers to look for other well-known brand names. The issue over age-appropriate gaming devices was inevitable, since so many of the public's best-loved trademarks come from childhood: Monopoly, Betty Boop, the Three Stooges, and Elvis Presley have all been used on slot machines. The whole point of branded slots is to tap into commercially exploitable feelings of nostalgia. Such selling-by-association is certainly nothing new. Movies may make more money from toys and other related products than from the movie itself. But this marketing technique is new to legal gambling.

Regulators face myriad problems when an issue like kiddie-theme slots is raised in the press. It would be natural to think the first question to be resolved is whether the problem really exists. This is not as easy as it seems. Exactly how does one discover whether children are being unduly enticed into gambling by machines with themes? What is the standard? Would it be enough to show that merely one child in the country put money into a particular slot machine? How do we prove that the child would not have made the bet, but for the lure of the brand name? It is very difficult to show that something is true beyond any doubt, like the claim that certain games create underage gambling. But it is nearly impossible to prove the opposite, that something is not true. What evidence would you use to show a slot machine is not unduly attractive to children? Regulators are therefore forced to deal with probabilities, rather than with verifiable fact.

Should lawmakers be concerned if there is only a slim possibility the claim is true? For a politically explosive issue like this, regulators will, often unconsciously, follow the path with the least risk to themselves. If regulators ban certain slots that should not have been banned, the loss to casinos, manufacturers, and players is small and difficult to measure; but if they allow a device they should have outlawed, there is the possibility of scandal—such as nationally televised pictures of children playing slots—that will raise questions about the regulators' own competence.

Although there may be a bias in favor of imposing new standards in the name of protecting children, there is also a bias against making any new rule. The first question a good regulator, or lawyer representing an interested party, will ask is whether these regulators have the power to issue rules such as these. Major constitutional challenges make news. But the day-to-day world of making regulations involves questions of procedure and delegation.

What procedures should the regulators use to guarantee due process—that all interested parties have a fair and equal opportunity to have their say—not just now, but whenever new machines are invented? The easiest format is to allow presentations of evidence and arguments at hearings open to the public.

The delegation doctrine is also fundamental to our democratic system. Regulators are appointed, not elected. The only power they have is the specific, limited power given them by the legislature or governor. The NGC found a law passed by the Nevada Legislature to justify its action. It is already a crime for a licensed operator to allow anyone under 21 to gamble.[52] The NGC declared its new rules "will further the enforcement of [this law] by establishing standards for gaming device themes."

Is it necessary to have a prohibition on these games at all? Regulators of riverboat casinos, which can easily prevent any child from boarding, will probably find it unnecessary to issue new rules about gaming themes. In other cases self-regulation will work: There will not be any Pokemon slot machines, because these cartoons are clearly designed only for children.

How does a regulator define what games are prohibited? A rule that simply lists cartoon characters and other kiddie attractions will not work: There are too many, and they are constantly changing. The NGC had to take three pages to describe what themes it was making illegal. The regulators used a mix of general statements and specific examples. Banned are themes "based on a product that is currently and primarily intended or marketed for use by persons under 21." These include television programs, cartoons, books, board games, movies, and video games less than 21 years old with "G" and similar ratings. Exceptions are allowed where "the theme is attractive to adults because of its nostalgic appeal." The regulators also gave themselves the power to "restrict the time, place and manner in which an approved gaming device may be displayed." And they grandfathered in "any themes that were used in connection with gaming devices" already approved.

Underage Winners and Losers

Gambling is different in one major respect from all other activities for which there are age limits: Sometimes the minor wins money from the adult. Does allowing minors to collect their gambling winnings encourage underage gamblers? Does prohibiting the minor from collecting gambling money encourage gambling operators to exploit children? Since it takes two to make an illegal wager, should underage gamblers be allowed to sue to recover their losses?

South Carolina law imposed a minimum age of 21 on its tens of thousands of video gaming devices. (The machines were outlawed in 2000). The issue received national attention during hearings of the National Gambling Impact Study Commission. One of the commissioners was Dr. James Dobson, head of the conservative

Christian "Focus on the Family," who proclaimed himself radically opposed to gambling. Dobson used his newsletter to proclaim:

> In South Carolina, children stumble across video poker machines (called the "crack cocaine of gambling") in convenience stores, pizza parlors and bowling alleys. With more than 30,000 video poker devices scattered across that state, elementary school children can stop by on their way to and from school to pump money into these machines—legally! The law in South Carolina does not prevent children from playing, it only prohibits them from collecting any winnings![53]

Obviously no child would actually put money into a video poker machine if he or she knew they would not get paid. The legislative history shows it was merely sloppy drafting: In June 1993 the state legislature passed the Video Games Machine Act, which licensed machines, so long as they were approved by local voters and paid no more than $125 per day.[54] The act provided: "No person under twenty-one years of age may receive a payout as a result of the operation of the machines,"[55] indicating the legislature intended to exclude everyone under 21 from playing.

Still, the question remains whether the law should prohibit minors from collecting winnings when they have gambled illegally. To obtain any public policy impact, the rule would have to be widely publicized. In fact, even the general law of gambling debts is not well known.

Gambling debts are not normally collectible in court, even between adults and licensed operators.[56] Licensed operators are made to pay through administrative, not judicial, processes: When an adult wins, a casino pays or loses its license; but when a minor wins, the bet is technically illegal. Regulators typically do not order gambling operators to pay illegally obtained winnings. However, some underage gamblers have won money by making a bet against the state itself, through the state lottery. It has been considered at the very least to be unseemly for a state government to sell a lottery ticket to a minor and then not pay if the minor wins.[57] As shows by the cases involving Caesars Palace, licensed casinos have not always shown such qualms.

Conclusion

Children gamble in part because it is fun, but also because they feel they are omnipotent and cannot lose. "Risk-taking with body safety is common in the adolescent years, though sky diving, car racing, excessive use of drugs and alcoholic beverages, and other similar activities may not be directly perceived as a kind of flirting with death. In fact, in many ways, this is counterphobic behavior—a challenge to death wherein each survival of risk is a victory over death."[58] If anyone needs the law's protection, it is those individuals who society feels are not fully competent and who tend to think of themselves as immortal.

The situation is even worse for gambling, since it, by definition, requires money, and most minors do not have funds to spare. But just as the proliferation of gambling has been without plan, the setting of age limits has been without reason. The televised war in Vietnam brought the age of majority down from 21 to 18. The well-publicized carnage caused by drunk drivers demonstrated the danger of treating 18-year-olds as full adults and brought the drinking age back up to 21. But the minimum age for many other activities remains at 18.

Is gambling as dangerous as drinking? In some cases gambling is not treated seriously, and the games are open to any child who can acquire the money to enter. Most gambling games are closed, at least in law if not in practice, to anyone under the age of 18, since that is the generally accepted age of adulthood. But there is a growing recognition that some forms of gambling are more dangerous than others. Casino games in general and slot machines in particular are often limited to players who are at least 21. Establishing a minimum age of 21 is relatively easy when a game is being first introduced. As policymakers in states like New York, Wisconsin, and Minnesota are discovering, it takes much greater political effort to raise an established gambling age from 18 to 21.[59] There is no "right" minimum age for gambling, just as there is no such age for drinking. But the lawmakers of every state have decided that to protect people from themselves, a person must be at least 21 to buy alcoholic beverages.

The visible impact of minors' drinking can be seen on the nation's roads. The impact of minors' gambling is invisible. If we could see what happens to individuals and society when gambling is set at various ages, would we continue to allow 18- to 20-year-olds to spend their discretionary dollars, and perhaps their life savings, on gambling? Perhaps 18 is the best age for adulthood. But I, personally, would put gambling right next to alcohol on the danger scale and raise all minimum gambling ages to 21.

Gambling and the Law
MINIMUM LEGAL AGE TO PLACE A BET

This list of states, provinces, and countries illustrates the tremendous variations found in the way the law treats issues involving the minimum age to place a legal wager, particularly in the United States.

Until the mid-1960s, American society conventionally viewed 21 as the most appropriate age for full adult status, as reflected in most state and federal laws. The Vietnam War brought the age of majority status into the spotlight. Eighteen-year-olds were sent off to kill or be killed, but they could not vote. The result was the 26th Amendment to the United States Constitution, which lowered the voting age to 18 for all elected positions, federal and state. After the 26th Amendment was ratified in 1971, it seemed logical to change all minimum age limits to 18.

The explosion of legal gambling, which the author has labeled "The Third Wave," occurred during this period. So, most U.S. state lotteries, almost all of which were created between 1971 and the present, put the minimum age at 18.

Most legal minimum ages are still at 18, with one significant exception: In every state in America, the drinking age has been raised from 18 to 21. Because casino gaming is usually associated with the availability of alcoholic beverages, most states put the minimum age for gambling in a casino at 21. Casino-style games, including slot machines, are also the most dangerous forms of gambling.

In other countries, the trend is exactly the opposite. In France, the minimum age was 21, until 1987, when parliament lowered it to 18.[60] Similarly, in 1969 the government of the Bahamas set the minimum age for gambling at 21, but the minimum is now 18.[61] Twelve of the sixteen states (*Länder*) in Germany have also lowered the age for casino gambling from 21 to 18.[62] Portugal has different rules for tourists and locals: Casinos are open to foreigners over 18, but citizens of Portugal may not enter Portuguese casinos unless they are over 21, and some casinos restrict local play to residents over 25.[63]

Countries outside the United States seem to be more internally consistent: They usually have one minimum age that applies throughout that nation; the legal consequences when an underage minor is involved in otherwise legal gambling do not vary from one province to another; and the same minimum age applies to different forms of legal gambling. Lawmakers in other nations also have concluded that maturity is reached at a younger age. For example, in Canada, casinos are open to 18- and 19-year-olds, while in the United States, the minimum age is almost always 21. Similarly, in England anyone over 16 may buy a lottery ticket; in America, the minimum age for lotteries is never less than 18, and a dealer who knowingly sells a ticket to a 16-year-old faces loss of his license and a criminal fine.

Historically, outside the mainland United States, casinos were restricted to resorts and spas, far from major population centers, and play was limited to foreigners, especially foreign tourists. The idea was to import the money and export the social problems. Restrictions on locals gambling can still be found throughout the world. In Puerto Rico, for example, it is against the law for local licensed casinos to advertise to the local population; this restriction was upheld by the U.S. Supreme Court, even though no such similar restrictions were placed on any other form of the Commonwealth's extensive legal gambling.[64] Casinos limited to foreigners still have minimum legal age limits, to preserve the adult atmosphere and to protect foreign children and avoid bad press. For example, the law in Nepal expressly restricts casino gambling to foreign visitors 21 years of age and older.

ANTIGUA AND BARBUDA: Minors younger than 18 are not allowed where casino gaming is taking place; casino employees must be at least 21.[65]

ARGENTINA: The minimum gaming age is 18 years.[66]

ARUBA: No one under 18 years old is allowed in casinos.[67]

AUSTRIA: Section 25 of the Gaming Act restricts attendance of casinos to persons who have reached the age of majority (19 years).[68]

THE BAHAMAS: The Lotteries and Gaming Act of 1969 required players to be at least 21, but the minimum age has been lowered to 18.[69]

BELGIUM: Casinos are technically "private clubs," limited to "members" at least 21 years old.[70]

BULGARIA: Casinos opened in 1967, limited visitors from countries outside the Communist bloc. Since 1990, casinos have been open to anyone over 18 years old.[71]

BRITISH COLUMBIA, CANADA: Casinos, 19 years old; bingo, minimum age set by bingo licensee.[72] There is no minimum age to buy a provincial lottery ticket; however, the British Columbia lottery has set a policy of discouraging sales to minors, and there is movement to codify the minimum age into statutory law.

CHILE: The gaming laws require the exclusion of persons under 21 from casinos.[73]

DENMARK: Casino guest must be at least 18 years old.[74]

ECUADOR: Persons under age 21 cannot gamble in casinos.[75]

FINLAND: The minimum age limit is 18 for Finland's various casino-style games, including true casinos, slot machines in restaurants and bars, and low-stakes table games in arcades.[76]

FRANCE: Parliament lowered the minimum gaming age for casinos from 21 to 18 on May 5, 1987.[77]

GERMANY: The national government under Hitler passed laws in 1933 and 1938 prohibiting gaming by minors under 21. This age limit remained until the 1980s. Today, state (Länder) governments set their own age limits, and twelve of sixteen states in the united federal republic have lowered the minimum from 21 to 18.[78]

GREAT BRITAIN: Casinos are technically membership clubs and no one under 18 may join.[79] Regular slot machines are commonly called "fruit machines." By law, however, fruit machines and other gaming devices, which have a maximum prize of under £8, are defined as "Amusement With Prizes" (AWP) and not gambling. Children of any age may thus legally play AWPs for money, although operators in London voluntarily restricted use to players over 18. The U.K. national lottery, considered to be the largest in the world, has an unusual minimum age: Anyone over 16 may buy a ticket.

GREECE: An unusual age restriction: Individuals must be at least 23 years old to enter a casino.[80]

HUNGARY: Casinos cannot be visited by persons under 18 years of age.[81]

KENYA: Persons under 18 cannot enter casinos. Patrons between 18 and 21 years are allowed to use the slot machines, but a casino guest must be at least 21 to engage in live (table) gaming.[82]

MALTA: Players in the casinos must be at least 18 years old.[83]

MAURITIUS: The minimum casino admittance age is 18 years.[84]

NEPAL: Only foreign visitors 21 and over may gamble in the casinos.[85]

THE NETHERLANDS: Anyone 18 years and over may be permitted to enter casinos.[86]

NEW SOUTH WALES, AUSTRALIA: "A person under the age of 18 years cannot place a bet in any form of gaming and betting, except in sweepstakes and calcuttas where persons between the ages of 16 and 18 years can participate."[87] (Calcuttas are a primitive form of parimutuel wagering, where the bettors bid against each other at an auction for the right to "own" a horse in a race. The highest bidder for each horse "owns" that horse and pays the bid money into a pool. Whoever "owns" the winning horse gets the pool.)

NEW ZEALAND: No one under 20 years old may enter the gaming area of a casino.[88]

NOVA SCOTIA, CANADA: "No person under the age of 19 years may participate in casino gaming."[89] Bingo has a minimum age of 16.

ONTARIO, CANADA: An individual must be at least 19 to enter or gamble in a casino, and casinos are prohibited from advertising that "is specifically directed at encouraging individuals under nineteen (19) years of age to play games of chance in a casino." However, casino employees may be 18.[90]

PARAGUAY: The minimum age for gaming is 18.[91]

PHILIPPINES: The minimum gaming age is 21 years.[92]

POLAND: Any person under 18 is not allowed in casinos.[93]

PORTUGAL: A unique system: Casinos are open to foreigners over 18 years old, but Portuguese nationals are barred unless they are over 21, and in some casinos over 25.[94]

PUERTO RICO: Persons under 18 are not permitted in casino gaming areas.[95]

QUEBEC, CANADA: Most of Canada sets the age of majority at 19; Quebec sets it at 18. No one under 18 years old may enter a casino.[96] There had been no statutory minimum age to buy a lottery ticket, although Loto-Quebec had established its own restrictive policy. In 1999, Jeff Derevensky and Rina Gupta of McGill University's Youth Gambling Research and Treatment Clinic gathered information on the dangers of youth gambling and presented it to a leader of Quebec's national parliament. Russell Williams, vice-chairman of the Committee on Public Finance, authored legislation, which went into effect in February 2000, making it a crime to sell a lottery ticket or pay lottery winnings to anyone under 18.[97] Loto-Quebec is providing funding for more research and treatment programs and has removed lottery vending machines from most places accessible to minors under 18. The minimum age for betting on horse races or playing bingo for money is also 18.

QUEENSLAND, AUSTRALIA: "Persons under the age of 18 years are not permitted in the casino."[98]

SECHELLUS: No person under 18 is admitted in casino gaming areas.[99]

SLOVENIA: Casino guests must be at least 18, but some casinos prescribe an age requirement of 21 years.[100]

SOUTH AFRICA: The National Gaming Act regulates gaming by province. All persons under 18 years are prohibited from casino gambling.[101]

SPAIN: "Minors under 18 are not allowed to gamble or enter into casinos, bingo halls, or slot machines parlors."[102]

TASMANIA, AUSTRALIA: Minors, under 18, may not legally gamble. Casinos, on their own, have imposed a policy of not allowing minors in the main casino areas, though they may, if accompanied by an adult, be in other gaming areas.[103]

TURKEY: In live gaming areas, the minimum age to gamble is 18, but new regulations in 1992 provided that game patrons must now be at least 25 years old.[104]

UGANDA: The minimum casino entrance age is 18 years.[105]

VICTORIA, AUSTRALIA: Individuals under 18 years old may not enter casinos.[106]

State-by-State Analysis of Gambling Laws
ALABAMA
An adult who bets with a minor commits a misdemeanor. According to the Commentary section of the State Code, entitled "Relationship to Existing Law," the Criminal Code was amended 30 years ago to leave "such subjects as adults gambling with minors to other controls such as the juvenile laws."[107]

Lottery: Religious activists won an upset victory in November 1999, making Alabama only the third state in the twentieth century to fail to vote in a state lottery.

Parimutuel betting: Alabama Code §11-65-44 sets the minimum age as 19 throughout the state. Previously, the minimum age for betting at horse and greyhound racetracks was 18 in some cities and counties, 19 in others: Greene and Mobile—18, Birmingham and Macon—19.[108]

Table 7.1. *The United States: Minimum Legal Age to Place a Bet*

State	Lottery	Parimutuel Betting	Casinos & Slot Machines	Charity Bingo & Pull-tabs
Alabama		19		None/19
Alaska			18	19/21
Arizona	18→21	18→21	18→21	18→21
Arkansas		18		
California	18	18	18/21	18
Colorado	18	18	21	18
Connecticut	18	18	18/21	18
Delaware	18	18	21	16/18
District of Columbia	18		18	18
Florida	18	18	?	18
Georgia	18			None
Hawaii				
Idaho	18	18	?	None/18
Illinois	18	17	18/21	18
Indiana	18	18	21	18
Iowa	21	21	18/21	None/21
Kansas	18	18	?	
Kentucky	18	18		None/18
Louisiana	18→21	18	18→21	18
Maine	18	18	16	16
Maryland	18	18?	21	16/18
Massachusetts	18	18		18
Michigan	18→21	18→21	18/21	18
Minnesota	18	18	18	18
Mississippi			21	None/18
Missouri	18	18	21	16
Montana	18	18	18	None/18
Nebraska	18/19	18		18
Nevada	21?	21	21	21?
New Hampshire	18	21		18
New Jersey	18	18	21	18
New Mexico	18	18/21	21	None?
New York	18	18	18	None
North Carolina	18		18→21	None?
North Dakota		18/21	21	None/18/21
Ohio	18	18		18/60

Table 7.1. *continued*

State	Lottery	Parimutuel Betting	Casinos & Slot Machines	Charity Bingo & Pull-tabs
Oklahoma		18	?	?
Oregon	18	18	18/21	?
Pennsylvania	18	18	18	None/18
Puerto Rico	18	18	18	18
Rhode Island	18	18	18	18
South Carolina	18		21	?
South Dakota	18	18	21	?
Tennessee				
Texas	18	21		None/18
Utah				
Vermont	18	18		18
Virgin Islands	18		21	?
Virginia	18	18		None/18
Washington	18	18	18	None/18
West Virginia	18	18	18/21	18
Wisconsin	18	18	18→21	None/18
Wyoming		18		18?

A question mark ("?") without a number means that particular form of gambling is legal in that state, but the minimum age requirements, if any, are not known. A number with a question mark means there is a state limit, but it is unclear whether it applies. This is usually the case with Indian gaming, where tribes are often free to set their own limits. An arrow (18→21) indicates the minimum age is in the process of being raised from 18 to 21.

Bingo: Nonprofit organizations can run bingo games for charitable or educational purposes. The state has separate statutes for various counties and at least one city. All set at 19 the minimum playing age as well as the minimum age for conducting or assisting bingo. There is no age limit, however, for children accompanied by their parents: Alabama Constitutional Amendment No. 506, "Bingo Games In Etowah County," states, "No person under the age of 19 shall be permitted to play any game or games of bingo, unless accompanied by a parent or guardian."

ALASKA
Alaska has been considering allowing casino gambling on cruise ships between ports in the state, during the course of an international voyage.

Slot machines: Alaska Statutes sets the minimum age at 18 and forbids the location of coin-operated amusement and gaming devices within a radius of 100 yards of a school building.[109]

Bingo and pull-tabs: State statutes set the minimum age for bingo at 19, but the age for pull-tabs was raised from 19 to 21 on June 26, 1993.[110]

ARIZONA

Arizona is the only state attempting to implement a comprehensive plan for dealing with the minimum age for gambling. On March 14, 2000, House Bill 2131 became law, raising the gambling age from 18 to 21, effective June 1, 2003, for all wagers, including commercial, charitable, tribal, and even social gambling.

Lottery: It is a misdemeanor to sell a lottery ticket to anyone under 18 (raised to 21 on June 1, 2003).[111] Before the passage of H.B. 2131, it was clearly not unlawful to give a lottery ticket to a minor as a gift. Section 5-520 contains a prohibition: "no prize may be paid on any winning ticket or share to any person who is under eighteen years of age [raised to 21 on June 1, 2003]." But section 5-515 contained the following sentence: "This section does not prohibit the purchase of a ticket or share for the purpose of making a gift by a person eighteen years of age or older to a person less than eighteen years of age." H.B. 2131 repealed that sentence, making it a crime to give a lottery ticket to someone under 18 [21 on June 1, 2003], and the minor cannot collect if the ticket wins.

Parimutuel betting: "A permittee shall not knowingly permit a minor [changed to "a person who is under twenty-one years of age" on June 1, 2003] to be a patron of the parimutuel system of wagering."[112] The addition of the word *knowingly* in the statute allows an operator to raise the defense that it did not know a child was underage.

Casinos: Charities can operate casino nights. The state has entered into compacts with many tribes, authorizing the operation of slot machines and nonbanked, revolving deal, card games, primarily poker. The minimum age for Indian casinos in Arizona is 18 as of the date this is written. However, the compacts begin expiring in 2003, so the governor is negotiating to raise the gambling age to 21 in all tribal casinos, pursuant to the mandate of the state legislature that all "tribal-state gaming compacts shall prohibit persons under twenty-one years of age from wagering on gaming activities." H.B. 2131, effective March 14, 2000.

Bingo: At present, there is no statutory minimum age; however, the Bingo Section of the Department of Revenue has issued this rule: "No bingo card shall be sold or bingo prize awarded to any person under 18 years of age."[113] Like every other form of gambling, the minimum age will be 21 beginning on June 1, 2003, pursuant to H.B. 2131.

ARKANSAS

Parimutuel betting: Arkansas's horse-racing statute expressly prohibits "any person under eighteen (18) years of age to be a patron of the parimutuel or certificate system of wagering conducted or supervised by it." But it is unclear if such persons are prohibited from attending horse races. The dog-racing counterpart prohibits employing a minor or allowing "any minor to be a patron at the racetrack." This language seems closer to prohibiting the presence of children.[114]

CALIFORNIA

Lottery: California has a complete set of restrictions, typical of the state lotteries that have addressed youth gambling:

(a) No tickets or shares in Lottery Games shall be sold to persons under the age of 18 years. Any person who knowingly sells a ticket or share in a Lottery Game to a person under the age of 18 years is guilty of a misdemeanor. Any person under the age of 18 years who buys a ticket or share in a Lottery is guilty of a misdemeanor. In the case of Lottery tickets or shares sold by Lottery Game Retailers or their employees, these persons shall establish safeguards to assure that the sales are not made to persons under the age of 18 years. In the case of the dispensing of tickets or shares by vending machines or other devices, the Commission shall establish safeguards to help assure that the vending machines or devices are not operated by persons under the age of 18 years. All tickets or shares in Lottery Games shall include, and any devices which dispense tickets or shares in Lottery Games shall have posted in a conspicuous place thereupon, a notice which declares that state law prohibits the selling of a Lottery ticket or share to, and the payment of any prize to, a person under the age of 18 years.[115]

"No prize shall be paid to any person under the age of 18 years."[116]

Parimutuel betting: The age limit of 18 for horse races was established by regulations of the Racing Control Board, not by the legislature in a statute.

Casinos: On March 7, 2000, voters approved Proposition 1A, amending the state constitution, to allow federally recognized Indian tribes to have a monopoly on full casinos (banking card games, like blackjack, and all forms of slot machines). Governor Gray Davis signed a model compact with a majority of the state's tribes (there are more than 100), which allows 18-year-olds to gamble in Indian casinos. Patrons have to be over 21 only if alcohol is served at the gaming tables and slot machines. A tribe is free to place higher age limits on its patrons and employees and can change the age limits whenever it wishes. For example, the Cabazon Band of Mission Indians announced in September 1995 that it was raising the minimum age from 18 to 21 for its casino near Palm Springs and that it was firing all casino workers under 21; Harrah's will run the Rincon casino with a minimum gambling age of 21.

California law also allows cities and counties the local option of licensing gaming clubs, limited to nonbanked table games, without slot machines. There are more than 300 gaming clubs operating throughout the state; most age limits appear to be 21. The only state limit is a restriction requiring operators and owners to be at least 18.[117]

Bingo: Minors (currently, those under age 18) are not allowed to participate in bingo games.[118]

COLORADO

Lottery: It is illegal to sell a lottery ticket to anyone under 18 or for any person under 18 to purchase a ticket; however, a lottery ticket may be given as a gift to a person under 18.[119] The difference can be significant: The minor who receives a winning lottery ticket as a gift is allowed to collect the prize on a winning ticket; but a minor who uses an adult to buy a ticket is not so allowed. "Any prize won by a person under 18 years of age who purchased a winning ticket . . . shall be forfeited. If a person otherwise entitled to a prize or a winning ticket is under 18 years of age, the director may direct payment of the prize by delivery to an adult member of the minor's family or a guardian of the minor of a check or draft payable to the order of such minor."[120]

Parimutuel betting: It is a petty offense (maximum fine $100) to sell a parimutuel ticket to any person under the age of 18, or for anyone under 18 to purchase, redeem, or attempt to purchase or redeem a parimutuel ticket.[121]

Casinos: Privately owned casinos are limited to three little mountain towns, with $5 maximum bets. Colorado has also signed compacts with two Indian tribes. The age limit for casinos is 21. Minors may pass through the casino but not place wagers, collect or share winnings, or even "sit on a chair or be present" at a gaming table or slot machine. Both the minor and the casino would be committing misdemeanors. If the child is under 18, the adult can also be prosecuted for contributing to the delinquency of a minor. (Employees may be under 21).[122]

Bingo and pull-tabs: State law prohibits anyone under 18 from playing bingo or buying pull-tabs. However, it also allows anyone 14 or older to "assist in the conduct of bingo or pull-tabs."[123]

CONNECTICUT

Connecticut's off-track betting operation, owned and operated by a private, publicly traded company, Autotote, is taking telephone wagers from around the nation. Tribally owned Foxwoods is probably the largest casino in the world.

Lottery: Games are limited to players over 18. "No person shall sell a lottery ticket to a minor and no minor shall purchase a lottery ticket. Any person who violates the provisions of this subsection shall be guilty of a class A misdemeanor. A minor may receive a lottery ticket as a gift."[124] As with many gambling enabling statutes, Connecticut requires the regulators of its state lottery to "adopt regulations which shall include limitations on advertising and marketing content to assure public information as to the odds of winning the lottery and the prohibition of sales of tickets to minors."[125]

Parimutuel betting: Connecticut allows betting on jai alai, as well as on racing. "Any person who knowingly permits any minor to wager in any gambling activity and any minor who places a wager shall be guilty of a class A misdemeanor."[126] Connecticut not only bars anyone under 18 from betting but also prohibits "the presence of any minor under the age of 18 being present in any room, office, building or establishment when off-track betting takes place."[127] The fine is only $25, but it is imposed both on the operator and on minors over the age of 16.

Casinos: Charity "Las Vegas Nights" are limited to patrons over 18.[128] The state prohibits anyone under 16 from even being present in a room where gambling is taking place. Connecticut has signed compacts with two Indian tribes, and more are seeking federal recognition. The Mashantucket Pequot Tribe apparently felt that 18 was too young and put its age limit at 21. The tribe's casino, Foxwoods, is the most profitable casino in the world, with blackjack, craps, and 5,000 slot machines.

Bingo and pull-tabs: In its "Sealed tickets" statute, Connecticut prohibits the sale to any person less than 18 years of age.[129]

DELAWARE

Lottery: Delaware has one of the strongest set of restrictions of any state lottery: It locked its 18-year-old age limit into the state constitution.[130] However, state statutes, while prohibiting the sale of lottery tickets to persons under 18, expressly allow the purchase of a ticket for the purpose of making a gift by a person 18 years of age or older to a person less than that age.[131]

Parimutuel betting and slot machines: While racetracks appear to put the limit at age 18, the state recently amended its laws to allow video lottery machines in racetracks, with an age limit of 21.

Bingo: A person has to be 18 or over to participate in any charitable gambling, the prize for which is money; yet anyone over 16 may participate in bingo and other charitable games. This must limit 16-year-olds and 17-year-olds to games where prizes are merchandise.[132]

Casinos and slots: The state lottery has video lottery terminals at racetracks; age limit is 21.[133]

DISTRICT OF COLUMBIA

Lottery: Limited to players over 18, but the lottery will pay minors who win prizes.[134]

Casinos and bingo: Charities in the District of Columbia can run "Monte Carlo Night" parties as well as bingo. The minimum age to participate as well to be present is 18, but minors under 18 may be present if accompanied by an adult.[135]

FLORIDA

Social, small-stakes gambling is legal, but minors under the age of 18 may not participate in one of these "penny-ante games," defined as "a game or series of games of poker, pinochle, bridge, rummy, canasta, hearts, dominoes, or mah-jongg in which the winnings of any player in a single round, hand, or game do not exceed $10 in value."[136]

Lottery: Minors under age 18 are prohibited from purchasing lottery tickets.[137]

Parimutuel betting: Florida has dog and horse tracks as well as jai alai. State statutes prohibit wagering by a person under the age of 18 but permit admittance if the minor is accompanied by a parent or legal guardian.[138]

Bingo: State law prevents anyone under 18 from being allowed to play any bingo game or be involved in the conduct of a bingo game in any way.[139]

Casinos and slots: Age limits at tribal casinos and cruises to nowhere (casino games opened in international waters, three miles out in the Atlantic, 12 miles in the Gulf of Mexico), are up to the operators. Florida allows commercial card clubs, limited to poker and $10 pots.

GEORGIA

The state legislature has enacted a unique law creating civil liability along with the more common criminal punishments. "A parent shall have a right of action against any person who shall play and bet at any game of chance with his minor child for money or any other thing of value without the parent's permission."[140]

Lottery: State statutes not only prohibit anyone under 18 from buying lottery tickets but also require conspicuous labels prohibiting minors from using any electronic or mechanical devices related to the lottery.[141]

Bingo: State law allows a person under 18 to play bingo if accompanied by an adult.[142]

HAWAII

Hawaii, Tennessee, and Utah are the only states that have not legalized some form of commercial gambling. Hawaii, like many other states, does allow "social gambling"—the minimum age is 18.[143] The legislature has been considering allowing casino gambling, either in selected areas or on cruise ships.

IDAHO

The Coeur d'Alene Tribe made the most serious attempt of any federally recognized tribe to set up nationwide Internet and telephone lotteries. The tribe's "U.S. Lottery" was discontinued after adverse court decisions.

Lottery: No one may knowingly sale tickets to anyone under 18.[144]

Parimutuel betting: Minors are prohibited from using the parimutuel system.[145] The Idaho State Racing Commission promulgated rules expounding the restriction: "No person under eighteen (18) years of age shall be allowed to wager [or] be granted a license to work in the parimutuel department."[146]

Bingo: A person under 18 may not play bingo for a cash prize or games where the prize exceeds $25 worth of merchandise.[147] Therefore, children under 18 may play bingo for money for smaller prizes.

Casinos and slots: Age limits at tribal casinos not known. The governor signed a compact with Coeur d'Alenes allowing a federal judge to decide whether gaming devices will be allowed. Other tribes are protesting, because they did not agree to this test case.

ILLINOIS

Illinois is unique in defining a minor (at least under the horse-racing statutes) as "any individual under the age of 17 years."[148] The state also makes a distinction between casino gambling run by charities—age 18—and casino gambling run for profit on riverboats—age 21.

Lottery: In 1997 the state legislature made it more difficult for anyone under 18 to play the state lottery. It repealed a statute that had allowed adults to purchase tickets as gifts for children and added a provision forbidding payment of prizes to minors under 18.[149] Selling a ticket to anyone under the age of 18 is a Class B misdemeanor for the first offense, a Class 4 felony for subsequent violations. A minor who buys a lottery ticket is guilty of a petty offense.[150]

Parimutuel betting: Minors (defined as those under 17) are forbidden from being admitted as a patron during a racing program unless accompanied by a parent or guardian. Exceptions are made for employees, licensees, owners, trainers, jockeys, or drivers.[151]

Casinos and slots: The state has both riverboat and charity casinos. The state Riverboat Gambling Act prohibits any person under 21 from being on an area of a riverboat where gambling is being conducted. A riverboat casino operator was fined and a guard fired for allowing a mother with her infant in a baby carriage onboard. It is a Class B misdemeanor to permit "a person under 21 years to make a wager."[152] An exception is made for employees, but workers must be at least 21 to perform any function involved in gambling.[153] Illinois charitable casinos do a multimillion dollar business. The Charitable Games Act allows the following games: roulette, blackjack, poker, pull-tabs, craps, bang, beat the dealer, big six, gin rummy, five card stud poker, chuck-a-luck, keno, hold-em poker, and merchandise wheel with a $10 maximum bet. Unlike for-profit riverboat casinos, charity casinos are open to anyone over 18.[154]

Bingo and pull-tabs: Minimum age for bingo and pull-tabs is 18.[155] In fact, persons under 18 may not be in the area where bingo is being played unless accompanied by a parent or guardian.

INDIANA

Lottery: Minimum age is 18. Prizes may not be paid to anyone under 18, unless the ticket was received as a gift.[156]

Parimutuel betting: Minimum age to bet seems to be always 18, although the law sets slightly different ages for being present at tracks and off-track betting outlets.

(a) A person less than eighteen (18) years of age may not wager at a horse racing meeting.

(b) A person less than seventeen (17) years of age may not enter the grandstand, clubhouse, or similar areas of a racetrack at which wagering is permitted unless accompanied by a person who is at least twenty-one (21) years of age.

(c) A person less than eighteen (18) years of age may not enter a satellite facility.[157]

Minimum age to work at a racetrack is 16, but the racing commission can license even younger children who are working for their parent or legal guardian.[158]

Casinos: Indiana has riverboat gambling; the current controversy is whether the boats actually have to sail. Anyone under 21 is prohibited from being in the area of a riverboat where gambling is being conducted; the minimum age for an occupational license, however, is 18.[159]

Bingo and pull-tabs: Players must be 18 or older.[160]

IOWA

Iowa may have more forms of legal gambling than any state, other than Nevada—everything from bingo and amusement games to casinos and sports pools. Most are low-stakes and limited to players over 21, but not all.

Lottery: Iowa raised the minimum age from 18 to 21 in 1994. Present law prohibits the sale of a lottery ticket to persons under the age of 21 but allows adults to buy tickets for them as gifts. A licensee or a licensee's employee who knowingly offers to sell a lottery ticket to anyone under 21 is guilty of a simple misdemeanor and the seller's license is suspended. As for the minor: "A prize won by a person who has not reached the age of twenty-one but who purchases a winning ticket or share[s] in violation of this subsection shall be forfeited."[161]

Parimutuel betting: Iowa raised the minimum age here as well, from 18 to 21, in 1994.[162] Permitting a person under 21 to make a parimutuel wager is a simple misdemeanor.[163]

Casinos: In 1989 riverboat casinos became the first area where Iowa raised the minimum gambling age from 18 to 21.[164] It is against the law for a licensee to knowingly allow a minor to participate in gambling, or even to be in the area of the excursion boat where gambling is being conducted, unless the minor is an employee 18 years or older. Indian tribes assert they are not bound by this state law, and one lowered the minimum age to 18 in 1999. The minimum age for low-stakes social gambling, including card games and sports pools, was raised from 18 to 21 in 1994.[165]

Bingo: Iowa makes some specific exemptions to its general prohibition on gambling by anyone under 21. Charitable gambling, bingo and raffles, has no age limits. There are no age limits at all for games of chance at carnivals, as long as only non-cash merchandise worth no more than $50 is given as prizes.[166] The Iowa state lottery, but not charities, can sell pull-tabs; legal age is 21.

KANSAS

The general law of Kansas defines a minor as "a person under 21 years of age," yet the age of 18 is used for both legal and illegal gambling statutes.[167]

Lottery: Kansas goes further than most states in preventing children from participating in its state lottery. Besides the usual restriction that licensees must be at least 18, the state legislature has prohibited the Kansas lottery from "recruiting for employment or as a volunteer any person under 18 years of age for the purpose of appearing, being heard or being quoted in any advertising or promotion of any lottery in any electronic or print media."[168]

Parimutuel betting: The legislature put the same ban on the Kansas racing commission, prohibiting the use of children in commercials. It is a crime to sell a parimutuel ticket to a person knowing such person to be under 18 years of age. Those under 18 are also specifically barred from buying tickets.[169]

Casinos: The state is in the middle of a protracted fight over Indian casinos. Although the state legislature created a detailed system for negotiating compacts, including a joint committee on gaming compacts, no mention was made of minimum age limits.[170] The legislature's main concern was precluding slot machines and electronic gaming devices. "'Tribal gaming' does not include games on video lottery machines . . . that the Kansas lottery is prohibited from conducting."[171]

Bingo and pull-tabs: A person must be at least 18 to participate in the management, operation, or conduct of any game of bingo.[172] This would appear to put the minimum age at 18 to work in a bingo hall, but not to be a patron there.

KENTUCKY

Lottery: It is a violation to knowingly sell a lottery ticket to someone under 18 and a misdemeanor to do it a second time. This would not prohibit adults from buying lottery tickets for minors.[173]

Parimutuel betting: Although Kentucky statutes dealing with age limits do not expressly mention parimutuel wagers, the state places an age restriction of 18 on all similar activities (except drinking); therefore, it is safe to assume that it is illegal for anyone under 18 to bet at racetracks.[174] The state's racing commissioners also report the minimum age as being 18.[175]

Bingo: Kentucky has a Charitable Gaming Act, which controls bingo games. The age limit is 18. A charitable organization may permit persons under 18 to play bingo if they are accompanied by a parent or legal guardian and if only non-cash prizes are awarded.[176]

LOUISIANA

Louisiana is the latest state to raise the minimum age for some forms of gambling. Casino gaming was always limited to players over 21, but in 1998 the state legislature raised the age from 18 to 21 for the state lottery and privately owned video poker machines. A 19-year-old and the owner of a bar with video poker machines filed a lawsuit in January 1999. The trial judge agreed with their claim that the new law violated the state constitution. But the State Supreme Court reversed, in a split decision, on January 29, 2001.[177] The court looked to its precedent, where it upheld raising the drinking age from 18 to 21, to protect both the young adults and society.

Louisiana law permits virtually every form of gambling except sports betting: The state has riverboat casinos, two Indian casinos, America's first urban land-based casino in New Orleans, video poker machines in many parishes, with large numbers at truck stops and racetracks, electronic bingo machines, parimutuel betting, and a state lottery.

Lottery: Knowingly selling a ticket to anyone under 21 leads to a fine of $100 to $500: The minor is fined up to $100. Adults, however, may purchase lottery tickets for children as gifts.[178]

Parimutuel betting: The state legislature told the State Racing Commission to adopt rules and regulations to exclude and eject "persons who are not of age."[179] Anyone 6 or above may, with the permission of the racing association, be allowed to attend any race meeting if accompanied by a parent, grandparent, or legal guardian, but minors are never allowed to engage in wagering. Applicants for licensure as a jockey, etc., must be at least 16.[180] Because "minor" is defined as anyone under 18, that is the minimum age for parimutuel betting.

Casinos and slot machines: Although 21 is the age limit for the widespread video poker machines, riverboat casinos, and Louisiana's one very large land-based casino in New Orleans, there is an extraordinary difference in the details. In all cases, underage patrons cannot collect; winnings are paid to the state. Punishments vary; the video poker law adds an additional penalty if the patron is under 15; but the most dramatic differences are in the ability of an operator to raise a "good faith" ("I thought he was over 21") defense.

The riverboat law reads as follows:

Any licensee, employee, or other person who intentionally violates or permits the violation of any of the provisions of this Section may be imprisoned for not more than six months or fined not more than five hundred dollars, or both.

In any prosecution or other proceeding for the violation of any of the provisions of this Section, *it shall be no defense that the licensee, employee, or other person believed the person to be twenty-one years old or over.*[181]

The law for the land-based casino:

Any casino operator, licensee, or other person who intentionally violates or permits the violation of any of the provisions of this Section and any person under twenty-one years of age who violates any of the provisions of this Section may be punished by imprisonment of up to six months or a fine of up to one thousand dollars, or both.

In any prosecution or other proceeding for the violation of any of the provisions of this Section, *it shall be a defense that the casino operator, employee, dealer, or other person had a reasonable factual basis to believe and in good faith believed the person was twenty-one years old or over.*[182]

The video poker law:

(1) Violations shall be penalized by the division as follows:

    (a) For allowing a person under the age of twenty-one to play or operate a video draw poker device at a licensed establishment, unless the licensee, his employee, or agent reasonably believed that the person was twenty-one years old or older:

        (i) For a first or second violation, a fine of one thousand dollars shall be imposed.

        (ii) For a third or subsequent violation, license revocation shall be imposed.

    (b) For allowing a person under the age of twenty-one to play or operate a video draw poker device at a licensed establishment when the licensee, his employee, or agent is shown to have known or reasonably believed he was allowing a person under the age of twenty-one years old to play or operate a video draw poker device, or for allowing a person under the age fifteen years old to play or operate a video draw poker device at a licensed establishment regardless of what the licensee, his employee or agent knew or reasonably believed about the age of that person:

(i) For a first or second violation, license revocation may be imposed.

(ii) For a first or second violation, a fine of one thousand dollars shall be imposed if the license is not revoked.

(iii) For a third or subsequent violation, license revocation shall be imposed.[183]

Bingo and pull-tabs: Louisiana has an 18 year age limit on bingo, but not on charity raffles: "No licensee shall allow any person under eighteen years of age to assist in the holding, operation, or conduct of any game of chance. Charitable raffles . . . shall be exempted from requirements of this Subsection."[184]

MAINE

Lottery: Maine has one of the weakest regulatory schemes for its state lottery. Tickets may not be sold to anyone under 18 but may be bought by adults as gifts for minors. The minor who buys illegally is subject to no punishment. In addition, there is no penalty for unintentionally selling to a minor. The only punishment comes into affect when a lottery agent knowingly sells to a minor, but this is punished as a civil, not criminal, violation, with a maximum fine of only $200.[185]

Parimutuel betting: Off-track betting facilities are open to children under age 16 when accompanied by a parent, legal guardian, or custodian. A person under the age of 18 not only is prohibited from participating in a parimutuel pool, but may not come within 15 feet of a betting window or other place for accepting wagers.[186]

Bingo and pull-tabs: No one under the age of 16 years is permitted to take part in the conduct of, nor participate in, the game of beano or bingo, nor shall such minor be admitted to the playing area unless accompanied by parent, guardian, or other responsible person.[187]

Casinos: Charities can operate low-limit "games of chance" (limited dice and card games, including blackjack) and up to five "electronic video machine," but not roulette or slot machines.[188] Players and employees are limited to persons 16 and over, though minors under 16 years may sell chances "in relation to charitable, religious or recognized youth associations."[189]

MARYLAND

Maryland's gambling laws contain a number of unique quirks.

Lottery: The state follows most other states with state lotteries, in requiring that no ticket be sold to a person the seller knows is under 18, while allowing adults to buy tickets for minors as gifts. Lottery sellers must be at least 21.[190]

Parimutuel betting: Age unknown.

Casinos and slot machines: Charities used to be able to operate slot machines in some counties. Now they are limited to a few dice games and card games, including blackjack. The age limit is 21.[191]

Bingo: Maryland's bingo laws are unique in two aspects: The state legislature has passed specific statutes for individual counties rather than a single law covering the entire state, and some statutes explicitly allow 16-year-olds to play bingo.[192]

MASSACHUSETTS

Lottery: Massachusetts follows many other states in requiring that no ticket be sold to a person the seller knows is under 18, while allowing adults to buy tickets for minors as gifts. Lottery sellers must be at least 21.[193]

Parimutuel betting: Massachusetts does not allow minors (those under age 18) to attend its horse and dog races, let alone make bets. But the penalties are small. First-time violators are fined no more than $100. Even permitting a minor to make wagers subjects a track to a fine of no more than $100.[194]

Bingo and pull-tabs: In Massachusetts, bingo is called beano. State law requires "that no person under 18 years of age shall be permitted in that portion of any building or premises of the licensee during such time as such game is being played."[195]

Casinos and slots: Political negotiations are continuing to allow an Indian tribe to own a casino, with a minimum gambling age of 21, and for horse and dog tracks to get slots; so far, however, the necessary legislation has not been passed.

MICHIGAN

Lottery: It is a misdemeanor to knowingly sell, or offer to sell, a lottery ticket to anyone under 18. Although tickets may not be sold to minors, an adult may buy one as a gift for someone under 18. State law also requires a person to be at least 18 in order to acquire a lottery resale license.[196] House Bill 5819 was introduced in Michigan on May 23, 2000, to raise the minimum age to 21 to purchase or receive a lottery ticket, but it was defeated.

Parimutuel betting: "A holder of a race meeting license shall not knowingly permit a person less than 18 years of age to be a patron of the parimutuel wagering conducted or supervised by the holder."[197] A bill to raise the age here was defeated as well.

Casinos and slot machines: Commercial casinos in Detroit have a minimum gaming age of 21.[198] The minimum age for playing at high-stakes tribal Indian casinos throughout the state appears to be mostly 18, but not necessarily because 18-year-olds to 21-year-olds are a large market. For example, in July 2000, the Grand Traverse Band of Ottawa and Chippewa Indians lowered the gambling age from 21 to 18, as it was allowed to do under its tribal-state compact, at the request of parents who wanted their young adult children to be able to attend concerts in the casino. The biggest problem now is keeping those under 21 from drinking. Charities are also allowed to run "millionaire parties," i.e., casino nights, with a minimum age of 18.[199]

Bingo and pull-tabs: Charity game tickets may not be sold to anyone under 18. However, like lottery tickets, adults may buy charity pull-tabs for minors as gifts.[200]

MINNESOTA

Minnesota tried to become the second state (along with Arizona) to have a comprehensive plan for dealing with the minimum age for gambling, but the effort failed. Unlike Arizona's tribal-state compacts, which have sunset provisions, Minnesota's compacts have no expiration dates, giving the state no power to make additional demands on its tribes. The compacts allow tribes to put the minimum age at 18. The state legislature passed a statute mandating that Indian casinos be restricted to adults 21 and over and added that the minimum age for all other forms of legal gambling in the state be raised from 18 to 21 if more than half the tribes agreed to that limit. The tribes, however, took this as a trick to get them to reopen compact negotiations on other matters and rejected the move to 21.

Lottery: Minnesota is unusual in setting up a complex system for dealing with underage lottery players, including prohibiting minors from receiving prizes. This would seem to preclude gifts by adults.[201] Prohibited acts include: "Purchase by minors. A person under the age of 18 years may not buy nor redeem for a prize a ticket in the State Lottery," and "Sale to minors. A lottery retailer may not sell and a lottery retailer or other person may not furnish or redeem for a prize a ticket in the State Lottery to any person under the age of 18 years."

It is an affirmative defense, meaning the burden is on the lottery retailer to prove by a preponderance of the evidence that he reasonably and in good faith relied upon the minor's identification for proof of age.

Parimutuel betting: The age restrictions are identical to those for the state lottery.[202]

Casinos: The number of legal, full-scale, tribal-run casinos in this state exceeds the number of casinos in Atlantic City. Minimum age limits are currently at 18.

Bingo and pull-tabs: No one under 18 may buy a pull-tab, tipboard ticket, paddle-wheel ticket, or raffle ticket, or a chance to participate in a bingo game other than a bingo game exempt or excluded from licensing; violation is a misdemeanor. A licensed organization or employee who allows a person under age 18 to participate in lawful gambling is guilty of a misdemeanor.[203]

MISSISSIPPI

Mississippi is one of the toughest states on both casinos and minors who violate the law: The underage gambler may not keep the winnings, and the casino may not use the excuse that it thought the minor was over 21.

Casinos: Although it has no state lottery, Mississippi is third nationwide (after Nevada and New Jersey) in the number of commercial casinos in the state, with true riverboat casinos as well as dockside casinos that are technically over water but cannot move.

(1) A person under the age of twenty-one (21) years shall not:
   (a) Play, be allowed to play, place wagers, or collect winnings, whether personally or through an agent, from any gaming authorized under this chapter.
   (b) Be employed as a gaming employee.
(2) Any licensee, employee, dealer or other person who violates or permits the violation of any of the provisions of this section, and any person under twenty-one (21) years of age who violates any of the provisions of this section shall, upon conviction, be punished by a fine of not more than One Thousand Dollars ($1,000.00) or imprisoned in the county jail not more than six (6) months, or by both such fine and imprisonment.
(3) In any prosecution or other proceeding for the violation of any of the provisions of this section, it is no excuse for the licensee, employee, dealer or other person to plead that he believed the person to be twenty-one (21) years old or over.[204]

Bingo and pull-tabs: Charity bingo operators are given the unusual (for bingo) option of excluding anyone under 18, merely by posting a written notice. The state charitable bingo law provides that no licensee shall allow anyone under 18 to play a bingo game unless accompanied by his or her parent or legal guardian.[205] The state allows video pull-tab and video bingo machines.

MISSOURI

Lottery: Tickets may not be sold to anyone under 18; however, gifts by adults to minors are permitted. No one under 21 may be licensed as a lottery game retailer.[206]

Parimutuel betting: A strangely worded statute prohibits minors from "*knowingly* making or attempting to make any wager on any horse race." I do not know how a minor could *accidentally* make a bet. The other possible interpretation, that the minor know that the wager was illegal, is almost never accepted by courts, due to the maxim that ignorance of the law is no excuse. Racetrack licensees may not knowingly permit anyone under 18, unless accompanied by a parent or guardian, into any parimutuel wagering area. Licensees are also prohibited from knowingly permitting any individual under 18 to place a wager.[207]

Casinos: Missouri has two unusual provisions for its large boat-in-a-moat casino industry: The state legislature explicitly gave cities the option to completely exclude minors from riverboat casinos, and according to a statute passed decades before the legalization of casinos, a minor's parent or conservator may sue to recover any money lost while gambling. The other provisions of the Excursion Gambling Boat Statute are typical:

A person under twenty-one years of age shall not make a wager on an excursion gambling boat and shall not be allowed in the area of the excursion boat where gambling is being conducted; provided that employees of the licensed operator of the excursion gambling boat who have attained eighteen years of age shall be permitted in the area in which gambling is being conducted when performing employment-related duties, except that no one under twenty-one years of age may be employed as a dealer or accept a wager on an excursion gambling boat.

It is a misdemeanor to permit a person under 21 to make a wager.[208]

Bingo and pull-tabs: Children as young as 16 may play or participate in the conducting of bingo, and even those under 16 may attend when accompanied by a parent or guardian, although a child under 16 is not supposed to be allowed to play for money: "No person under the age of sixteen years may play or participate in the conducting of bingo. Any person under the age of sixteen years may be within the area where bingo is being played only when accompanied by his parent or guardian."[209]

MONTANA

The state has legalized video poker and keno machines. Montana also has card clubs and allows calcutta betting on sports events. Indian tribes are operating casinos. The state legislature has imposed a blanket minimum age of 18 for anyone involved with gambling, with one exception: Children may buy and sell raffle tickets.[210]

Lottery: Tickets may not be sold to or by anyone under 18.[211]

Parimutuel betting: Licensees may not permit a minor to use the parimutuel system.[212]

Casinos and slots: An operator shall not purposely or knowingly allow a person under 18 years of age to participate in a gambling activity. This allows an operator to claim it did not know the patron was underage. A little stranger is the statute, similar to Missouri's, prohibiting persons under 18 from "purposely or knowingly" participating in a gambling activity. It is difficult to imagine how a minor could prove he or she placed a wager not on purpose or unknowingly. The Video Gaming Machine Control Law requires operators to place gaming devices in such a way as to prevent access by persons under 18.[213] It appears that the state's many tribal casinos also put 18 as the minimum-age limit.

Charity bingo and pull-tabs: Montana allows commercial bingo, making it tough for a charity game to survive. The statewide minimum of 18 applies, although the only specific statute is one defining a "bingo caller" as a person 18 years of age or older.[214] Pull-tabs are prohibited by statute. The state explicitly allows minors to sell and buy raffle tickets for charitable purposes.[215] The state legislature apparently faced problems with Little Leaguers selling raffle tickets to their friends, so it just made the whole thing legal. Raffles are also the only form of gambling in the state where players can pay with a check rather than with cash.[216]

NEBRASKA

Nebraska has a state lottery but also allows cities and counties to run their own lotteries. It is also unique in allowing privately owned for-profit keno games. The lottery law contains a strange age distinction.

Lottery: Villages, cities, and counties can operate lotteries in Nebraska; the minimum age to buy a ticket is 19. However, for charity lotteries and raffles, the minimum age to buy a ticket is 18.[217] It is a minor misdemeanor for anyone under 19 to knowingly buy a governmental lottery ticket and a more serious misdemeanor to knowingly sell one. The addition of the word *knowingly* for the buyer makes little sense, unless it is to cover the rare case of someone over 18, but under 19, who buys a local government lottery ticket thinking he or she was buying a charity lottery ticket. While most states either allow adults to buy lottery tickets as gifts or are silent on the issue, Nebraska explicitly prohibits anyone from buying a ticket for the benefit of a person under 19.

Parimutuel betting: Knowingly aiding or abetting any minor to make a parimutuel wager is a misdemeanor.[218]

Bingo and pull-tabs: The minimum age is 18; lotteries are allowed to sell "pickle cards," i.e., pull-tabs. The state also allows keno, which has become a big business.

NEVADA

Lottery: The Nevada Constitution still prohibits all lotteries except charity raffles. The enabling statute does not mention a minimum age for buying a raffle ticket. The age limit of 21 for casinos probably applies.

Casinos and parimutuel betting: Almost complete prohibition for everyone under 21. Notice the statutory prohibition on "loitering" or allowing minors to pass through casinos. Also note that the minor is not allowed to collect; nothing is said to prevent casinos from keeping children's money, win or lose.

A person under the age of 21 years shall not:

Play, be allowed to play, place wagers at, or collect winnings from, whether personally or through an agent, any gambling game, slot machine, race book, sports pool or parimutuel operator.

Loiter, or be permitted to loiter, in or about any room or premises wherein any licensed game, race book, sports pool or parimutuel wagering is operated or conducted.

Be employed as a gaming employee except in a counting room. Any licensee, employee, dealer or other person who violates or permits the violation of any of the provisions of this section and any person, under 21 years of age, who violates any of the provisions of this section is guilty of a misdemeanor.[219]

There are many additional specific restrictions, all set at age 21. A minor may be judicially emancipated and legally become an adult for all purposes, with a few significant exceptions, including remaining barred from gaming or being employed at gaming.[220] Nevada has extensive, detailed laws against anything to do with phoney age identification cards that might allow a minor to gamble.[221] In a section entitled "Employing or Exhibiting Minor in Injurious, Immoral or Dangerous Business," Nevada has made it a misdemeanor to employ a minor in a casino (except as an entertainer). The penalty applies both to the gaming operator and the child's parent, if the parent "in any way procures or consents to the employment of the minor."[222]

NEW HAMPSHIRE

Lottery: Tickets may not be sold to anyone under 18; however, gifts by adults are allowed.[223]

Parimutuel betting: Limited to bettors 21 and over.[224]

Bingo and pull-tabs: State law prohibits anyone under 18 to be admitted to or play bingo games.[225]

NEW JERSEY

Mostly as the result of historic accidents, New Jersey has chosen a different standard for each type of gambling permitted by law: for parimutuel wagering the excluded class is "minors"; for bingo it is anyone under age 18, with no exceptions; for the state lottery it is also anyone under 18 years of age, but tickets may be received by children as gifts; for casinos the barrier is set at the drinking age (21).

Lottery: Tickets may not be sold to anyone under 18; gifts by adults are allowed. Minimum age for lottery agents is 21.[226]

Parimutuel betting: Strict restrictions on minors, legally defined as those under the age of 18.[227]

Casinos: Atlantic City casinos must exclude anyone not old enough to drink alcoholic beverages, currently 21.[228] The state allows a casino to claim it did not know the minor was under 21 only when the casino is charged with a criminal offense. Strict liability is imposed for all noncriminal procedures, including administrative fines.

Bingo: Prohibited to anyone under 18.[229]

NEW MEXICO

The governor signed compacts to allow tribes in the state to operate full casinos, but the State Supreme Court ruled them all unconstitutional. The legislature solved the problem, in part, by approving a model compact, with a high tax rate. The legislation was probably illegal, because federal law prohibits the states from demanding tax revenue from tribes during compact negotiations. The governor, legislature, and tribes are working out the problem by negotiating a lower rate. As part of the legislative deal-making, the legislature and governor agreed to let racetracks and fraternal organizations also have slot machines. The state is unique in allowing betting on bicycle races.

Lottery: Tickets may not be sold to anyone under 18, but gifts by adults are permitted. Lottery retailers must be at least 18.[230]

Parimutuel betting: Betting on bicycle races is limited to age 21. The horseracing statutes do not give a minimum age for placing a bet.

Casinos: Although the original compacts, signed in February 1995, contained no minimum gaming age, tribes that have agree to the current compacts prohibit patrons under 21. Political pressure from non-Indians forced the legislature to include a requirement that tribal gaming agencies, which regulate tribal casinos, enact regulations "prohibiting participation in any Class III gaming by any person under the age of twenty-one (21)."[231]

Bingo and pull-tabs: The state legislature has decreed that minors may not participate in "recreational bingo" offered by senior citizen groups, although there is no similar statutory age limit on any other form of bingo.[232]

NEW YORK

New York has signed compacts with some of its federally recognized Indian tribes, resulting in casinos that are supposed to be without slot machines. The Oneida's Turning Stone was probably the most profitable table-games-only casino in the world; it now has installed hundreds of gaming devices. New York was one of the first states to allow its off-track betting operators to take telephone wagers from gamblers in other states, in possible violation of federal law.

Lottery: Tickets may not be sold to anyone under 18; however, adults may buy tickets for the purpose of making a gift to a minor. The New York courts upheld the right of underage recipients to collect if their ticket wins.[233]

Parimutuel betting: Tracks and off-track betting operations are required to prevent betting by anyone who is actually and apparently under 18 years of age. This gives racing operators the excuse that the minor looked to be over 18.[234]

Casinos: New York has signed compacts with at least two tribes and allows charities to run casino nights.

Bingo and pull-tabs: Anyone under 18 may neither participate in nor conduct a bingo game.[235]

NORTH CAROLINA

Lottery: "No ticket or share shall be given as a gift or otherwise to any person under the age of eighteen years. Any person who knowingly gives a lottery ticket or share to any person under the age of eighteen years is guilty of a Class 3 misdemeanor."[236]

Casinos: In late 1999, the state and Cherokee Tribe renegotiated their 1994 compact. Beginning January 1, 2001, the minimum age was raised from 18 to 21.[237]

Bingo: State bingo statutes do not specify a minimum age for players.

NORTH DAKOTA

Lottery: North Dakota is one of only three states in which voters refused, in the twentieth century, to authorize a state lottery, in part because the state already has so many other forms of gambling, including charity casinos.

Parimutuel betting: North Dakota allows calcutta pools on all sporting events other than high school contests. The age limit 18.[238] North Dakota is apparently the only state to put a higher limit on parimutuel wagering at off-track betting establishments than at the track. According to the state's racing commissioners, the minimum age for wagers made at an off-track betting outlet is 21; the same wager may be made at the track by anyone over 18.[239]

Casinos: No one under 21 may directly or indirectly play games of pull-tabs, punchboards, twenty-one, Calcuttas, sports pools, paddlewheels, or poker.[240] Medium-limit blackjack ($25) for charity is common throughout the state. Tribes operate full-scale casinos under compacts.

Bingo and pull-tabs: Although pull-tabs are restricted to players over 21, bingo is limited to players over 18 unless accompanied by an adult.[241]

OHIO

Lottery: It is illegal to sell a lottery ticket to a person under 18 years of age.[242]

Parimutuel betting: "Any minor sixteen years of age or under shall not be admitted to the grandstand, club house or similar areas of any racetrack at which wagering is permitted unless accompanied by an adult member of his/her family. This provision shall not apply to state, county or independent fairs. No person under the age of eighteen years shall be permitted to wager at any horseracing meeting."[243]

Bingo: A wonderful minimum age provision: Participants and operators in bingo games conducted by multipurpose senior centers must be at least 60 years old. Employees at other bingo halls must be over 18.[244]

OKLAHOMA

Lottery: A proposal for a state lottery failed at the polls in 1996. Governor David Walters' pro-lottery forces were far outspent by horseracing interests.

Parimutuel betting: Licensed organizations may not knowingly permit any minor to be a patron of the parimutuel system of wagering.[245]

Casinos: The state is in a heated dispute with tribes over their right to operate casinos. Age limits unknown.

Bingo: The state has no mention of bingo in its statutes.

OREGON

The state lottery operates video poker machines and takes bets on sports events. Tribes in the state are operating full-scale casinos pursuant to compacts.

Lottery: The state has a strict scheme for dealing with minors. Lottery tickets may not be sold to anyone under 18. If someone under 18 wins the lottery, the winner may not be paid the prize. This effectively eliminates adults buying tickets as gifts.[246]

Parimutuel betting: If a track has a reasonable doubt that a patron is over 18, it must require the bettor to make a written statement of age and furnish evidence of his true age and identity. The state statutes prevent any person under 18 from entering a racecourse except when accompanied by a person 18 years of age or older who is the person's parent, guardian, or spouse, or when in the performance of a duty incident to employment. It further prohibits any person under 12 from entering after 6 P.M. This statute also prohibits any person under 18 from loitering in the wagering area of a racecourse.[247]

Casinos and slots: Video poker is limited to players age 21 and older because the devices are limited to establishments with liquor licenses. However, the first tribal-state casino compact put the minimum age at 18 for video poker machines;

all later compacts put the age at 21. Compacts were also signed putting the minimum age at 18 for bingo and blackjack. So the present situation allows one Indian casino to let 18-year-olds gamble at all of its games; the other tribal casinos must restrict machine gambling to age 21, but may allow 18-year-olds to play every other game. The compacts for blackjack are only temporary, and the state will insist that the age for that game be raised to 21. The state operates cardrooms for poker and blackjack under a vaguely worded statute allowing "contests of chance." It is a crime called "endangering the welfare of a minor" to knowingly induce, cause, or permit a person under 18 to participate in gambling.[248]

PENNSYLVANIA

Lottery: Lottery tickets may not be sold to anyone under 18, but adults may give tickets as gifts to minors. Lottery agents must be over 21.[249]

Parimutuel betting: The same restriction (age 18 minimum) is phrased in two different ways. For on-track wagers: "No licensed corporation shall permit any person who is actually and apparently under 18 years of age to wager at a race meeting conducted by it."[250] For off-track betting: "No licensed corporation may permit a person who is 17 years of age or younger to wager at a nonprimary location."[251] Similarly worded restrictions are placed on the rights of 17- and 18-year-olds to be attend the locations.

Casinos: Charities can operate casinos under Pennsylvania's Small Games of Chance Act; minimum age is 18.[252]

Bingo: Persons under 18 are not permitted to play bingo unless accompanied by an adult.[253]

PUERTO RICO

Puerto Rico allows cockfight betting and various other forms of gambling, including full-scale casinos. Until recently, casino slot machines were owned and operated by the commonwealth government itself.

Lottery: Sales are prohibited to persons under 18.[254]

Parimutuel betting: No age limit is mentioned in the statute. The state's racing commissioners report the minimum age as being 18.[255]

Casinos: "No gambling room shall be permitted to advertise or otherwise offer their facilities to the public of Puerto Rico; or to admit persons under 18 years of age."[256] Despite the obvious infringement on free speech, this statute was declared constitutional by the U.S. Supreme Court.[257]

Bingo: Puerto Rico Law equates bingo with other gambling games such as roulette, dice, and cards; thus, bingo would be governed under the 18-year-old age limit.[258]

RHODE ISLAND

The Rhode Island State Lottery operates video lottery terminals at racetracks.

Lottery: "No person under the age of eighteen (18) years may play a video lottery game authorized by this chapter, nor shall any licensed video lottery retailer knowingly permit a minor to play a video lottery machine or knowingly pay a minor with respect to a video lottery credit slip. Violation of this section shall be punishable by a fine of five hundred dollars ($500)." Lottery tickets may not be sold to anyone under 18, but adults may give tickets as gifts to minors. Lottery agents must be over 21.[259]

Parimutuel betting: Licensees may not admit anyone under 18 into a building where parimutuel betting or simulcasting is taking place, nor may they knowingly permit any minor to be a patron of the parimutuel system or any other betting system.[260]

Bingo and pull-tabs: Anyone under 18 is not permitted to play.[261]

SOUTH CAROLINA

Lottery: The state's approved a state lottery in November 2000. In September 2001 the legislature passed the South Carolina Education Lottery Act, which makes it a misdemeanor to knowingly sell a ticket to a person under 18. Minors may receive tickets as gifts, but minors who buy tickets are committing misdemeanors and will not be paid if they win.[262]

Casinos and slot machines: Until the middle of the year 2000, South Carolina had tens of thousands of video gaming machines, with a minimum age limit of 21. The state legalized and then prohibited video gaming machines, with offbeat restrictions, through a series of strange statutes and court decisions. In July 1999 the state legislature passed Act No. 125, which eliminated video gaming devices effective July 1, 2000, unless voters approved letting the machines remain. But on October 14, 1999, the State Supreme Court ruled the legislature could not delegate any power to the state's voters, so there would be no election; yet the court upheld the repeal of the Video Games Machine Act.[263] So the last word from the State Supreme Court was that the legislature's attempt to have voters decide whether they wanted to have slot machines violated the state constitution, because South Carolina does not allow initiatives or referenda. But the court found that part of the same bill passed by the legislature was valid—the part that said the gaming devices could not continue without a vote of the people (which, of course, the court would not allow). So slot machines are out, for the moment.

Bingo: It appears that all South Carolina bingo legislation was repealed.

SOUTH DAKOTA

South Dakota was one of the first states to allow its state lottery to set up video lottery terminals, slot machines without coin drops. The state also allows full-scale, low-stake casinos in Deadwood and on Indian land.

> *Lottery:* Lottery tickets may not be sold to anyone under 18. However, to play a video lottery terminal, a gambler must be at least 21.[264]
>
> *Parimutuel betting:* Racetrack licensees may not permit any individual under the age of 18 to place a bet on a race.[265]
>
> *Casinos and slots:* Participation in casino games is limited to gamblers 21 and older.[266] Video lottery terminals are limited to patrons over 21.
>
> *Bingo:* Charity bingo is legal, but there is no mention in the statutes of an age limit.[267]

TENNESSEE

> *Parimutuel betting:* Tennessee legalized parimutuel wagering on horse races. However, the statute had a sunset provision, causing it to expire by its own terms when no track was opened in time. If betting on races would have remained legal, the age limit would have been 18: "No person under eighteen (18) years of age shall be permitted to wager at any race meeting."[268]

TEXAS

The state legislature has enacted some unique laws to deal with underage gambling.

> *Lottery:*
> (a) A sales agent or an employee of a sales agent commits an offense if the person intentionally or knowingly sells or offers to sell a ticket to an individual that the person knows is younger than 18 years of age.
> (b) A person 18 years of age or older may purchase a ticket to give as a gift to another person, including an individual younger than 18 years of age.
> (c) An offense under this section is a Class C misdemeanor.[269]
>
> *Parimutuel betting:* The Texas Legislature wanted to impose different minimum ages for betting, as opposed to merely attending races. Rather than merely stating what those ages are, the legislature, probably for political reasons, decided to create two sets of underage individuals: Children and Minors. The Texas Racing Act defines "Child" as "a person younger than 16 years of age," while "Minor means a person younger than 21 years of age."[270] The legislature then required the state's racing commission to adopt rules "to prohibit wagering by a minor and to prohibit a child from entering the viewing section of a racetrack unless accompanied by the child's parent or guardian."[271] The law cleanly lays out how the

penalty increases for a willful violation of the law as opposed to a merely negligent act, and which party has the burden of proof:

(a) A person commits an offense if the person with criminal negligence permits, facilitates, or allows:

  (1) wagering by a minor at a racetrack facility; or

  (2) entry by a child to the viewing section of a racetrack facility.

(b) An offense under Subsection (a) of this section is a Class B misdemeanor.

(c) A person commits an offense if the person is a minor and intentionally or knowingly engages in wagering at a racetrack.

(d) An offense under Subsection (c) of this section is a Class C misdemeanor.

(e) It is an affirmative defense to prosecution of an offense under Subsection (a)(2) that a child was accompanied by and was in the physical presence of a parent, guardian, or spouse who was 21 years of age or older.

(f) It is an affirmative defense to prosecution of an offense under Subsection (a) of this section that the minor falsely represented the minor's age by displaying to the person an apparently valid Texas driver's license or identification card issued by the Department of Public Safety that contains a physical description consistent with the minor's appearance.[272]

Bingo and pull-tabs: Individuals under 18 may not play bingo, unless accompanied "by his parent or guardian." However, bingo operators are free to set their own limits, to keep out younger players or parents with very young children: "a licensee may prohibit all persons under the age of 18 or an age younger than 18 years of age as determined by the licensee from entering the licensed premises by posting a written notice to that effect at the place where the game is conducted."[273]

UTAH

Utah, Tennessee, and Hawaii are the only states prohibiting all forms of commercial gambling. Utah does not even allow social bets.

VERMONT

Lottery: Vermont limits its state lottery to persons who have "attained the age of majority," currently 18. However, minors may receive lottery tickets as gifts.[274]

Parimutuel betting: Minors may not participate in any parimutuel pools or even be admitted to any parimutuel enclosure.[275]

Bingo and pull-tabs: Like the lottery, these games are limited to age of majority. The statute focuses on workers rather than patrons: "A nonprofit organization shall not permit any person who has not attained the age of majority to organize or execute a game of chance. A person who has not reached the age of majority may work performing services at a game of chance which are not related to the execution of the game of chance."[276]

VIRGIN ISLANDS

The Virgin Islands is the most recent American jurisdiction to legalize casinos. Land-based casinos are limited to St. Croix. Casinos onboard cruise ships may remain open, but only in St. Thomas and only if the ship remains docked beyond 6 P.M.

Lottery: Tickets may not be sold to anyone under the age of 18. This does not prohibit gifts by adults to minors.[277]

Casino: The Virgin Islands Casino and Resort Control Act of 1995 states: "No person under the age of twenty-one (21) years of age shall be admitted into, nor be permitted to place any wager in any casino hotel licensed to operate in St. Croix."[278]

VIRGINIA

Lottery: "No ticket shall be sold to or redeemed from any person under the age of 18 years. Any licensee who knowingly sells or offers to sell or redeem a lottery ticket or shares to or from any person under the age of 18 years is guilty of a Class 1 misdemeanor."[279]

Parimutuel betting: No one under 18 may wager on or conduct any wagering on the outcome of a horse race.[280]

Bingo and pull-tabs: Instant bingo is limited to players 18 and over.[281] The Charitable Gaming Commission has promulgated detailed regulations covering minors and bingo:

Individuals under 18 years of age may play bingo provided such persons are accompanied by a parent or legal guardian. It shall be the responsibility of the organization to ensure that such individuals are eligible to play. An organization's house rules may limit the play of bingo by minors.

Individuals under the age of 18 may sell raffle tickets for a qualified organization raising funds for activities in which they are active participants.

No individual under the age of 11 may participate in the management, operation or conduct of bingo games. Individuals 11 through 17 years of age may participate in the conduct or operation of a bingo game provided the organization permitted for charitable gaming obtains and keeps on file written parental consent from the parent or legal guardian and verifies the date of birth of such youth. An organization's house rules may limit the involvement of minors in the operation or conduct of bingo games.[282]

WASHINGTON

The state has entered into compacts allowing tribes to open casinos with gaming terminals that technically are video lottery terminals and electronic bingo games but play like slot machines. One tribe's true slot machines were grandfathered in through the federal Indian Gaming Regulatory Act.

Lottery: Tickets may not be sold to anyone under 18. This does not prohibit gifts by adults to minors.[283]

Casinos and slots: Besides Indian casinos, Washington allows cardrooms, where poker and casino-style banked blackjack are played; minors are prohibited from wagering.[284]

Bingo and pull-tabs: The state Gaming Commission has issued rules prohibiting anyone under 18 from making wagers, with exceptions for bingo: e.g., children can play bingo "at agricultural fairs or school carnivals" and "in licensed bingo games if accompanied by an adult member of his/her immediate family or guardian."[285] The regulation has the unique provision: "All bingo advertisements that are directed to minors shall include language indicating that all minors must be accompanied by a member of their immediate family or guardian, who is at least 18 years old."[286]

WEST VIRGINIA

The West Virginia State Lottery operates video lottery terminals in racetracks.

Lottery: Tickets may not be sold to anyone under the age of 18. This does not prohibit gifts by adults to minors.[287]

Parimutuel betting: The state's racing commissioners report the minimum age as being 18.[288]

Bingo: Bingo operators are prohibited from allowing anyone under 18 to participate in the playing of any bingo game with knowledge or reason to believe that the individual is under the age of 18. However, an individual 18 may attend the playing of a bingo game when accompanied by and under the supervision of an adult relative or a legal guardian.[289]

Casinos and slots: Video lottery terminals are at racetracks. The West Virginia Racetrack Video Lottery Act[290] says that the State Lottery Act[291] shall apply unless the two conflict. Because the Racetrack Video Lottery Act is silent as to an age limit for wagering, the minimum age of 18 set by the Lottery Act applies. The Limited Gaming Facility Act, which would allow registered guests of a hotel to gamble at casinos in "historic resort hotels" if county voters approve, sets the minimum age at 21.[292] The only local election held so far, in Greenbrier County, failed in November 2000. An attempt will undoubtedly be made again to put a casino is this historic structure—a bomb shelter designed for top federal officials in case of nuclear war.

WISCONSIN

Lottery: Wisconsin has a comprehensive statutory scheme for handling minors and lottery tickets. Like many other states, the minimum age is 18, although minors may receive tickets as gifts. Wisconsin is one of the few states to specifically go after a minor's adult agent: The state makes it a crime to sell a lottery ticket not only to a minor but to an adult who is buying on behalf of the minor and not as a gift.[293]

Parimutuel betting: Anyone under 18 is prohibited from being "admitted to a racetrack, unless accompanied by a parent, grandparent, great-grandparent, guardian or spouse who is at least 18 years of age, or unless accompanied by another person at least 18 with the written permission of the minor's parent or guardian." Even at the track individuals under 18 may not make a wager or receive any payout on a wager, and no licensee may knowingly accept a wager or pay out winnings to anyone under 18. No one under 16 may work in any parimutuel wagering activity.[294]

Casinos: The state entered into compacts allowing tribes to open full-scale, high-stake casinos—with expirations dates beginning in 1998. When the compacts came up for renewal, the state asked for more money and insisted that the age limit be raised from 18 to 21; thirteen of the state's fifteen tribes agreed. Two tribes renewed before the state made its demand, so their compacts have no minimum age for gambling, though the tribal casinos require players to be at least 21 anyway because they serve alcoholic beverages.

Bingo and pull-tabs: Persons under 18 may not play bingo unless accompanied by their parent, guardian, or spouse.[295]

WYOMING
The state allows limited sports betting.

Parimutuel betting: "No person under the age of eighteen (18) years shall place or be allowed to place a bet."[296]

Bingo: Charity bingo is legal. The statutes do not set a minimum age, but the age limit of 18 for parimutuel betting probably applies.

Notes

1. *State of Nevada v. Rosenthal,* 93 Nev. 36, 559 P.2d 830 (1977) (footnote omitted).
2. E.g., *United States v. Goldfarb,* 464 F.Supp. 565 (E.D. Mich. 1979).
3. SB33, introduced by state Sen. Jay Dardenne and passed in a special session, was signed into law by Gov. H. M. "Mike" Foster on May 6, 1998, raising the age from 18 to 21 to play the state lottery or the thousands of privately owned video poker machines. (Amending La.R.S. §§27:319, 47:9025(B)(2), and 47:9070).
4. AP Newswire J5840 (Jan. 7, 1999).
5. *Latour v. State,* 2000-1176, 778 So.2d 557 (La. Jan. 29, 2001).
6. *Manuel v. State,* 692 So.2d 320 (La. 1996).

7. Ibid.

8. *U.S. v. Edge Broadcasting Co.*, 509 U.S. 418, 113 S.Ct. 2696, 125 L.Ed.2d 345 (1993).

9. J. E. Coons, R. H. Mnookin, S. D. Sugarman, "Deciding What's Best for Children," *Notre Dame J.L. Ethics & Public Policy* 7 (1993): 465.

10. Ibid.

11. For a more detailed discussion of the history behind this third wave of legal gambling, see I. Nelson Rose, "Gambling and the Law: Endless Fields of Dreams," *Journal of Gambling Studies* 11 (1995): 15.

12. The burden of proof is also often higher than in normal civil cases, requiring a finding by clear and convincing evidence that the adult is incompetent, rather than the lesser standard of a preponderance of evidence.

13. M. A. R. Kleinman and A. J. Saiger, "Drug Legalization: The Importance of Asking the Right Question," *Hofstra Law Review* 18 (1990): 527, 550.

14. For example, M. A. Guara, "Card Club Boom Puts Asians at Loss," *San Francisco Chronicle* (March 3, 1995): A1.

15. Mark Griffiths, *Adolescent Gambling* (London: Routledge, 1995), chap. 2, pp. 34–74.

16. "Bay Area Casino Would Limit Gaming to 21 and Up," *Casino Journal's National Gaming Summary* (March 19, 2001), 4.

17. "Age Limit to be Raised at Cherokee Casino," NC News, http://www.journalnow .com/news/local/local/northcarolina/casino24.htm (Dec. 29, 2000).

18. If you asked these legislators, they would probably say that they did not realize there was no age restriction in the bill legalizing bingo, "and anyway, bingo is not gambling."

19. U.S. Constitution, Art. II, §1.

20. Former North Carolina Statute §51-2(b) (marriage allowed at age 12 for pregnant females; raised to age 14 in 2001, §51-2.1); New Hampshire Statute §457:4 (marriage allowed at 13 for females, 14 for males); Tennessee Statute §40-17-121 (13-year-old girl capable of giving consent to sexual intercourse); Washington Statute §71.34.030 (13-year-olds may request outpatient treatment of mental health services without parental consent).

21. Rabbi Joseph Telushkin, *Jewish Literacy: The Most Important Things to Know About the Jewish Religion, Its People, and Its History* (New York: William Morrow and Co., 1991), 611–12.

22. "The argument has been advanced that 'children' did not exist in medieval society—that 'childhood' as a temporal phase of personal development separating infancy from adulthood is largely an invention of the industrial mind and of the school and family institutions to which industrialization gave rise." L. H. Tribe, "Childhood, Suspect Classifications, and Conclusive Presumptions: Three Linked Riddles," *Law and Contemporary Problems* 39 (1975): 8.

23. William N. Thompson and Lawrence Dandurand, "The Bahamas," in *International Casino Law*, 2d ed., Ed. Anthony N. Cabot, William N. Thompson, and Andrew Tottenham (Reno: Institute for the Study of Gambling and Commercial Gaming, University of Nevada, Reno, 1993) (hereinafter cited as *International Casino Law*, 2d ed.).

24. Francois Roux, "France," ibid.

25. The sex offenses show the widest range of penalties, with the penalties increasing dramatically in inverse proportion to the age of the child. Even consensual sexual intercourse can range from a major felony, when committed with a child under 14, to no crime at all, when both parties are over 21.

26. N.J. Rev. Stat. §5:5-65 (1988).

27. N.J. Rev. Stat. §5:8-32 (1988).

28. N.J. Rev. Stat. §5:9-15 (1988).

29. N.J. Rev. Stat. §9:17B-1(c) (1988).

30. 23 U.S.C. §158 (1996).

31. NTSB 93-05/5977 News release: "Stronger state laws and vigorous enforcement needed to save teen lives" (March 3, 1993).

32. Iowa Code §99B.6 (1994).

33. Two tribes signed compacts before the request was made, so they can legally offer casino gambling to 18-year-olds. However, they also limit casino gaming to 21-year-olds, because they serve alcoholic beverages. For more information, see "Wisconsin: New Compacts Guarantee State Tribal Payments," *Casino Journal's National Gaming Summary* (January 4, 1999), 12.

34. Ibid.

35. For example, *Poppen v. Walker*, 520 N.W.2d 238 (S.D. 1994); *West Virginia v. Mountaineer Park, Inc.*, 190 W.Va. 276, 438 S.E.2d 308 (1993).

36. Delaware Code tit. 29, §4810.

37. *Thompson v. Oklahoma*, 487 U.S. 815, 835, 108 S.Ct. 2687, 101 L.Ed.2d 702 (1988) (footnotes omitted). In this death penalty case, the U.S. Supreme Court tried to determine the contemporary standards of morality in relation to age. The dissent noted that in Blackstone's *Commentaries on the Laws of England,* published in 1769, capital punishment could theoretically be imposed upon a 7-year-old. The dissent decried the plurality's finding of "evolving standards of decency which mark the progress of a maturing society," stating that "[o]f course the risk of assessing evolving standards is that it is all too easy to believe that evolution has culminated in one's own views." *Thompson v. Oklahoma,* 487 U.S. 815, 108 S.Ct. 2687, 101 L.Ed.2d 702, Appendix A (1988), 487 US: 864–865. By a slim majority, the court prohibited the execution of a man who committed first-degree murder when he was 15 years old.

38. *Erickson v. Desert Palace, Inc.*, 942 F.2d 694 (9th Cir. 1991); *Erickson v. Caesar's Palace,* 106 Nev. 1021, 835 P.2d 36 (Table) (1990).

39. Torstar News Service http://www.thestar.com/NASApp/cs/ContentServer?pagename=thestar/Layout/Article_Type1&c=Article&cid=993766640366&call_page=TS_Ontario&call_pageid=96825628982 (accessed July 4, 2001).

40. Ibid.

41. 48 CJS Intoxicating Liquors §259.

42. "Every person who *knowingly*: (a) Sells, gives, or otherwise furnishes an alcoholic beverage to any person under 21 years of age . . . is guilty of a misdemeanor." Nevada Rev. Stat. 202.055 (1995) (emphasis added).

43. Compare *State, Dept. of Law and Public Safety, Division of Gaming Enforcement*

v. Boardwalk Regency Corporation, 227 N.J. Super. 549, 548 A.2d 206 (1988) (upheld New Jersey Casino Control Commission fine based on a theory of strict liability against the Caesar's Palace Atlantic City casino for allowing two minors in gambling area), with *Erickson v. Caesar's Palace*, 106 Nev. 1021, 835 P.2d 36 (Table) (1990) (upheld Gaming Control Board ruling allowing Caesar's Palace to avoid paying underage winner, based in part on testimony that minor appeared to be over 21).

44. N.J. Rev. Stat. §5:12-119 (1988).

45. *State, Dept. of Law and Public Safety, Division of Gaming Enforcement v. Boardwalk Regency Corporation*, 227 N.J. Super. 549, 548 A.2d 206 (1988).

46. Miss. Code. Ann. §97-33-21 (1993).

47. Ibid.

48. *Carver, Inc. v. Dixon*, 759 So.2d 316 (La.App., 2d Cir. 2000).

49. Louisiana Revised Statutes 33:4862.19 [now designated 27:319]. The administrative rules in effect at the time of these events were even more explicit: "Licensees of licensed establishments and/or device owner(s), if applicable, shall be subject to immediate revocation if minors are allowed, whether intentionally or unintentionally, to operate devices." Louisiana Administrative Code 42:XI:2417(A)(5).

50. "Casino Questions Abound," *L.A. Times*, June 3, 2000, p. B13, col. 1.

51. Anti-gambling activists like Dr. James Dobson and Congressman Frank Wolf (R-Va.) helped bring the issue to the attention of the press. Sen. John McCain (R-Ariz.), chairman of the Senate Commerce Committee, sent a letter to Federal Trade Commission chairman Robert Pitofsky, stating: "I am deeply concerned that the use of these images may negatively impact children. . . . I question the propriety of companies using child-based themes in an obviously adult industry." "'Kiddie Slot' Controversy Reaches Capitol Hill," *Casino Executive* 6, no. 2 (February 2000): 10.

52. Nevada Gaming Control Act §463.350.

53. *Family News from Dr. James Dobson* (April 1999): 2.

54. South Carolina Statutes §§32-1-10, 12-21-2791, 61-9-410.

55. Ibid., §12-21-2804.

56. For a more detailed discussion of the law of gambling debts, see I. Nelson Rose, *Gambling and the Law* (Los Angeles: Gambling Times, Inc., 1986), chaps. 11 and 12.

57. Cf. *Pando v. Fernandez*, 485 N.Y.S.2d 162, 127 Misc.2d 224 (1984), affirming that the minor's age is no bar but reversing on other grounds, 499 N.Y.S.2d 950, 118 A.2d 474 (1986).

58. *Thompson v. Oklahoma*, 487 U.S. 815, n. 43 (1988), quoting Gordon, *The Tattered Cloak of Immortality, in Adolescence and Death* (1986), 16, 27.

59. Editorial, "Adulthood Is a Gamble," *(Madison) Capital Times* (February 16, 1996), 10A. (Editorial opposes attorney general's attempt to raise gambling age in Wisconsin from 18 to 21.)

60. Roux, "France," in *International Casino Law*, 2d ed., 275, 276, 284.

61. Thompson and Dandurand, "The Bahamas," in *International Casino Law*, 2d ed., 210.

62. Joseph Kelly, Christian Marfels, and Hartmut Nevries, "Germany," in *International Casino Law*, 3d ed., Ed. Anthony N. Cabot, William N. Thompson, Andrew Tot-

tenham, and Carl G. Braunlich (Reno: Institute for the Study of Gambling and Commercial Gaming, University of Nevada, Reno, 1999) (hereinafter cited as *International Casino Law*, 3d ed.), 379.

63. William N. Thompson, "Portugal," ibid., 458.

64. *Posadas de Puerto Rico v. Tourism Co.* 478 U.S. 328 (1986).

65. William N. Thompson and Lawrence Dandurand, "Antigua and Barbuda," ibid., 237.

66. William N. Thompson and Andrew Tottenham, "Argentina," ibid., 284.

67. Lawrence Dandurand and William N. Thompson, "The Lesser Antilles," in *International Casino Law*, 2d ed., 221.

68. Leo Wallner, "Austria," in *International Casino Law*, 3d ed., 333.

69. Thompson and Dandurand, "The Bahamas," in *International Casino Law*, 2d ed., 210.

70. Joris J. De Smet and Andrew Tottenham, "Belgium," in *International Casino Law*, 3d ed., 341.

71. Andrew Tottenham, "Bulgaria," ibid., 342.

72. J.A. Villa-Arce, "British Columbia," in *International Casino Law*, 2d ed., 181.

73. William N. Thompson, "Chile," in *International Casino Law*, 3d ed., 288.

74. Hartmut Nevries, "Denmark," ibid., 353.

75. William N. Thompson, "Ecuador," ibid., 300.

76. Esko Romppainen, "Finland," ibid., 355–56.

77. Roux, "France," in *International Casino Law*, 2d ed., 275, 276.

78. Kelly, Marfels, and Nevries, "Germany," in *International Casino Law*, 3d ed., 379.

79. David Miers, "Great Britain," ibid., 401.

80. John Andrews Anagnostaras and Harry Melvani, "Greece," ibid., 422.

81. Magdolna Kocsis, "Hungary," ibid., 431.

82. Lawrence Dandurand, Anna Mukonambi, and Charles Mayaka Mong'oni, "Kenya," ibid., 487.

83. William N. Thompson, "Malta," ibid., 440.

84. Lawrence Dandurand and William N. Thompson, "Mauritius," ibid., 490.

85. Joseph Kelly, Atam Uppal, and William N. Thompson, "Nepal," ibid., 527.

86. Chris Hoogendoorn, "The Netherlands," ibid., 451.

87. Phil Bennett, "New South Wales," ibid., 557.

88. Robert Falvey and Tony Nagel, "New Zealand," ibid., 592.

89. Christian Marfels, "Nova Scotia," ibid., 190.

90. Jacquie Castel, "Ontario," ibid., 200.

91. Lawrence Dandurand and William N. Thompson, "Paraguay," ibid., 309.

92. Frederic E. Gushin and William J. Callnin, "Philippines," ibid., 531.

93. Malgorzata Rogowicz-Angierman, "Poland," ibid., 454.

94. William N. Thompson, "Portugal," ibid., 458.

95. Daniel Schiffman and Maria Milagros Soto, "Puerto Rico," ibid., 258.

96. Loto-Quebec, Casino Montreal at http://www.caschar.com/francais/montreal/dhtml/index_montreal_IE.html (accessed April 26, 2001).

97. Bill 84, which went into effect Feb. 1, 2000. The Trésors de la Tour website: http://www.ingenio-quebec.com/TT1/html/anglais/home.html (accessed April 26, 2001).

98. Kev Leyshon, "Queensland," ibid., 569.

99. Steve Donoughhue, "Seychellus, Africa," ibid., 491.

100. Carl Braunlich and William N. Thompson, "Slovenia," ibid., 464.

101. Hendrik Brand, "South Africa," ibid., 509.

102. Carlos Lalanda Fernández and Ana López de Lemos y Gallego, "Spain," ibid., 473.

103. Paul E. S. Horne, "Tasmania," ibid., 581.

104. William N. Thompson and Jerry Johnson, "Turkey," ibid., 539.

105. Lawrence Dandurand, "Uganda," ibid., 492.

106. Peter Caillard, "Victoria," ibid., 588.

107. See Commentary to Alabama Code §§13A-12-21 and -22 ("Commentary"), discussing former §13-7-25; see also §15-8-150 for pleading.

108. Alabama Code §11-65-44; Association of Racing Commissioners International, Inc., *Pari-Mutuel Racing: 1996* (hereinafter cited as *Pari-Mutuel Racing: 1996*), 59.

109. Alaska Statutes §43.35.040.

110. Alaska Statutes §§05.15.180, 05.15.187.

111. Arizona Revised Statute §5-515; H.B. 2131.

112. Arizona Revised Statute §5-112.

113. Arizona Administrative Code R15-7-223.

114. Arkansas Statutes §§23-110-405 and 23-111-308.

115. California Government Code §8880.52.

116. Ibid., §8880.32.

117. California Business and Professions Code §19809.

118. California Penal Code §326.5.

119. Colorado Revised Statute §24-35-214.

120. Ibid., §24-35-212(4).

121. Ibid., §12-60-601.

122. Ibid., §12-47.1-809.

123. Ibid., §12-9-107.

124. Connecticut General Statute §12-813(d).

125. Ibid., §12-568a.

126. Ibid., §12-576(a).

127. Ibid., §12-576(b).

128. Ibid., §186a.

129. Ibid., §7-169h.

130. Delaware Constitution art. 2, §17.

131. Delaware Code, tit. 29, §4810.

132. Ibid., tit. 28, §1139.

133. Ibid., tit. 29, §4810.

134. DC Code §2-2535.

135. Ibid., §§2-2522.1, 2-2534.

136. Florida Statute, tit. XLVI, §849.085.

137. Ibid., tit. VI, §24.1055.

138. Ibid., §550.0425.

139. Ibid., §849.0931.

140. Georgia Code §51-1-18.

141. Ibid., §50-27-10.

142. Ibid., §16-12-58.

143. Hawaii Revised Statute §712-1231.

144. Idaho Code §67-7413.

145. Ibid., §54-2512.

146. Idaho Administrative Code 11.04.01.901.21, .22.

147. Idaho Code §67-7703.

148. Illinois Revised Statutes ch.230, §5/3.08.

149. HB1802, amending 20 ILCS §1605/15 and repealing 1605/18.

150. Ibid., §1605/15.

151. Ibid., chap. 230, §5/26.

152. Ibid., chap. 230, Act 10, §18.

153. Ibid., §10/11.

154. Ibid., §30/8.

155. Ibid., chap. 230, §§20/4, 25/2.

156. Indiana Code §§4-30-9-3, 4-30-11-3, 4-30-12-1, 4-30-13-1.

157. Ibid., §4-31-7-2(2).

158. Ibid., §4-31-6-5.

159. Ibid., §§4-33-8-3, 4-33-9-12.

160. Ibid., §4-32-9-34; Indiana Administrative Code tit. 45, regulation 18-3-2 (Department of State Revenue).

161. Iowa Code §99E.18(2).

162. Ibid., §99D.11(7).

163. Ibid., §99D.24.

164. Ibid., §99F.9(5).

165. Ibid., §99B.6(1)(k).

166. Ibid., §99B.7.

167. Kansas Statutes §41-2601(l), (m).

168. Ibid., §§74-8708, 74-8718, 74-8722.

169. Ibid., §§74-8810, 74-8839.

170. Ibid., §§46-2301 et. seq.

171. Ibid., §74-9802.

172. Ibid., §79-4706.

173. Kentucky Revised Statute §154A.990.

174. Ibid., §2.015.

175. *Pari-Mutuel Racing: 1996*, 59.

176. Kentucky Revised Statute §238.545.

177. *Latour v. State*, 2000-1176, 778 So.2d 557 (La. Jan 29, 2001)

178. Louisiana Revised Statutes §§47:9025, 47:9070.

179. Ibid., §4:193.

180. Ibid., §§4:150, 4:157.

181. Ibid., §27:85.

182. Ibid., §27:260.

183. Ibid., §14:90.4.

184. Ibid., §4:714.

185. Maine Revised Statutes tit. 8, §§374, 380.

186. Ibid., tit. 8, §§275-D, 278.

187. Ibid., tit. 17, §319.

188. Ibid., tit. 17, §§332, 341.

189. Ibid., tit. 26, §773, tit. 17, §340.

190. Maryland State Government Codes §§9-112, 9-124.

191. Maryland Statutes, Code of 1957, art. 27, §255.

192. Maryland Criminal Law Code art. 27, "Gaming."

193. Massachusetts General Laws chap. 10, §§24, 29.

194. Ibid., chap. 128A, §§9, 10.

195. Ibid., chap. 10, §38.

196. Michigan Compiled Laws §§432.11, 432.29.

197. Ibid., §431.317.

198. Ibid., §432.209 (9).

199. Ibid., §432.110a.

200. Ibid., §432.107a.

201. Minnesota Statute §349A.12.

202. Ibid., §§240.13, 240.25.

203. Ibid., §349.2127.

204. Mississippi Code §75-76-155.

205. Ibid., §97-33-67.

206. Missouri Revised Statutes §§313.260, 313.280.

207. Ibid., §313.670.

208. Ibid., §§434.060, 313.817.

209. Ibid., §313.040.

210. Montana Code §23-5-158, see §23-5-158(3).

211. Ibid., §§23-7-110, 23-7-301.

212. Ibid., §23-4-301.

213. Ibid., §23-5-603.

214. Ibid., §23-5-112.

215. Ibid., §23-5-158(3).

216. See also Department of Justice, Gambling Control Division: www.doj.state.mt.us/gcd for detailed information on laws and regulations.

217. Compare Nebraska Revised Statutes §§9-646, 9-810, 9-814 with §§9-345, 9-430, 9-426.

218. Ibid., §2-1207.

219. Nevada Revised Statute §463.350.

220. Ibid., §129.130.

221. Ibid., §205.460.

222. Ibid., §609.210.

223. New Hampshire Revised Statute §287-F:8.

224. Ibid., §284:33.

225. Ibid., §§287-E:7, 287-E:10, 287-E:12.

226. New Jersey Revised Statutes §§5:9-15, 5:9-7.

227. Ibid., §5:5-65.

228. Ibid., §5:12-119.

229. Ibid., §5:8-32.

230. New Mexico Statutes §§6-24-14, 6-24-15, 6-24-32.

231. Ibid., §11-13-1.

232. Compare New Mexico Statutes §30-19-7.2 with the New Mexico Bingo and Raffle Act, at §§60-2B-1 to 60-2B-14.

233. New York Tax Law §1610, *Pando v. Fernandez* 485 N.Y.S.2d 162, 127 Misc.2d 224 (1984), affirming that the minor's age is no bar but reversing on other grounds, 499 N.Y.S.2d 950, 118 A.D.2d 474 (1986).

234. New York Racing and Parimutuel Law §104.

235. New York General Municipal Law §486.

236. North Carolina General Statutes §58.1-4016.

237. "Age Limit to be Raised at Cherokee Casino," NC News, http://www.journalnow.com/news/local/local/northcarolina/casino24.htm (Dec. 29, 2000).

238. North Dakota Century Code §53-06.1-07.3.

239. *Pari-Mutuel Racing: 1996*, 59.

240. North Dakota Century Code §53-06.1-07.1.

241. Ibid., §53-06.1-07.1.

242. Ohio Revised Code §3770.08.

243. Ohio Administrative Code §§3769-4-07, 3769-14-06.

244. Ohio Revised Codes §§173.121, 2915.09.

245. Oklahoma Statute, tit. 3A, §208.4.

246. Oregon Revised Statutes §§461.250, 461.300, 461.600.

247. Ibid., §§462.190, 462.195.

248. Oregon Revised Statute §163.575.

249. Pennsylvania Consolidated Statutes, tit. 72, §§3761-6, 3761-10.

250. Ibid., tit. 4, §325.228.

251. Ibid., tit. 58, §189.71; 58 Pennsylvania Administrative Code §171.71.

252. Pennsylvania Consolidated Statute, tit. 10, §320.

253. Ibid., tit. 10, §305.

254. Puerto Rico Laws, tit. 15, §§809, 814.

255. *Pari-Mutuel Racing: 1996*, 59.

256. Puerto Rico Law, tit. 15 §77.

257. *Posadas de Puerto Rico Assoc. v. Tourism Co.*, 478 U.S. 328 (1986); repudiated in part in *Greater New Orleans v. United States*, 527 U.S. 173 (1999).

258. Puerto Rico Law, tit. 15, §§71, 77.

259. General Laws of Rhode Island §§42-61.2-5, 11-19-32, 42-61-9.

260. Ibid., §§41-4-2, 41-11-4.

261. Ibid., §11-19-32.

262. South Carolina Statutes §§59-150-210 and -250.

263. *Joytime Distributors and Amusement Co. v. State,* 338 S.C. 634, 528 S.E.2d 647 (1998).

264. South Dakota Codified Laws §§42-7A-13, 42-7A-32, 42-7A-44, 42-7A-48.

265. Ibid., §42-7-76.

266. Ibid., §§42-7B-35, 42-7B-4, 42-7B-25.

267. See ibid., §22-25-25.

268. Tennessee Code §4-36-310.

269. Texas Government Code §466.3051.

270. Texas Civil Statutes art. 179e, §1.03(68) and (69).

271. Ibid., §11.06.

272. Ibid., §14.13.

273. Texas Civil Code, tit. 6, art. 179d, §17.

274. Vermont Statutes, tit. 13, §2143, tit. 31, §§654, 661.

275. Ibid., tit. 31, §613.

276. Ibid., tit. 13, §2143.

277. Virgin Islands Statutes, tit. 32 §254.

278. Ibid., tit. 32, §453.

279. Code of Virginia §58.1-4015.

280. Ibid., §59.1-403.

281. Ibid., §18.2-340.5.

282. Virginia Admin. Code, tit. 11, §15-22-40.

283. Revised Code of Washington §67.70.120.

284. Ibid., §9.46.0305.

285. Washington Administrative Code §230-12-027.

286. Ibid.

287. West Virginia Code §29-22-11.

288. *Pari-Mutuel Racing: 1996,* 59.

289. West Virginia Code §47-20-4.

290. Ibid., §§29-22A-1 et seq.

291. Ibid., §§29-22-1 et seq.

292. Ibid., §§29-25-1 et seq.

293. Wisconsin Statutes §§565.17, 565.30, 565.12, 565.10.

294. Ibid., §444.09.

295. Ibid., §563.51.

296. Wyoming Statute §11-25-109.

Chapter Eight

Economic, Social, and Policy Observations on Youth Gambling

William R. Eadington

Economics, Wisdom, and Youth

The logic of economics—as presented to college students in principles of economics courses throughout America—is often wasted on the young. Economics involves the study of how individuals achieve material well-being through the exchange of one's time for a wage or salary, the exchange of tangible property for more liquid forms of wealth, or the exchange of money for desired goods and services.

For many youths, however, experiences regarding money and well-being really center more around negotiation and bargaining than on true exchange. Children negotiate for allowances, privileges, or special favors beyond normal grants bestowed by parents or other authority figures; teens negotiate with their dates for affection and acceptance. Moreover, bad behavior by preteens and teens is often punished by restrictions on existing rights and privileges. When caught violating parental rules, adolescent perpetrators can only plead mercy or try to negotiate out of an unpleasant circumstance. At this stage of life, the politics of the household and the playground are far more real and understandable to youths than is the somewhat arcane science of economics.

True appreciation of economics and economic relationships does not come until later in life, when—once out of the family home—there are no obvious benefactors remaining with whom to negotiate. One then realizes that in order to achieve a satisfactory standard of living, an income must be earned through the sale of something of value—time or property—in the marketplace. Furthermore, the largesse of parents tends to disappear as adolescents develop into adults. Symbolic umbilical cords are cut; no longer can the young adult negotiate his or her way into a desirable situation. Instead, young people must acknowledge economic realities and deal with them. At this stage in life, many people realize that economics is not so irrelevant after all; often they wish they had studied the subject more diligently.

In much the same spirit, Charlotte Olmstead commented on the symbolic dimensions of the casino game of blackjack in her book *Heads I Win, Tails You Lose* (1962):

> [Twenty-one] seems to symbolize mostly dominance-dependency conflicts, and the attainment of full adult status without assuming adult responsibilities. . . . Twenty-one, the traditional age of attaining adult status, is aimed for. . . . Family ties are not desired or required, simply independent adulthood with no ties. . . . The dealer, backed by the house, represents the family figure. . . . Twenty-one is played for, but it is even more dangerous to go over this figure than to fall short of it. Independence, adult status, is aimed for, but no responsibilities.

Thus, being the Black Jack, the randy young son of the King and Queen who has none of the responsibilities of adulthood, is the ultimate objective of the game. Come as close to 21 as you can, but if you go over, you are busted. The burdens of adulthood are unavoidable if you exceed 21.

Youthful Omnipotence, Fantasy, and Reality

There is another element of youth that diminishes and ultimately disappears as a person grows to adulthood: the belief in magic and omnipotence. Edmund Bergler (1958) noted this factor as part of his Freudian explanation of compulsive gambling:

> In our culture . . . the family setup fosters the child's misconception of his omnipotence. This is the result of the parents' effort to fulfill the infant's every demand for food, love, attention. The child misconceives causality; he sees these wish fulfillments, not as a consequence of the mother's or mother-representative's love and kindness, but as a fruit of his own omnipotence. Education is an attempt to adapt the child to a reality far different from the fantasy world in which he can feel omnipotence.

In short, during childhood, you can believe that your powers allow you to accomplish magic. Even more fundamentally, a belief arises that as a child, you are the center of the universe. Things happen because you are to be rewarded or punished. Megalomania is not a mania; it is a life view before—and sometimes throughout—puberty.

Of course, one of life's great disappointments is growing up and realizing that you are not the reason things happen. Rather than being the center of the universe, you come to realize you are just a cog—a rather irrelevant one at that—in the complex and impersonal machinery of modern life. Freud referred to this transition as a shift from the "pleasure principle" to the "reality principle" (Bergler, 1958, p. 17).

Bergler noted that one of the appeals of gambling is that it permits an adult to temporarily forego the reality principle and all the responsibilities it implies and regress to the pleasure principle, where one controls causality and can revel in megalomaniac dreams, at least temporarily.

In modern parlance, we speak of the "escapist" value of gambling; it permits us to "dream luxurious dreams" about what we will do with our winnings. The reality will shortly come back into dominance for most people, but while in the casino, in front of the video poker machine, or while waiting for the lotto numbers to be drawn, fantasy and escape are welcome diversions. Problem gamblers often have trouble returning to the reality principle; the pleasures of childhood beliefs in magic, mysticism, and self-centeredness may be too difficult to give up. One can make a case that many people who struggle with excessive gambling have found themselves "stuck" in the fantasy world they have created around gambling.

Gambling and Human Development: Maintaining Youthful Bliss by Regressing Intelligence

Older people usually share the belief that the process of aging brings about, among other transitions, an evolution from foolishness and stupidity to knowledge and wisdom (though we are all aware of the many exceptions to this principle). Bergler and others have suggested that part of the appeal of gambling is the consequent regression to a childlike mental state, to a bliss of stupidity and foolishness.

Thorstein Veblen touched on this theme in his classic *The Theory of the Leisure Class* (1899). Veblen argued that industrialization and the pursuit of industrial efficiency make people and society more intelligent, that is, less stupid, by replacing superstitions and a "belief in luck" with greater understanding of scientific principles that underlie the cause and effect of modern production. The role of education is to increase industrial efficiency by removing stupidity from the workplace. According to Veblen, gambling works in the opposite direction of education. Through a belief in good luck charms or symbols, the gambler tries to impute causality where only chance is at work. The belief that one's side of a wager in a sporting event will win because an individual is providing spiritual support for the team or that one side will prevail over another because its cause is just and the opponents' is not, are examples of the gambler's muddled thinking about causality.

In this sense, gambling contributes to a collective stupidity, to a regression in the progress of intelligence necessitated by the industrial imperative. "Through its cumulative effect upon the habitual attitude of the population, even a slight or inconspicuous bias towards accounting for everyday facts by recourse to other ground than that of quantitative causation may work an appreciable lowering of the collective industrial efficiency of a community" (Veblen, 1899, pp. 284–85). In short, gambling makes us stupid by making us superstitious and illogical. In a sense, this argument is equivalent to Bergler's theory that gambling causes the rational adult to regress to the foolish belief systems of youth.

Values and Attitudes of Youths

Modern teenagers and young adults are already confronted with various challenges, misconceptions, and confusions regarding the realities of life. Permitted and legitimized gambling may further contribute to the complexities of growing up. Young males in particular are subject to peer pressures that dictate they should be "cool," "macho," "risk-taking," and that they should rebel against their parents' lifestyle and work ethic. Adolescents and young adults have been confronted with a mixed bag of role models in recent years, offering a confusing array of lifestyle options. These include Bill Clinton, Madonna, Michael Jackson, River Phoenix, Jerry Garcia, Ice-T, Pete Rose, Britney Spears, the Spice Girls, and Dennis Rodman—individuals who have put forward, by word or act, their own personal and social commentary on sexual activity, gender and racial identity, drug use and self-realization, respect for authority, and high-stakes gambling.

Increasing concerns over the solvency of the Social Security system and of health care funding in recent years have provided credibility and support for the German adage that it is the duty of the old to lie to the young. A few years ago, youth were confronted with the feeling that all the good jobs had been taken by the previous generation, especially the boomers; all that was left to them were "McJobs." The strong economy of the 1990s diminished that anxiety, but has replaced it with others. Ongoing concerns about global warming, terrorist threats, and collapsing economies once again give youths reason to question the world being endowed to them by their elders.

There has been some discussion in the media about predictions that this will be the first generation unable to attain their parents' standard of living. Some projections on the costs of retirement plans and Medicare for seniors, for example, suggest that upwards of 70 percent of income will be needed to support Social Security and Medicare programs by the year 2040 if population and demographic trends continue and laws are not changed. A convincing case can be made for the assertion that younger generations will pay heavily for the indulgences of their parents and grandparents who, as health-conscious and politically savvy retired seniors, will divert large portions of future earnings from twenty-first-century workers to fund their own lifestyles well into their 80s and 90s.

Given this perspective among modern youths, what is wrong with a little nihilism? Why not gamble, why not do drugs, why not party all night? Why worry about the long-term consequences of smoking, drinking, or promiscuity? In economic terms, the angst of youth created by a pessimistic outlook for their long-term prospects encourages a high rate of personal and social discount. This outlook encourages young people to "live for the moment" because the future looks bleak regardless of sacrifices made now. This is not the first generation to be pointed toward the philosophy of "Eat, drink, and be merry, for tomorrow we die." Today's adults have been providing a lot of support material to make nihilism a reasonable alternative for some adolescents.

Youth, Gambling, and Public Policy Questions

The scenario described above provides the context within which we can begin to discuss important policy questions surrounding youth gambling. As stated elsewhere, an explosion of permitted commercial gaming throughout America and throughout the world occurred during the 1980s and 1990s (Eadington, 1999). There is considerable evidence to support the theory that as commercial gaming becomes more available and acceptable, gambling behavior and problems associated with gambling will also increase among the adult population (Final Report, 1999; Gambling Review Report, 2001; Productivity Commission Report, 1999). There are some obvious incongruities here. Gambling is an adult activity that invites childish behavior; it allows adults to "play" and to behave frivolously and irresponsibly with money, and as foolishly as children.

For children and teens striving to become adults and attain the privileges and perquisites of adulthood, gambling provides some strange messages. In the eyes of many youths, the conventional means of acquiring wealth—hard work, savings, accumulation—do not appear promising because of future economic uncertainties and various financial commitments to older generations. However, extensive gambling by adults sends the message that they have enough extra money to allow them to throw away significant amounts of it in casinos, on slot machines, on lotteries, and at the races. Thus, to adults, money is critically important to earn and to protect, especially from the taxing power of the government. But at the same time it is the vehicle for frivolous and childlike play in casinos and other gambling venues. The message conveyed to youths seems to be "Fight like hell to get and keep what is rightfully yours, then do as you damn well please—wasteful or not—in disposing of it."

The irony of bitter political battles against tax increases, Social Security cuts, and Medicare cuts—in juxtaposition to the growing popularity of gambling among seniors—is not wasted on the young. At a time when many special interest groups in society were exerting tremendous efforts to protect either their disposable incomes or their existing benefits packages, it seems somewhat incongruous that the popularity and revenue base of commercial gaming grew so rapidly in the late twentieth century. Through the eyes of youths, the battle for Social Security benefits might appear as a means for senior citizens to turn their backs on future generations.

An alternative message to youths is that gambling indeed provides a realistic path by which one can attain a higher level of wealth. Through common sense or hard-learned lessons, most adults know that this claim is false, but the absence of experience among youths makes them more susceptible to this false promise. Furthermore, the erosion of other pathways to a good life increases the appeal of getting there by winning the lottery or by becoming a professional gambler.

All these lines of discussion suggest that there are a number of policy issues related to youth gambling that we need to address in the years ahead. The continuing acceptance of commercial gaming will clearly make youth gambling an increasing phenomenon, whether or not it has negative consequences. For purveyors of gaming services—whether we are considering casinos, lotteries, racing, or other legal forms of gambling—it is unlikely that youth gambling will be terribly important from a revenue perspective. Young people just do not have access to the amounts of spending money that adults command, and for those under 18 or 21, the activity in commercial establishments is illegal anyway. Nevertheless, gaming companies have been investing in youth as their future customers by increasing the allure of casinos to young people through the addition of thrill rides, amusement arcades, and fantasy environments, and slot machine manufacturers have borrowed cartoon characters and other popular youthful icons for their themed entertainment-oriented gaming device offerings.

However, there is good reason to believe that the issue of youth gambling may create its share of problems. First, young people, especially males, may have more difficulty than adults separating reality from the fantasy associated with gambling. From Bergler's perspective, youths do not have to regress so far—compared with adults—to revert to the fantasy world of the pleasure principle. Indeed, some young people may not yet have left this state. Teenage males often consider themselves immortal, invulnerable, or bulletproof in their approach to risky situations. Adolescents often believe that the laws of physics and probability do not apply to them. Examples of this behavior are abundant; we see it demonstrated in driving, sporting activities, and unsafe sex. It is reasonable to expect that such attitudes and beliefs will carry over, at least for some, into gambling as well.

In addition, a lot of socialization around gambling takes place among young males. Wagering on sports teams, Friday night poker games, and personal contests of skill or intelligence are part of life for many young men. The desire to win is strong among teenage males and young adults, and wagering can rectify a person's commitment to his own side. Providing some forms of legal and accepted gaming, thus commercializing the social activity, can certainly provide the temptation for young men to participate actively at a higher financial level.

Alcohol, Tobacco, and Gambling: The Issue of Age Restrictions

As with alcohol and tobacco, almost all jurisdictions have placed age restrictions on gambling, where it is permitted. These policies derive from the belief that children and teenagers need some paternalistic protection from their own lack of knowledge or experience. These age restrictions can turn prohibited behavior—in this case, gambling—into the "forbidden fruit" and increase its allure, as well as provide the prestige of one's being able to "get away with" gambling in commercial venues. Wherever age limits are set, underage gambling becomes a challenge to those who fall just below the limit. The actual social consequences of underage gambling—as opposed to the legal implications—probably relate most to the issues of present or future gambling abuse resulting from underage gambling.

There has been considerable discussion of the linkage of an adolescent's positive gambling experiences—a big win, for example—and later bouts with pathological gambling (Custer, 1982). To the extent that adolescents are more impressionable to seductive fantasies that can surround gambling and are less able than adults to sort out realities from such fantasies, they might warrant a greater degree of protection than adults.

However, if a jurisdiction chooses to implement and enforce age restrictions that limit gambling, a series of policy concerns involving violations of the law rapidly emerge. These policy issues include the same considerations that must be weighed when establishing policy regarding violations of laws by adults. For example, should underage gambling be considered a criminal or a civil violation? Should penalties be financial (fines, forfeitures), time constraining (jail time, mandated public service work), or stigmatizing (misdemeanor or gross misdemeanor status, loss of civil rights)? One approach might be to revoke certain "adult" privileges that are meaningful to teenagers, such as drivers' licenses or preferred insurance rates. On balance, it is important that the punishment fit the crime. It is still unclear, however, how heinous a "crime" society should consider underage gambling to be.

Positive Potentials of Youth Gambling

There is little doubt that gambling can be fascinating for many people, including adolescents and young adults. For some, this fascination will be quite destructive. For others, it will be temporarily but memorably expensive. For the majority, it will probably be relatively neutral in its overall effect on their lives and lifestyles. As with adult pathological gambling, knowledge of the prevalence rates of in-transition and pathological gambling among adolescents is important if we wish to appreciate the extent of social costs surrounding this issue. However, our current understanding of the incidence of underage problem gambling is not yet definitive (Shaffer & Hall, 1996).

Since gambling is apparently more acceptable to the general public than ever before and many people now consider it one of their entertainment and leisure options, commercial gaming is likely to remain a pervasive presence in society for the foreseeable future. Given this social reality, we must ask ourselves whether there are positive ways to take advantage of gambling's changing status. One such arena of opportunity is education, especially in the field of mathematical skills. Mathematics education in America has been slanted toward deductive fields such as algebra, geometry, and calculus. A field that receives much less attention in most mathematics curricula is probability and statistics.[1]

Although the inferential logic of probability and statistics is underemphasized in most curricula, its value in terms of providing useful life skills is substantial. A good understanding of decision making under conditions of uncertainty, negotiation skills, and strategies for problem solving and winning contests can be gained by studying these mathematical disciplines. There is a clear opportunity to exploit the interest in and obsessions with legal gambling to enhance the skill level of students in probability and statistical analysis. Veblen does not have to be correct; perhaps gambling can make (some of) us smart rather than stupid. Knowledge regarding statistics and probability also has the ability to dissipate the magic of gambling and to help people put gambling into its proper perspective—that of a minor digression from the important elements of life.

The spread of commercial gaming in America has been a powerful force with good and bad side effects. With regard to youths, the best way to harness the good of gambling and limit the bad is through education. Youthful consumers and potential consumers of gambling activities must understand the risks and costs, as with alcohol and tobacco. They should know that for some people, gambling can be terribly destructive; they should also know how to spot problems in their own lives or the lives of their friends.

Conclusion

Young people should understand gambling from the standpoint of knowledge, science, and logic. Adolescents do not need misinformation, nor do they need to hear about superstitions and belief in luck. Gambling does induce fantasy, which is not bad in itself. Fantasy is fun in moderation, and moderation suggests that reality always be kept in sight. If young men and women become fascinated with gambling as a result of its presence and popularity among adults, then the challenge is to use that fascination as a means to an end: to teach youths to become more analytical and realistic adults and to better understand and control the allure of gambling in their own lives.

Notes

1. For an innovative approach to teaching probability through gambling, see chap. 4, "What Are My Chances? Using Probability and Number Sense to Educate Teens About the Mathematical Risks of Gambling," by Terry W. Crites.

References

Bergler, E. (1958). *The psychology of gambling.* London: Bernard Hanison Ltd.
Custer, R. L. (1982). An overview of compulsive gambling. In P. A. Carone, S. F. Yolles, S. N. Kieffer, & L. W. Krinsky (Eds.), *Addictive disorders update,* vol. 7 (pp. 107–124). New York: Human Sciences Press, Inc.
Eadington, W. R. (1999). The spread of casinos and their role in tourism development. In D. Pearce & R. Butler (Eds.), *Contemporary issues in tourist development: Analysis and applications.* London and New York: Routledge.
Final Report (United States). (1999). National Gambling Impact Study Commission. (Available at http://www.ngisc.gov)
Gambling Review Report (United Kingdom). (2001). (Available at http://www.culture.gov.uk/index_noflash.html)
Olmstead, C. (1962). *Heads I win, tails you lose.* New York: Macmillan Company.
Productivity Commission Report (Australia). (1999). (Available at http://www.indcom.gov.au/inquiry/gambling/index.html)
Shaffer, H. J., & Hall, M. N. (1996). Estimating the prevalence of adolescent gambling disorders: A quantitative synthesis and guide toward standard gambling nomenclature. *Journal of Gambling Studies, 12,* 193–214.
Veblen, T. (1899). *The theory of the leisure class.* New York: Macmillan Company.

Chapter Nine

Youth Gambling
The Casino Industry's Response

Philip G. Satre

Introduction

As chairman and chief executive officer of Harrah's Entertainment Inc., I would like to present our company's views, as well as our company's course of action, on the problem of underage gambling. However, I also write from my perspective as a parent: I am the father of four children, all of whom are native Nevadans. My children spent their formative years in Reno, where my family lived within walking distance of the casinos.

Casino entertainment is woven into the social fabric where my children grew up. Casinos were as close as the nearest McDonald's. Many parents of my children's friends also worked in the industry. Like most children, my children went to work with their dad on occasion and walked through the casino floor. And children can ask the most innocent, yet most penetrating, questions. Mine have asked me more than once why the bright lights, ringing bells, and exciting games that look like so much fun are only for grown-ups. That question has been in the back of my mind for a long time. So I bring a very personal, as well as a professional, interest to the subject.

Casinos, Adolescents, and Responsibility

Why *is* casino gaming just for grown-ups? What are we, at Harrah's and others in the industry, doing to make sure casino gaming stays that way? And how can industry representatives, researchers, treatment providers, and policymakers work together to formulate a blueprint to effectively address underage gambling? These are some of the questions I will address in this chapter.

I cannot say that we have all the answers, but I believe we are asking the right questions. Fifteen years ago, most casino executives would have immediately dismissed the notion of underage gambling—or any kind of problem gambling, for that matter. The idea that a minor could play undetected in our casinos or that some of our customers gambled not out of choice but out of something akin to compulsion was considered heretical by the casino industry. Today we know better.

There are many responsible casino operators who actively seek ways to increase public awareness about the existence and consequences of problem and underage gambling. I am proud to lead a company that has been on the forefront of this issue for more than a decade. Tom Brosig of Park Place Entertainment is also an executive with such a company. We may have a long way to go, but Harrah's managers and our many like-minded colleagues at other companies are committed to making a difference.

The job of industry representatives, researchers, treatment providers, and policymakers in the field of youth gambling is to develop a strong plan of action for a collaborative, cohesive effort. My personal pledge is that Harrah's will support an effort that involves more proactive involvement by the casino entertainment industry.

Underage Versus Problem Gambling

As I read the mission for the North American Think Tank on Youth Gambling Issues, two distinct issues emerged: underage gambling and problem gambling. While these issues can be intertwined, they are often very different. Underage gambling is a problem regardless whether the underage gambler meets particular diagnostic criteria indicating that he or she may be a "problem gambler." Thus, I am going to separate the two topics in this chapter to focus on underage gambling as it relates to casinos.

At Harrah's, our wake-up call on underage gambling came in 1989. A 14-year-old checked into Harrah's Atlantic City, ordered beer from room service, and then gambled on our casino floor. When our senior management became aware of the incident, we realized that we needed to take a very serious look at underage gambling. Jim Butler, who was our general counsel in Atlantic City at the time, spearheaded that effort. Although we felt that the presence of one 14-year-old in a casino was more than enough motivation to take immediate action, we also saw four other compelling reasons to treat underage gambling as a significant problem: (1) legal status; (2) consequences for the youthful offender; (3) consequences for the casino; and (4) public health concerns.

LEGAL STATUS

First, underage gambling is, by definition, illegal. Society has determined that casino entertainment is an activity much like driving a car, purchasing alcohol, casting a vote, serving in the military, or entering a legal contract. Society has set a threshold of intellectual and emotional maturity that young people must be reach before they can decide for themselves whether to engage in these behaviors. For better or worse, maturity level is measured in terms of age. However, simply establishing an age threshold for driving has not ensured that all people above the threshold will exercise good judgment while behind the wheel. Even though people have flawed driving records, we still do not outlaw cars.

CONSEQUENCES FOR THE YOUTHFUL OFFENDER

Underage gambling has far-reaching consequences for those who are caught and arrested. Although prison terms are an option in many jurisdictions, it is unlikely that an underage gambler will actually serve time; fines are a more typical sanction. Having to admit to a conviction for underage gambling may adversely affect a young person's college admission or job prospects. Harrah's supports the efforts of state gaming agencies and local law enforcement officials in enacting and enforcing appropriate sanctions against the underage gambler.

CONSEQUENCES FOR THE CASINO

Underage gambling has consequences for casino companies: Casino companies and their employees risk fines and even the revocation of gaming licenses for permitting underage gambling. Furthermore, companies that fail to police underage gambling betray the trust that casino regulators and the public have placed in us. In addition, Harrah's views the effort to combat youth gambling as a sound business decision. Underage gambling is against the law. Like any good company in any industry, we obey the law. But more important, preventing underage gambling is the right thing to do. Casinos are in business to provide entertainment, not to take advantage of youthful gamblers. We want our product to be used responsibly and by adults.

PUBLIC HEALTH CONCERNS

Finally, while we recognize that only a tiny fraction of underage gambling takes place in casinos, we treat underage gambling as a significant problem because it may be a significant public health risk. According to one researcher (Lesieur et al., 1991), every major study of pathological gambling shows that the vast majority of adult male pathological gamblers started gambling in their teens. However, this observation does not mean that all underage gamblers are pathological gamblers or will become pathological gamblers in the future. Studies also show that nearly all young men and many young women wager in some form and that the vast majority of these young people grow up to be responsible citizens. Nevertheless, it is conceivable that, for some, preventing underage gambling will prevent pathological gambling later in life.

The Development of Project 21

Spurred on by a 14-year-old and four fundamental beliefs, Harrah's Atlantic City put to work a task force representing twelve areas of casino and hotel operations. The group made initial recommendations that became the essential elements of Project

21, a program Harrah's developed to combat underage gambling.[1] In the course of its work, the task force uncovered three auxiliary issues that contributed to the problem under examination. First, minors were confused by the gaming laws. In New Jersey, an 18-year-old can vote, drive a car, buy a lottery ticket, wager on a horse race, and play bingo, but the minimum age for casino gambling is 21. Second, the general public—even some parents—seemed to view underage gambling as "harmless fun." Third, our employees were unclear about who was responsible for deterring and apprehending underage gamblers. Some thought this task was solely the responsibility of Harrah's security department. The task force recognized that each of these issues would need to be addressed for Project 21 to succeed.

Project 21 focused on each of these factors in its efforts to more effectively deny underage gamblers access to Harrah's casinos. We made each employee responsible and accountable for detecting and apprehending underage gamblers. This sustained effort included seminars, training sessions, inserts into paycheck envelopes, reminders in internal publications, and a back-of-house advertising campaign. Posters reminded employees, "If you don't check their license, we could lose ours." As a result of this initiative, our security officers are backed by informed and prepared slot mechanics, cocktail servers, and pit bosses, as well as every other employee on the casino floor. Our message to those under 21 is that they may get past our security at the casino entrance, but they will not get past the several hundred employees who are trained and empowered to identify them.

For the general public, Harrah's worked with the media to generate awareness of underage gambling. We also created signs and public service announcements about underage gambling. Figure 9.1 presents an example of a sign created for this program.

For minors, we held a student press conference to announce Project 21. Our executives met with school principals, superintendents, and teachers, as well as with professional groups such as the New Jersey Principals and Supervisors Association. We created a flyer for high schools and colleges, and we developed a public service announcement. At the casino, we posted a pointed warning at each entrance and in the parking garage (see fig. 9.2).

Perhaps most important, we created the Project 21 Scholarship Program. This program awards scholarships for the best student articles or public-awareness posters on underage gambling. To be eligible for submission, articles by the students must be published in a high school or college newspaper and posters must be displayed for at least a week. In this way, students communicate with and educate their peers on the message that casinos and the law will not tolerate underage gambling.

The following excerpt is a sample from a recent winning entry:

Gary decided to try his luck at getting into the casinos. Gary was greeted by a Security Officer and escorted from the floor under the suspicion of underage

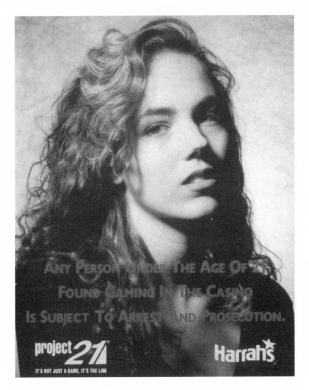

Fig. 9.1. Underage Gambling Sign

gambling. This should have served as a wake up call for Gary, but it didn't. Gary was interviewed by an officer from the DGE, his parents were called, and he was ultimately charged with a Disorderly Persons Offense for gambling underage. He pled guilty at his trial, and was fined $1,250 and 80 hours of community service. In addition, he had been denied four scholarships and rejected from three colleges. What he thought was no big deal, and just a little fun, would affect the rest of his life.

What happened to Gary has happened to many other underage persons who attempt to gamble in the casinos. It is a criminal offense that has lasting consequences. It will give you a criminal record, which will most definitely affect you later in life. It will hinder your chance to attend a good college, get a scholarship and/or get a good job. Don't tempt fate. If you gamble underage, you are destined to be caught, sooner or later. Wait until you're 21. (Vey, 2000)

This is the kind of powerful message and positive peer pressure that students share with their schoolmates through the scholarship program. We estimate that

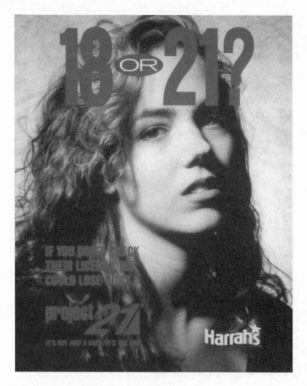

Fig. 9.2. Underage Gambling Sign

these messages about underage gambling reach approximately twenty thousand students each year through student newspaper circulation and poster exhibits.

Evaluating the Success of Project 21

When Project 21 began in 1990, twenty-three students in ffiteen schools submitted articles, and we awarded five $1,000 scholarships. The poster contest began the following year. The program now reaches the entire region, and today hundreds of students from New Jersey, Pennsylvania, and New York have participated in the Project 21 scholarship campaign.

Another measure of the program's success is that Project 21 opened a truly public dialogue in which all sides began to participate. The dialogue and the awareness it generated have met our objective of educating those in New Jersey and throughout the region about the legal age for casino gaming. And in a sense, the project has come full circle: The 14-year-old who was the catalyst for the awareness effort submitted an article for the scholarship program.

Beyond the New Jersey Initiative

We next worked to extend each facet of Project 21 to all Harrah's markets by inviting other members of the casino industry to join these projects as their counterparts did in Atlantic City. During March 1995, we initiated a Nevada campaign. Scholarship program information was sent to every principal, guidance department, art department, and school paper at every high school and college in Nevada. We have reached out, and other Nevada casinos have joined the program. In other states we have made similar efforts.

For example, the Missouri riverboat casino industry adopted a comprehensive, three-pronged program to promote responsible gambling, which became fully operational in spring of 1995. Project 21 is the basis for the underage gambling segment of this program. The Missouri campaign is funded by annual contributions from the state's riverboat gaming association, which includes the casinos currently operating in the state as well as nongaming companies that provide products or services to the industry. The Show-Me State is certainly showing the rest of the country what a model program should look like. This is exactly the type of broadly focused effort that I would like to see adopted in all casino jurisdictions.

In addition, the National Council on Problem Gambling established a nationwide twenty-four-hour toll-free help line for problem gambling, with seed money provided by Harrah's and technical assistance provided by AT&T. This help line may be the ultimate "winning number" for which problem gamblers—including underage gamblers—have been looking.

Most recently, Harrah's and other members of the American Gaming Association, in conjunction with the National Center for Missing and Exploited Children, developed guidelines to prevent and address potential problems associated with unattended minors in the casino environment. The guidelines outline ways to encourage parents to take responsibility for their children when they visit a casino destination, and they identify appropriate means of resolving situations when children may be unattended, should such situations arise.

Moving Forward: Industry Commitments

All of these efforts demonstrate that the casino industry has made strong strides regarding underage gambling. To move even further ahead, however, the industry needs a united front on four major issues. The following are commitments I would like the entire casino entertainment industry to make:

- Target advertising carefully to ensure the message focuses only on legal-age audiences.
- Design casino special events and casino promotions to attract only legal-age customers.

- Promote responsible gaming through internal programs like Project 21 and outreach vehicles like the toll-free help line established by the National Council on Problem Gambling.
- Invite an objective, comprehensive study of the youth-gambling issue on a national level.

Despite the steps the casino industry can take, there are certain things the industry cannot do. We cannot take the place of parents; they must exercise parental responsibility. In addition, the casino industry cannot shoulder the burden of addressing those types of gambling in which young people more commonly participate (such as illegal bets on athletic events, card games with friends and family, lottery games, and bingo games at the local community center). However, we can focus on our piece of the issue, support others as they identify their responsibilities, and collaborate on a comprehensive, synergistic approach to solving the problems associated with underage gambling.

Conclusion

Those of us who have spent our careers in the casino industry have seen a great deal of change over the past decade. One of the most significant areas of change, in addition to the explosive growth of our industry, has been the substantial progress made by the industry regarding underage and problem gambling. The industry has moved from denial to acceptance and then from reaction to proaction. It will take time before the public information programs that Harrah's and other casino companies advocate achieve dramatic effects. However, the industry deserves the plaudits it received recently from members of the National Gambling Impact Study Commission for its efforts to date. Still, much is left to be done. Like so many other industries faced with choices of responsibility, the casino industry stands at a crossroads. We can take the initiative to establish programs to encourage responsible gaming by adults, or we can have onerous programs placed upon us by politicians and activists who do not understand our business or who simplify the complex issues surrounding problem and underage gambling.

The gaming industry has found that it is easy for our opponents to sensationalize the issues of problem and underage gambling. We are well aware that some small percentage of people may use our products irresponsibly. This fact makes our industry no different from the alcohol industry, the automobile industry, the fireworks industry, or even the stepladder industry. The key tasks are to ensure that our customers are adults, that we encourage adults to use our products responsibly, and that we discourage irresponsible behavior.

Although Harrah's is dedicated to preventing underage gambling, we cannot accomplish this task alone. Representatives from other forms of gambling, such as the states that run lotteries and organizations that sponsor horse racing, have an obligation to ensure responsible use of their products as well. Likewise, parents, educators, lawmakers, and organizations such as the National Council on Problem Gambling and its many state affiliates also have a responsibility. That responsibility includes promoting awareness of the issue of youth gambling, keeping young people out of casinos, discouraging other forms of youth gambling, and offering help when it is needed.

If we act now, we can seize the opportunity to work together and make a difference. I am optimistic that the North American Think Tank on Youth Gambling Issues and the publication of this book are vital steps in this direction.

Note

This article was adapted from the author's keynote address at the North American Think Tank on Youth Gambling Issues, April 6, 1995.

1. Readers interested in learning more about Project 21 and other programs initiated by the gaming industry to address youth and problem gambling should consult the American Gaming Association's *Responsible Gaming Resource Guide* (1998). For ordering information, see www.americangaming.org.

References

American Gaming Association. (1998). *Responsible gaming resource guide.* 2nd edition. Washington, DC: Author.

Lesieur, H. R., Cross, J., Frank, M., Welch, M., White, C. M., Rubenstein, G., Mosely, K., & Mark, M. (1991). Gambling and pathological gambling among university students. *Addictive Behaviors, 16,* 517–27.

Vey, Michael. (2000, June). Wait until you're 21. *Wildwood Catholic High School Newsletter,* p. 3.

Chapter Ten

A Personal View from the Gaming Industry

Recognizing a Problem, Working Toward a Solution

Tom Brosig

An update on the progress made since this article was written in 1995–1996 is found at the conclusion of the chapter.

I wrote this chapter for two reasons. First, I am from the gaming industry, and I believe the industry can do a great deal to help prevent youth gambling problems. Second, I have taken a proactive posture regarding the gaming industry's response to problem-gambling issues involving young people and adults. I represent the new wave gaming executive, that is, one who does not have a long history working in the industry and who has taken steps to prevent problem gambling. In addition, my company's casino operations are located in regions not typically known to allow such enterprises, such as Mille Lacs and Hinckley in northern Minnesota, Gulfport and Biloxi in Mississippi, and Marksville and Kinder in Louisiana.

In the following sections, I tell how I became involved in the North American Think Tank on Youth Gambling Issues and discuss why initiatives of this type are important to the contemporary gaming industry. Some gaming industry executives have remained independent of social policy and research activities. In this chapter, I will demonstrate why that posture must change.

Background

I work for Grand Casinos Inc., which is headquartered in Minneapolis, Minnesota. Founded in 1991, the company now has more than ten thousand employees, operates six casinos in three states, and is constructing two additional casino resort properties. Our growth has been nothing short of phenomenal. In April 1995, we were identified by *Fortune* as the fastest growing company in America. If the company had selected Las Vegas as the location for its first casino, its arrival—and the five hundred new jobs it created—would have had little impact on that gambling mecca. In northern Minnesota, however, the opening of the first Grand Casino, in Mille Lacs, dramatically affected the communities within a forty-mile radius of the facility. This operation became responsible for a significant economic boom within the region, with similar results for the regions surrounding each of the other Grand Casinos. Yet not all of the effects of a new casino are positive. Our company's founders were experienced with community issues surrounding new casino development. Therefore, it was only natural for our company to face problems and controversies head-on. The problems associated with compulsive and underage gambling represent two of the issues that Grand Casinos Inc. has confronted and continues to confront directly.

My first exposure to problem gambling occurred during the summer of 1991, just three months after our first casino opened. I spent quite a bit of time on the casino floor in those early days. During that time, I began to notice some of the same faces again and again; these people were spending considerable amounts of time in the casino. I noticed that some of these people were poorly dressed and drove old cars, yet they would spend a great deal of time gambling. My initial attempts to slow their gambling habits were clumsy at best and generally ineffective. For example, I remember spending hours with tribal leaders discussing whether Native Americans living on or near the casino grounds would be at higher risk for developing compulsive gambling patterns. After all, there is a high incidence of alcohol abuse among this population, and some research has hinted there might be a high crossover rate among addictive behaviors. This possibility concerned me and the other executives at Grand Casinos Inc.

These initial concerns convinced us to seek advice from a professional in the field of compulsive gambling research, prevention, and treatment. Consequently, I called Betty George, executive director of the North American Training Institute (formerly, the Minnesota Council on Compulsive Gambling), and asked her to present a seminar to our executive staff. We wanted to educate our staff regarding the characteristics and attributes associated with compulsive gambling, expose them to the dramatic negative effects a gambling disorder has on personal lives, and educate them about the various stages of problem gambling. Finally, as a gaming company, we wanted to determine exactly what we could do to prevent gambling problems. We wanted to behave responsibly and do the right thing. However, we were unsure of what, exactly, the "right thing" was.

Observations from the Floor: Vignettes of Compulsive Gambling

Some of the seemingly illogical behavior we witnessed regularly made the feeling of uncertainty especially acute. There was that early Saturday morning in our Hinckley casino, for example, when a middle-aged woman sat down at one of our $25 minimum bet tables. She purchased chips worth $250 and began to play. Over the course of the day, she accumulated between $25,000 and $30,000 of net profit on the original $250 she put at risk. Yet the woman showed no signs of pocketing the winnings. Instead, she continued to play until, some twelve hours after she had started, she left broke. She had not preserved even the initial $250.

There was the 18-year-old high school senior who was an honor student and model athlete with a full college scholarship. Because he could not win at gambling, but also could not stop, he went from being a potential star athlete at a Midwestern university to being a criminal. After he lost all his money, the young man stole his parents' credit cards and burglarized some cabins near the casino. He ended up in jail. It was the blackjack dealer at the Hinckley casino who brought attention to this student, getting him away from the tables and out of the casino. Unfortunately, this stricture came too late.

The tragic story of this young man was the subject of a newscast video that I subsequently used to raise funds for gambling education programs. This story was particularly effective as a fundraiser, because the video depicted the young man as a "perfect kid." When I pleaded with executives to support the cause of gambling education and research, I sensed they were thinking that if this tragedy could happen to this kid from an upper-middle-class family, it certainly could happen to anyone—maybe even their own children.

By now, most people have heard of tragedies associated with excessive gambling. Yet I have witnessed thousands of people who enjoy casino gambling as a form of entertainment. I know there are more people who have a good time gambling than those who gamble themselves into ruin. From my observations, I know there are more people gambling responsibly than irresponsibly. These observations, by the way, directly parallel the justifications used by executives when discussing the negative aspect of businesses in which addictive ramifications surface.

I have been told, for example, that there are far more people who drink responsibly than people who drink irresponsibly. Similarly, I have been told that eating disorders affect only a small percentage of people, and we do not challenge a restaurant's right to exist even if thousands are affected by eating disorders. No one—at least not yet—is asking restaurants to bear the cost of dietary treatment for intemperate eaters. Bar owners are not asked to subsidize the cost of alcohol dependence. Yet today's prevailing public opinion is that casino operators are culpable for the problems and costs associated with their business. Some casino operators argue that gambling should not be treated differently from these other activities; they argue that gambling addiction affects only a small percentage of the total number of people who visit the casinos. I did not accept this logic when I first heard it in 1991, and I do not accept it today. I believe that the gaming industry must become more proactive in how it approaches gambling-related disorders.

Early Exposure to Facts

When I first called the North American Training Institute for information and educational materials in 1991, Betty George was surprised to receive such a request from a casino company executive. The seminar she presented began a relationship that culminated in progressive efforts by both our firms to better understand and prevent gambling-related problems. Many positive consequences emerged from our company's initial exposure to formal information about gambling addiction. In addition to raising awareness levels among employees and the community, this early education about gambling addiction lead to two tangible benefits. First, we were able to make more employees aware of binge cycles and how these cycles affect compulsive gamblers. Second, we developed brochures publicizing the "hotline" help number where support could be found.

Although the Grand Casino team was composed of experienced executives from the gaming industry, our core management team was recruited primarily from a variety of nongaming enterprises—principally retail and hospitality enterprises. Thus, it was necessary for us to address, head-on, the problems our industry created. I continued to pursue educational and consultative information about gambling problems for Grand Casino. During this time, I made three important discoveries. First, I realized that the majority of gaming operators never discussed the problems associated with pathological gambling. Rather, I found that the gaming industry took an "out of sight, out of mind" posture. Of course, there were exceptions. For example, Promus Companies, which owns Harrah's casinos, was very progressive and forthright about the issue of problem gambling. As industry pioneers on this issue, Promus has fought a lonely and mostly uphill battle. We decided that Grand Casinos Inc. needed to make the commitment to be at least as progressive as the Promus Companies.

The second discovery was that media representatives, legislators, and researchers consistently and narrowly defined the gambling industry as merely the casino operators. Charitable and church-sponsored bingo parlors had no culpability, at least from the public's perspective. The large numbers of state-run lotteries also had no culpability for gambling-related problems. I was shocked to hear state legislators—from states operating sizable lottery operations themselves—chastise casino operators while casting a blind eye toward their own state's compulsive-gambling issues. Once again, there are exceptions to this observation; the Massachusetts State Lottery, for example, has done fine work in this area with the assistance of the Massachusetts Council on Compulsive Gambling.

Finally, I discovered that recognition of the addiction issues existed only in relation to adult gambling; gambling problems associated with youths were never meaningfully addressed. Armed with new information, Grand Casinos Inc. would have liked nothing better than to divert sufficient management time and financial resources to pursue these issues. However, in 1991 neither the time nor the resources were available. Sadly, our newfound information and plans to act on it were put on hold.

Taking the First Steps

Unfortunately, the aggressive Grand Casinos expansion program overshadowed our interests in the area of compulsive and underage gambling. Despite our inability at that time to implement a comprehensive program to address these problems, we diligently followed the guidelines we learned from Betty George and others, implementing subtle safeguards to protect patrons from themselves. We set a limit, for example, on how much money a person could be advanced on any one visit to our casino. We decided that $1,000 would be the maximum cash accessible during a twenty-four-hour period, either by cashing a check or getting an advance on a credit card. We rationalized that if we limited someone's cash access, there would be a safeguard to prevent that person from losing more money than he or she could readily afford. At a minimum, we believed, the time it would take to leave the casino to get more cash might serve as a buffer that could break a "binge" cycle. Although we had no way of being certain whether this strategy was an effective deterrent to the addicted gambler, we sensed that it could help.

We also asked our training and employee development staff to work with the North American Training Institute to create formalized programs that could be taught to all Grand Casino employees. We made sure our employees knew of our concerns for the addicted gambler. The employees knew explicitly that management did not endorse an ideology of profit at any cost. We also aggressively validated the age of our younger guests. We publicized the fact that if someone under the age of 18 or 21 (depending upon the state in which the casino operated) did sneak in, he or she could never win, because jackpot payoffs require age checks. In retrospect, none of these efforts seems sufficient, yet they were revolutionary to the majority who worked in the gambling industry.

The Industry's Posture and the Health-Care System

Since these early efforts in 1991, I have come to understand the gaming industry's posture and health care providers' system of response to gambling problems. With the exception of a few companies or states, the gaming industry—using the broad definition of the industry I introduced earlier in the chapter—has remained noticeably silent on the issue of compulsive gambling. It is strange that an industry noted for innovation and aggressiveness has yet to make a focused effort to deal candidly and openly with the issues surrounding gambling addiction. Perhaps even more important is the observation that as this book goes to press, the gaming industry has no immediate plans to take a position on compulsive gambling.

The health-care community is not as coordinated and efficient as I originally had perceived it to be. The more I looked beyond the surface, the more disorganized things seemed to be. In Minnesota, for example, some of the money earned through the operation of the state's lottery had been earmarked, through legislation, for programs that provided public education on compulsive gambling—but when I tried, I could not identify anyone who had a clear idea about how to access these funds. Even worse, when someone did learn how to access these funds, bureaucrats put up so many roadblocks that no single agency could qualify to receive the funds.

There were, however, many organizations soliciting money from gaming operators. Consequently, Grand Casinos and other casino operators became the funding path of least resistance. As the then-president of what was quickly becoming a high-profile gaming company, I was overwhelmed with funding requests. As I evaluated requests, I noticed a redundancy and duplication of effort by the caregivers who were asking for resources. There seemed to be a multiplicity of perspectives on the who, what, when, where, and how. In short, there did not appear to be an overall plan for addressing the problem of compulsive gambling. Programs attempting to respond to the needs of problem gamblers were fragmented at best.

With these observations in mind, I once again called Betty George at the North American Training Institute and asked her to organize a symposium to discuss these concerns. We decided that this symposium should be attended by all of the stakeholders in the issue. It was not long, however, before we both realized that the list of prospective participants was rather extensive. Hosting a meeting of this magnitude would be not only costly but unwieldy as well.

The Minnesota Public Policy Think Tank

The idea of a Minnesota think tank emerged as a solution to our dilemma. The framework would be a comprehensive two- or three-day symposium attended by a limited, yet diverse, group of representative stakeholders. We assembled leaders from the various public- and private-sector segments who had something to gain or lose as a result of the potential and real problems associated with compulsive gambling. We focused on developing a collaborative process and settling our differences on the front end of this process.

There were many in the field of treatment who viewed gaming operators as a cross between their worst nightmare and the capitalistic purveyors of social destruction. Similarly, there were gaming operators who perceived treatment professionals as groping, unfocused, and searching for ongoing aid simply to perpetuate their own programs. While both perspectives were exaggerations, these views represented very real obstacles to progress.

The North American Training Institute took responsibility for organizing and facilitating the think tank, and I raised the funding to host the event. At that time in my career, I was too busy to solicit funds door to door, I simply put the "touch" on a few vendors (e.g., Pepsi-Cola, Monarch Foods, and Miller Schroeder Financial Services), and they, along with Grand Casinos Inc., provided the $45,000 necessary to support this event.

Held on two separate days in late 1993 and early 1994, the Minnesota Public Policy Think Tank was a success. The forum focused attention on youth gambling as the gambling problem most in danger of growing into a national catastrophe. Slowly but surely, the idea of an international think tank that would be focused solely on youth gambling issues began to emerge.

Personal Observations on the North American Think Tank

There are times when the anticipation of an event is so great that the reality cannot match the expectation. The Super Bowl game, for example, usually does not live up to the pregame hype. I was concerned that this would happen to the think tank as well. I can honestly say, however, that it lived up to expectations.

Early in the proceedings at the think tank, I wondered if I had made the correct decision by attending. As an executive and business professional, I am used to working in an environment with clear delineation of authority where protocols are understood and the decision-making process is apparent. This was not the case at the think tank. Quite frankly, I found it difficult to function in this unfamiliar environment. Diverse groups had gathered; but by meeting at the Harvard Medical School, their power bases had been neutralized. Instead, power was distributed, and compromise emerged quickly. The participants' focus on the youth gambling issue became the groups' common bond. Eventually, I stopped being so defensive and began to listen to the many perspectives represented by the participants. With all the egos "checked at the door," progress became possible. I believe the think tank's final report[1] reveals the diversity of the input and the give-and-take that went into the process. What I experienced at the think tank made me a better executive. I only wish more gaming executives would take the first step and open their minds to alternate perspectives.

The Gambling Addiction Industry[2]

As I became more aware of gambling addiction, I learned of the National Council on Compulsive Gambling and decided to attend its eighth annual conference, in Seattle. This experience was both enlightening and disappointing: It was enlightening to meet so many people from across the nation who were dedicated to this cause, and it was disappointing because the effort appeared to lack coordination and focus. Maybe my expectations were too lofty and I was naïve about the inherent complexities of trying to address the issues associated with such a broad-based problem.

As I planned to attend the National Conference on Gambling Behavior, I looked forward to exchanging ideas about gambling addiction with some of the gaming industry's key executives as well as with prevention specialists and caregivers. I was somewhat anxious about attending, and I wondered if I would have to defend Grand Casinos from accusations that it had not been proactive enough in the area of gambling addiction during its first three years of existence. I did not have to worry, however, because other than Promus, which was well represented, there were no other gaming executives present at the conference. Needless to say, I wondered why.

Like any other executive, when something good happens within my industry, I feel pride, and when something bad happens, I feel troubled. While in Seattle, I felt shame for the gaming industry. Before getting into the particulars, I would first like to commend Promus for its proactive stance on the issue of gambling addiction. Promus, along with Caesar's, provided financial support for the Eighth National Conference on Gambling Behavior. The company also conducted an interesting session on the role of casino operators in the prevention and treatment of compulsive gambling. It was gratifying to know that despite the lack of involvement by other gaming operators in this conference, Promus had provided a starting point for the rest of us.

Despite the respect I felt for Promus and Caesar's, other dynamics surrounding this industry continued to confound me. For example, the leaders of the gaming industry have been quick to seize opportunities present in new gaming jurisdictions to secure gaming sites. They have driven local land values to levels only dreamed of by the landowners. Yet this initiative and entrepreneurial vision has not been applied to solving the problems of compulsive and youth gambling.

Research indicates that roughly 5 percent of the adult population experiences some form of gambling problem (Volberg, 1996). As an industry, we have to acknowledge this fact and take responsibility for educating our customers, our employees, and lawmakers. Our message should be that responsible gambling is entertaining and that irresponsible gambling is destructive. As an industry executive, I believe this message is simply good business.

The gaming industry is often attacked for things over which it has little control. A few gaming companies have taken action and confronted the issues; unfortunately, others have elected to stay on the sidelines. It is time for the gaming industry to initiate responsible action, rather than to simply react to legislative mandates—usually a less effective and more costly approach. Other industries (state lotteries, organizers of horse racing, and the banking and insurance sectors, to name a few) that are negatively affected by the destruction wrought by an intemperate gambler should join forces with casino operators to educate the public in general and customers in particular.

I do not want to imply that, except for Promus and Caesar's, gaming operators do not support prevention programs. The Minnesota Indian Gaming Association, for example, recently received a national award for its efforts to prevent gambling problems, and gaming operators from the Mississippi Gulf Coast initiated a statewide think tank to develop a blueprint for the prevention and treatment of gambling addiction. These organizations, along with gaming operators from Tunica County, Mississippi, and representatives of the Mississippi banking and insurance industries, provided support for the North American Think Tank on Youth Gambling Issues, which stimulated the publication of this book. Mississippi, the newest of the country's major gaming markets, is leading the effort and deserves to be congratulated. This chapter should serve as a challenge to the gaming associations in Nevada, New Jersey, and elsewhere to join Mississippi and assist in prevention and education regarding gambling problems. It is the right thing to do.

Conclusion

In this chapter, I have outlined the history of Grand Casinos' involvement in efforts to prevent problem and youth gambling. Our concerns about problem gambling began with observations in our own casinos and in the communities surrounding them. Despite our concerns and our consultation with the North American Training Institute, our early efforts were limited. However, as our awareness of problem gambling grew, so did our dedication to prevent these problems. This dedication resulted in our role in the Minnesota Public Policy Think Tank and our ongoing collaboration with the North American Training Institute. In addition, our concern regarding youth gambling contributed to the founding of the National Advisory Board on Youth Gambling Issues and resulted in our involvement in the North American Think Tank on Youth Gambling Issues. The advisory board and the think tank promise to change the way policy, research, prevention, treatment, and funding regarding youth gambling issues are conducted.

Over the years, casino gambling has spread from Las Vegas and Atlantic City to diverse and far-flung regions of the country; state-sponsored gambling has spread at a similarly rapid pace. This expansion has created benefits for the gaming industry as well as the communities within which new gaming ventures are located. However, the expansion of gambling has also had negative effects, including increased youth gambling and increased compulsive gambling. As the expansion of commercial gaming continues, it will be vitally important that all members of the gambling industry, including casino corporations, Native American tribes, state governments, and parimutuel gaming organizations, recognize and address these problems. Now that strong connections have been established among members of the gaming industry, researchers, treatment providers, and policymakers, we have the opportunity to make unprecedented steps toward preventing problem gambling.

An Update from the Editors

Many dramatic and productive developments have occurred in the commercial casino industry since this article was written, thanks in large part to Tom Brosig and other enlightened casino operators, and through the activities of the industry's newly created trade association, the American Gaming Association (AGA). Brosig permitted us to include his candid assessment of the industry *at that time* (1995–1996) if we would also provide an update of the changes that have taken place.

Brosig, Philip Satre, and a few others were at the forefront of the industry's response to problem gambling. Their efforts were strengthened and expanded when the AGA, shortly after opening its doors in 1995, made a policy decision to address problem and underage gambling. As a first step, the AGA asked Brosig and others to join an industry task force on responsible gaming. Since its inception, that task force has worked to encourage the establishment of industrywide responsible gaming practices through the following activities:

- Developed and adopted comprehensive voluntary responsible gaming guidelines for problem and underage gambling as well as advertising and marketing guidelines and unattended minors guidelines through a unique collaboration with the National Center for Missing and Exploited Children;
- Spearheaded a responsible gaming national education campaign to increase awareness of this issue among employees and the public through various activities;
- Conducted numerous national seminars on problem gambling and responsible gaming; and
- Developed comprehensive tool kits, including sample brochures and posters, as well as training curricula, to help casino companies implement customized responsible gaming public awareness and employee education programs.

To encourage a better understanding of the causal factors related to problem gambling, Brosig assisted the AGA in founding the National Center for Responsible Gaming (NCRG) in 1996 to fund research on underage and pathological gambling. Twenty-two gaming companies and one foundation have committed more than $7 million to the NCRG. Since it was founded, the NCRG has awarded nineteen grants totaling nearly $2.6 million to respected universities and medical research centers such as Harvard Medical School, Washington University School of Medicine, and Massachusetts General Hospital.

While the casino industry itself is actively promoting responsible gaming initiatives at the corporate and property levels, several state regulatory bodies have implemented requirements related to responsible gaming practices. The Nevada Gaming Commission approved a regulation that requires casinos to provide written materials concerning the nature of problem gambling and the toll-free telephone number of an approved problem gambling help line; implement procedures and training for all employees who directly interact with gaming patrons; and implement a self-limitation program for customers who wish to limit their access to the issuance of credit, check-cashing, or direct-mail marketing.

Aside from making certain requirements of licensees, many states have taken measures to ensure there is adequate funding for treatment and education programs. Indiana, Iowa, Louisiana, Michigan, Missouri, and New Jersey are among the states that have enacted a tax, assessment, or other contribution to create a dedicated fund for the development and support of prevention, education, and treatment programs.

Finally, Brosig provided the original funding and support for the first broad-based health prevalence study among gaming industry employees in Mississippi. This groundbreaking research, which has now been expanded to include employees in other gaming jurisdictions, will help casino managers structure health promotion, education, and prevention programs.

Brosig remains active in his efforts to promote a better understanding of pathological gambling. He currently serves on the board of the Gaming Entertainment Research and Education Foundation that oversees the NCRG, and he continues to provide financial support to the organization. He is now the president of the mid-south region for Park Place Entertainment Corporation.

Notes

1. Readers interested in learning more about the North American Think Tank on Youth Gambling Issues should refer to the appendix, "The North American Think Tank on Youth Gambling Issues: A Blueprint for Responsible Public Policy in the Management of Compulsive Gambling."

2. Portions of this section were adapted from "Awakened," published originally in the September 1994 issue of the *Grogan Report*.

References

Volberg, R. A. (1996, July). *Gambling and problem gambling in New York: A 10-year replication survey, 1986–1996*. Roaring Spring, PA: Gemini Research.

Chapter Eleven

Social Policy and Youth Gambling
Perspectives from the Public Sector

Joseph D. Malone and Eric M. Turner

> *This chapter presents two special perspectives on gambling. During his two terms as the treasurer of the Commonwealth of Massachusetts (1991–1999), Joseph D. Malone also served as chairman of the Massachusetts State Lottery Commission.[1] Eric M. Turner served as the executive director of the Massachusetts State Lottery from November 1991 to October 1995. Together, they directed the most successful state-run gaming organization in the United States. They are both concerned about gambling and its potential effects on the youth of Massachusetts and the nation. This chapter reflects their personal perspectives on the nature of gambling and the complex issues that influence state lotteries.*

A View from the Treasurer's Office: Joseph D. Malone

I come from a blue-collar community, and my background has had a significant effect on how I view problem gambling. For example, I remember a specific instance, shortly after leaving high school, in which a young man I had known since grammar school abruptly left the state. He had incurred about $20,000 of debt from gambling and apparently saw no other option than leaving the state for his own safety. My schoolmate left in 1974. The next time I saw him was in 1994. At that point, he finally felt it was safe to come back home. During his absence, some of his family— he is one of ten children—had gone to visit him in California. Essentially, however, excessive gambling forced him to remain disconnected from his family during these years. In effect, he was out of control at an age when he lacked the necessary knowledge about the potentially dangerous activity in which he was engaging.

I also encountered gambling through my father's small trucking business. Every day, as far back as I can remember, a man who sold sandwiches from a catering truck would arrive, and the mechanics, bookkeeper, and other personnel would go out to buy their food. At my young age I was not sure what else they were doing, but I do remember the caterer writing down numbers and taking money in exchange for these numbers. Of course, this exchange represents the old style of running a lottery. Over time, I developed mixed emotions on this subject, realizing that prohibition certainly was not working. It seems that people will look for ways to vent their urge to gamble, and if there is not some legal way to satisfy that urge, there will be some sort of criminally organized way of doing so.

As chairman of the Massachusetts State Lottery Commission, I was in a very awkward position. Whenever I talked about my concerns about gaming and young people, there was a voice in my mind that said, "Joe, you oversee a $2.5 billion lottery. Sixty-five percent of the adults in Massachusetts play that lottery regularly." The message I received from the government is that the lottery should raise more money each year. In fiscal year 1994, the lottery generated $662 million in funds that the state distributed. About $442 million went to cities and towns, and the remaining $220 million went to state government.

Each year, as we went through our budget process, the folks who put the budget together would say, "Gee, revenues are tight. How are we going to get more money out of the lottery?" During 1991, the first year I was treasurer of the commonwealth, we thought informing the public of our accomplishments was a positive thing to do. We decided to tell people at regular intervals what had happened with the lottery during a recent period.

I remember the first such press conference announcing that lottery sales were essentially flat during the first six months of that year. Reporters responded by saying, "The cities and towns (primary beneficiaries of lottery profits) are depending on this money. What are you doing wrong? Your predecessor was always able to make the lottery grow." Six months later, lottery sales had increased, and those same reporters said, "You are exploiting people! What is the deal here? How do you sleep at night?" So, serving as chairman of a state lottery placed me in a very difficult position.

I congratulate the participants in the North American Think Tank on Youth Gambling Issues for the work they are doing. I wish I could say that after eight years in office I figured out this whole subject, but I have not done so yet. However, I do think the picture is becoming somewhat clearer. What the State Lottery Commission and its staff have been trying to do is find a way to manage the lottery's growth at a reasonable level while providing the necessary resources for compulsive gamblers who require treatment. We are also looking for ways to inform young people of the perils of gambling beyond moderation so that they do not get themselves into trouble.

One method that has proved helpful is the implementation of a program throughout Massachusetts schools, called "Saving Makes 'Cents,'" that emphasizes the importance of saving. We have stressed that people ought to achieve their

"American dream" through hard work and saving, as opposed to trying to strike it rich quickly through a lottery or similar device.

We started this program in 1994 in eleven schools, with the involvement of eleven local banks. Every two weeks a teller from one of the banks goes into the participating school to accept children's deposits into savings accounts, established without minimum balance requirements. In addition, the children learn the ABCs of our economic system so that they understand what mortgages, interest, and checking accounts are and how they work. They learn that on a per capita basis the Japanese save seven times as much as we do in the United States, and Germans save four and a half times as much. Other topics that we teach include the basics of budgeting and general financial decision making.

This project has grown from the original 11 schools and banks to include more than 400 schools and 175 banks. The biggest kick of all I get from my job is going into these elementary schools and seeing the satisfaction these children receive from having their own bankbooks and seeing their savings grow.

Another step was our effort to convey our seriousness about cracking down on those among our 8,000 retailer sales agents who sell lottery tickets to minors. In 1994, for the first time in the history of the Massachusetts lottery, we began suspending agents who were caught selling to minors.

In addition to these two steps, we started to display the toll-free telephone number for problem gamblers at the end of our new weekly television game show. An accompanying message suggests that if the viewer or someone the viewer knows has a gambling problem, he or she should call the number, which is staffed by the Massachusetts Council on Compulsive Gambling.

We also established an ad hoc committee on which Dr. Howard Shaffer, director of the Division on Addictions at Harvard Medical School, and Thomas Cummings, executive director of the Massachusetts Council on Compulsive Gambling, provided input on a continuing basis so that we could constantly refine our ideas. This committee, which also included a local police chief, a high school principal, a high school student, a priest, and a community activist, represented people from different walks of life, an attribute that proved tremendously valuable in helping come up with some answers. Although we did not have all the answers, I think the commitment to address this challenge was very important.

When I took office in 1991, the state was spending $13 million a year promoting the lottery. The advertising budget was reduced to $2.5 million for fiscal year 1995 and was further reduced to $400,000 for fiscal year 1996. In addition, advertisements were limited to point-of-sale promotions. Initially, this change was the result of our own initiative; later, legislative action directed the reduction in spending. The real dilemma, however, emerged when legislators and the governor would say, "Well, we need this much money because we need to meet our revenue demands. Therefore, maybe we should increase our advertising a little bit more."

The rationale for creating the lottery was that since organized crime was running lotteries anyway, why not have the government do it and use the proceeds for a good cause instead of letting the money go to illicit purposes? What was not discussed during the whole debate over whether the state should run a lottery was that the government would need to be tugging on the sleeves of the citizens of the state— and, as a by-product, on the sleeves of minors—and telling them: "This is how you can strike it rich. Just go out there and put one more dollar down and you are sure to be a winner next time. And God help you if you bet on Monday, Tuesday, and Wednesday, but not on Thursday, because Thursday is probably the night your number will be drawn." We were perpetually wrestling with the pressures to raise more money. At the same time, we did not want to do the sleeve pulling that is necessary to expand this activity. It remains unclear how policymakers will resolve this dilemma.

We ran the best lottery in the country in terms of operating efficiency. Approximately 2.5 percent of our gross sales went toward overhead; 8 percent is the national average for lotteries. Yet even though we felt our efficiency should have given us some credibility, our advice would go unheeded when we would go to the legislature, whether to say that the Massachusetts Council on Compulsive Gambling ought to get more money so that it could assist more people, or to say that keno, video poker, and other forms of gaming were not in the best interests of the citizens of the state.

We went through this debate almost every year I was in office. What strikes me as interesting, but also very dangerous, is that when I walked into the legislative hearing room to provide testimony, there were people who sold video poker machines, there were people who ran racetracks, there were lobbyists, there was a host of people who had particular vested interests in seeing these proposals advance; but there were few, if any, average citizens in that room telling the other side of the story.

Consequently, many lawmakers felt that there were a lot of people twisting their arms for support. In addition, lawmakers felt pressure to raise money for organizations that ran state-funded programs. When the time came to prepare the state's budget and there was not enough revenue to fund all of the state programs, some group had to be told that a program it considered important had to be cut or could not grow at the rate the group might have liked. Many states have seen gambling as a solution to budget problems and have justified it on the grounds that it is a "painless tax." The belief is that nobody is really going to get hurt from gambling, but this belief leads to the idea that we can get more revenues and pay for those programs by having just a little bit more gambling.

I foresee this situation continuing. As we look down the road, I think we are going to see that other sources of revenue are not available to meet budgetary needs. Instead, most states will continue to settle for this easy way out.

In Massachusetts, we fought off video gaming successfully for some time, but keno was legalized more than ten years ago. Now communities are asking, "Do we really want keno in a restaurant where kids walk in with their families? Do we really want keno in a convenience store where a child might go in to buy a candy bar or soft drink and see adults standing around waiting for numbers to be drawn every five minutes?"

My preference was to draw the line, to say that enough was enough, and just keep the lottery, which had already been part of the state's culture for twenty-two years. I think that if you had asked citizens throughout Massachusetts, for the most part they would have concurred. But unfortunately, it becomes a case in which a small group of people who are not necessarily interested in the greater, long-term good of the Commonwealth of Massachusetts drove hard to meet their own objectives.

One of the rationalizations offered is that the expansion of gambling is inevitable: "Every other state in New England is going to have these forms of gambling, and our citizens are going to visit those states anyway. So we may as well get it now and move on and live our lives." I do not accept that argument. I think lobbyists are selling that kind of message.

I congratulate the participants in the North American Think Tank on Youth Gambling Issues and commend them for this effort. The best thing we all can do is to communicate to those people who are involved in the budget-making side of government that more gambling and more revenue through gambling are not necessarily the solutions to the people's problems. What we need to do is to get back to sound fiscal management. We need to make governments more efficient and more effective and, by so doing, make people's "American dream" more attainable instead of saying we are going to take shortcuts.

Once young people hear that gambling is good, that is, gambling balances budgets, gambling is a winner for the people, gambling helps pay for programs, it will be difficult for adults to convince young people that gambling in fact has the potential to be very, very bad. When a young person sees churches running bingo parlors, how is he or she supposed to distinguish between good and bad gambling? We have a big challenge.

A Personal View from the Executive Director's Office: Eric M. Turner

April 6, 1995, marked the twenty-third anniversary of the Massachusetts State Lottery and the beginning of the North American Think Tank on Youth Gambling Issues. I am very pleased with this coincidence. Given some of the projects the lottery initiated around this time, I hope that we are embarking on a new era for both the organization and the Commonwealth of Massachusetts.

Like Treasurer Joe Malone, I was influenced by my background on issues related to gambling. When I was offered the opportunity to head the Massachusetts State Lottery, I was a bit reluctant to do so. I am the product of a devoutly Catholic mother and strongly Baptist father. In fact, my father was the son and grandson of Baptist ministers from Mississippi. Because my father was deceased at the time I was offered the position, I was able to consult only my mother regarding the decision to become the executive director of the Massachusetts State Lottery. To my surprise, she encouraged me to accept the offer, pointing out that without church-sponsored bingo, she might not have received early education in rural, then-segregated Louisiana. I often wonder what my father's opinion would have been.

Mixed personal feelings toward gambling reflect the same debate the larger society is now experiencing. Personal attitudes provide a great deal of perspective to managing an operation like the lottery in a responsible fashion. In this case, I believe that personal attitudes provide the foundation on which to build a healthy willingness to address concerns associated with problem gambling.

Approximately two-thirds of the adult population of Massachusetts play the lottery on a regular basis, that is, four to five times each month. This is an astounding statistic. Weekly per capita spending on lottery games in the state was more than $8.80 during the time I was executive director of the lottery. Although this figure does not account for the undetermined portion of lottery revenue from out-of-state sources, the conclusion is that substantial spending on lottery offerings occurs within Massachusetts. The lottery is very much a part of the fabric of life within the Commonwealth of Massachusetts.

As in most states, minors are prohibited from purchasing lottery tickets in Massachusetts. Yet immediately following this purchasing prohibition, the Massachusetts State Lottery's enabling legislation contains language allowing minors to be given lottery tickets as gifts. Therefore, minors may be restricted from purchasing lottery tickets, but they are not restricted from playing those chances or from winning. Young people in the state do take advantage of this provision.

At the Massachusetts State Lottery, we were shocked and stunned when we learned of the prevalence of underage gambling and gambling-related problems revealed by research conducted in Massachusetts (e.g., Shaffer, 1994; Shaffer, Hall, Walsh, & Vander Bilt, 1995; Shaffer, LaBrie, Scanlan, & Cummings, 1994; Shaffer, Stein, Gambino, & Cummings, 1989). As a result of this information, we initiated a variety of actions. We embarked on a new era of awareness and responsibility at the lottery. The following section outlines some of the specific actions we took relating to youth gambling.

THE MASSACHUSETTS LOTTERY: INITIATIVES FOR YOUTH

Prior to the implementation of the advertising reduction mentioned above by Treasurer Malone, we modified the content of lottery promotion. We attempted to focus this advertising more on the informational aspects of the games and much less on "enticements." While some may consider this a slight adjustment, we believe that this shift represents a meaningful change in both the substance and symbolism of lottery advertising.

In another initiative, we used Ernie DiGregorio, a former college and professional star basketball player, in a series of appearances aimed at youthful audiences. DiGregorio was an All-American basketball player at Providence College who went on to play for the Boston Celtics. He was named National Basketball Association Rookie of the Year in 1974. We enlisted DiGregorio to visit summer youth camps to deliver the message that, in life, success comes to those who work hard—not to those who look for instant luck.

DiGregorio still shoots free throws in the 80 to 90 percent range, even with his eyes closed, and has a wonderful routine in which he plays against five youngsters at a time. After competing with several teams—and almost never losing a game—DiGregorio addresses the young people, speaking of his accomplishments in life. He describes how he succeeded at several different levels of competition without many of the natural abilities other athletes possessed. In a very effective way he points to heroes and everyday role models such as parents, indicating that their successes stem from planning and hard work rather than gambling and other "quick-fix" approaches. The objective of this initiative is to convey that substantially more people in society achieve success through hard work than through luck.

Another commonwealth initiative requires that all lottery retail locations display signs noting the toll-free number for the Massachusetts Council on Compulsive Gambling. Going a step further, the lottery uses these signs to include reminders that minors are barred from purchasing tickets. To convey the serious nature of this issue and our growing concern, we require Massachusetts State Lottery field representatives to monitor compliance among retailers.

Another initiative involves instant-ticket vending machines. Like many state lotteries, the Massachusetts State Lottery installed instant-ticket vending machines, approximately 1,200 devices statewide. Initially, approximately 100 machines were placed on a trial basis in non-age-controlled environments. However, these machines were unattended, so we decided to remove them from these environments. Even though we required that the machines be placed in the line of sight of retailer personnel, we decided to locate them only in age-controlled establishments as a matter of policy.

Joseph Malone described above that one of the lottery's greatest efforts has been to significantly increase the enforcement of the regulation prohibiting ticket sales to minors. Since the recent implementation of statewide spot checks by the Massachusetts State Lottery, the Lottery Commission has conducted numerous hearings resulting in warnings, probations, and suspensions of retailers in violation of this regulation. To the best of our knowledge, this is the first time in the history of the Massachusetts State Lottery that agents have been sanctioned for selling lottery products to minors. To further reinforce vendor awareness, when sanctions are taken against retailers, these proscriptions are published prominently in the lottery's newsletter, which is sent to all licensed retailers.

To increase awareness still more and to emphasize our priorities, we have revised the training the lottery provides to newly licensed retailers. This training now emphasizes the issues associated with youth purchases of lottery tickets. The concepts addressed in the initial version of these efforts somewhat resemble the concepts used in cigarette and alcohol sales training. For example, during these training sessions, we address the methods of identifying underage individuals and discuss what obligations exist for owners and staff who have direct contact with underage customers.

Finally, a large part of our effort to prevent youth-gambling problems resided in the level of knowledge and awareness that lottery staff, players, and the general public have about the issue of youth gambling. This awareness campaign will require a sustained and vigilant effort. However, there were a number of plans to address this challenge. In fact, during the time this volume was in preparation, we designated a full-time staff member to deal with problem gambling as it relates to the many different activities of the lottery. Part of this person's responsibility is to help the entire staff to examine these problems and deal with them as a routine part of their jobs. To the best of our knowledge, this was a first within the U.S. lottery "industry."

In "Youth Gambling: The Casino Industry's Response" (chap. 9), Phil Satre describes a number of positive steps that one casino has initiated to prevent youth gambling in that industry. The Massachusetts State Lottery is probably in the same position that company found itself in back in 1989. We have a commitment, but we also have a long way to go before we can incorporate into the fabric of community life many of the concepts that emerged from the North American Think Tank on Youth Gambling Issues. We look forward to meeting that challenge.

Conclusion

We hope this discussion of the social policies of the Massachusetts State Lottery provides insight into some of the issues influencing public gaming in America. We believe the lottery should take an active role in gambling education and the prevention of problem gambling. Although the primary mission of the lottery is to raise money for the cities and towns of the commonwealth, we take our responsibility to the community on other issues, such as underage gambling, very seriously.

Note

1. The executive director of the Massachusetts State Lottery reports to the five-member State Lottery Commission, composed of two appointees of the governor, the secretary of public safety, the state comptroller, and the treasurer, who serves as chairman of the commission.

References

Shaffer, H. J. (1994). *The emergence of youthful addiction: The prevalence of underage lottery use and the impact of gambling* (Technical Report No. 011394-100). Boston: Massachusetts Council on Compulsive Gambling.

Shaffer, H. J., Hall, M. N., Walsh, J. S., & Vander Bilt, J. (1995). The psychosocial consequences of gambling. In R. Tannenwald (Ed.), *Casino development: How would casinos affect New England's economy? Special report no. 2* (pp. 130–41). Boston: Federal Reserve Bank of Boston.

Shaffer, H. J., LaBrie, R., Scanlan, K. M., & Cummings, T. N. (1994). Pathological gambling among adolescents: Massachusetts Gambling Screen (MAGS). *Journal of Gambling Studies, 10,* 339–62.

Shaffer, H. J., Stein, S., Gambino, B., & Cummings, T. N. (Eds.). (1989). *Compulsive gambling: Theory, research, and practice.* Lexington, MA: Lexington Books.

Chapter Twelve

Adolescent Gambling Research
The Next Wave

Henry R. Lesieur

Introduction

Research on teen gambling is still in its infancy. Nevertheless, a body of knowledge is emerging, with its base in the United States and the United Kingdom. This chapter reviews that literature, examines the data lacunae existing in the field, and makes suggestions for the direction of future research. Surveys of teen gambling (including rates of gambling, expenditure, and gambling problems) are discussed in light of allegations of epidemic teen gambling, as well as teen betting-ring hysteria. Some researchers have investigated gambling among teens in the gambling setting itself, but these studies have been limited to the United Kingdom. This chapter emphasizes studies of problem gambling, the range of gambling problems, definitional issues, and related problems; it reviews research on prevention and treatment of problem gambling among teens and outlines areas of needed research as well as a more inclusive multifactorial model of inquiry.

Prevalence of Adolescent Gambling

Beginning with an Atlantic City study where researchers found that 64 percent of the high school students surveyed had gambled in the casinos (Arcuri, Lester, & Smith, 1985), interest in teen gambling has mushroomed in the United States and elsewhere. Following that research, Lesieur and Klein (1987) examined four New Jersey high schools and learned that 86 percent of the students had gambled in the past year and 91 percent had participated in various forms of gambling during their lifetime. More recently, researchers have uncovered high rates of teen gambling in other parts of the United States, including Washington (Volberg, 1993), Minnesota (Winters, Stinchfield, & Kim, 1995), and Massachusetts (Shaffer, LaBrie, Scanlan, &

Cummings, 1994). Perhaps the most extensive studies come from the United Kingdom, where approximately two-thirds of young teens have played "fruit machines" (the term used in the United Kingdom for slot machines), with 15 percent to 21 percent playing at least once a week (Evans, 1989; Fisher, 1993b, 1995; Ide-Smith & Lea, 1988; Waterman & Atkin, 1985). Fisher (1993b) found that gambling was nearly universal (a 99 percent prevalence rate) among 11- to 16-year-olds. The data on rates of teen gambling are summarized in table 12.1. These studies reveal that rates of weekly gambling range from 9 percent to 38 percent, with most between 14 percent and 24 percent, while the typical lifetime gambling rate hovered around 75 percent to 85 percent.

Who are the teen gamblers? Of all the variables examined, gender is the most salient. Every study reviewed agrees that males are more likely to gamble (Griffiths, 1989; Wallisch, 1993) and/or gamble more frequently (Fisher, 1993b) than females. This disparity is more evident during the teen years than adulthood, where the ratio for past-year gambling in 1992 was seven male gamblers to five females (Hugick & Saad, 1994).

Gambling Expenditures

Children gamble. How much they spend gambling is another matter. Reported figures fluctuate widely. Wallisch (1993) reports adolescent gamblers spending approximately $23 a year on average (calculated from grouped data), Winters and Stinchfield (1993) counted $28 a year in 1990 and $32 in 1991/92, while Volberg (1993) reports adolescents gambling $10 a month. What explains this disparity? Quite simply, expenditure disparities exist because different researchers frame the issue differently. Both Wallisch (1993) and Winters and Stinchfield (1993) asked the same global questions about the total amount bet in a year. Wallisch (1993) stated:

> Adolescents who had gambled at all during the past year were asked, "If you think about all the times you have bet money in the past 12 months, how much total money would you estimate you have bet during that time?" They were asked to respond using the following dollar categories: $0, $1–9, $10–19, $20–49, $50–99, $100–199, and $200 or more. (p. 15)

Volberg (1993) asked subjects how much money they spent in a typical month for each form of gambling, for example, lottery or card games. Volberg's $10 per month was obtained by totaling the typical monthly expenditures. Males spent more per month ($13) than females ($7).

While requesting dollar amounts for specific types of gambling is more specific than asking the question globally, assessing expenditure is tricky business. Expenditure can be estimated three ways: the amount of money put at risk, the net cost to the player, or the total volume of money gambled with, including money won and

Table 12.1 *Studies of Gambling Behavior Among Adolescents*

Researcher(s)	Report Publication Year	Location	Sample size	Youth Age Range	Gambling Lifetime (%)	Gambling Past Year (%)	Gambling Weekly (%)
Arcuri, Lester & Smith	1985	N.J.	332	9–12 grade	64.0[a]	—	9.0[a]
Amati	1984	India	136	7–16 yrs. (offenders)	68.0	—	39.0[b]
British Market Research[g]	1986	UK	1,451	15–19 yrs.	67.0	—	—
Decision Sciences	1993	Ore.	121	14–18 yrs.	88.0	—	—
Evans	1989	UK	9,752	13–16 yrs.	64.0[c]	—	15.0[c]
Fisher	1993b	UK	460	11–16 yrs.	99.0	99.0	20.0
Huff & Collinson	1987	UK	100 males	15–21 yrs. (offenders)	—	35.0[c]	24.0[c]
Huxley & Carroll	1992	UK	1,332	11–12 & 14–15 yrs.	40.0[c]	—	—
Ide-Smith & Lea	1988	UK	51	14–15 yrs.	89.0	—	—
Insight Canada Research	1994[f]	Ontario	400	12–19	—	65.0	10.0[d]
Jacobs et al.[e]	1985	Calif.	843	9–12 grade	20.0[d]	—	—
Jacobs et al.[e]	1987	Calif.	257	9–12 grade	45.0[d]	—	—
Ladouceur et al.	1994a	Québec	1,320	8–12 yrs. 4–6 grade	86.0	—	38.0
Ladouceur et al.	1994b	Québec	1,471	college students	90.0	—	22.0
Ladouceur & Mireault	1988	Québec	1,612	9–11 grade	76.0	65.0	24.0
Lesieur et al.	1991	5 states	1,771	college students	85.0	—	23.0

Lesieur & Klein	1987	N.J.	892	11–12 grade	91.0	86.0	32.0
Omnifacts Research	1993[f]	Nova Scotia	300	13–17 yrs.	61.0	—	—
Oster & Knapp	1994	Nevada 1992	544	under 21	92.0	—	22.0
Oster & Knapp	1994	Nevada 1994	350.00	under 21	91.0	—	24.0
Shaffer et al.	1994	Mass.	856.00	13–20 yrs.	75.0	—	—
Steinberg	1988[e]	Conn.	573	high school	69.0	—	—
Volberg	1993[f]	Wash.	1,054	13–17 yrs.	83.0	71.0	11.0
Waterman & Atkin	1985	UK	451	14–18 yrs.	79.0	—	9.0
Winters et al.	1990[f]	Minn.	1,094	15–18 yrs.	90.0	—	—
Winters et al.	1993b	Minn.	702	15–18 yrs.	86.0	—	19.0
Winters et al.	1995	Minn.	532	16–20 yrs.	—	—	16.0
Wallisch	1993[f]	Tex.	924	14–17 yrs.	79.0	66.0	14.0

[a] Casino gambling only.
[b] "Frequent gambling."
[c] Fruit machines only.
[d] This is a figure that is close to the highest for specific forms of gambling; actual figure for "any gambling" is definitely higher.
[e] Unpublished data reported in Jacobs, 1989.
[f] Government-funded reports, unpublished data.
[g] As cited in Griffiths (1989).

lost (the handle). For example, people who bring $50 to the racetrack and lose it all would say they bet $50. However, if they bet all $50 and win $25 of it back, they may return with $25. In this case, they have two different figures: the amount bet ($50) and the net loss ($25). To confuse things further, if they start with $50 and win $200 but they lose that as well, they might say they bet $250 in all (the handle). New research will have to inquire into estimations of money bet and money won or lost. In addition, it would be useful to have an idea of what percent of their total available funds these adolescents are spending.

Epidemic or Not?

The question of whether there is an epidemic of youth gambling is an important contemporary issue. Journalists (Bruner, 1989; Harrah's Casinos, 1995; Levine, 1990) cite researchers who find that the accessibility of gambling venues is related to an increase in teen gambling. This finding implies that there is an association between the incidence of gambling and gambling addiction. While this association intuitively makes sense, we cannot be certain of its accuracy without objective investigation.

The first study to examine changes in youth gambling over time was conducted in Minnesota (Winters, Stinchfield, & Kim, 1995). By examining 532 adolescents' gambling behavior at two periods, 18 months apart, Winters et al. found that certain forms of gambling (lotteries and casino gambling) increased, while others (betting on games of skill and bingo) decreased. However, there was no significant change in problem-gambling levels during this interval. It is unclear why these levels did not change; too little time between questioning, sampling error, counterbalancing factors taking hold, and an alternative explanation are all possibilities.

Winters, Stinchfield, and Kim (1995) examined the same group of adolescents over time. One would expect that the type of gambling they engaged in would change, and this change did indeed occur. However, more trend data similar to the "Monitoring the Future" studies funded by the National Institute on Drug Abuse is necessary (Johnston, O'Malley, & Bachman, 1992). In those yearly studies, a national sample of eighth, tenth, and twelfth graders, college students, and young adults is asked about attitudes and behavior related to drug use. Researchers have collected data on twelfth graders since 1975, while data on eighth and tenth graders were first collected in 1991. We will be able to address many of the questions concerning the increase of gambling only after completing a similar series of youth-gambling studies.

Betting-Ring Hysteria

Periodically, authorities uncover teenage betting rings (MacFarquhar, 1995; Misseck, 1994; Murphy, 1994). The implication in newspapers is that these "rings" have the backing of organized crime or are somehow instigated by organized crime. "The financial backers of these bookmaking rings see high school students as a low-risk investment, according to police" (Murphy, 1994, p. 34).

Whether outcries over betting rings are the ramblings of overzealous law enforcement officers or are accurate representations of reality remains an area for research. For example, Misseck reports, "In May 1992, another investigation had revealed that a number of students at Scotch Plains–Fanwood High School [New Jersey] were part of a gambling operation that had involved bets ranging from $2 to as much as $1,500. Investigators said two students had confessed to taking bets and inventing a 'bookie' contact in New York to scare their youthful bettors into paying off their debts" (1994, p. 14). In any event, researchers need to treat the relationship between organized crime and betting rings with a critical eye. Interview-based studies of illegal betting patterns among youths would prove extremely valuable here.

Teen Gambling: Ethnographic and Field Studies

While researchers have commented on teens who gamble, only two researchers—Sue Fisher and Mark Griffiths in the United Kingdom—have studied teens systematically within the gambling setting. The research output of these two is astounding, both in its ambition and productivity. Fisher presents a more complete ethnographic picture of the gambling setting than any other researcher to date.

Fisher (1993a) worked for fourteen months as a video arcade cashier in a seaside resort in southern England. Her typology of video players included the following characters:

Arcade Kings—invariably males in their late teens and early 20s who played with a quasiprofessional status only to maximize winnings, and passed on whatever skills they had.

Apprentices—boys 9 to 11 years old who were part of the Arcade King's group and acted as his slaves by fetching drinks, food, and so on.

Machine Beaters—gamblers who played alone and interacted with the machine. These players were unable to sustain the discipline to rationalize play. They enjoyed beating the game and their behavior often led to truancy, spending school dinner money, selling possessions, theft, self-deprecation, and remorse.

Rent-a-Spacers—predominantly teenage females who had no skills or interest in acquiring them. Those in this group liked being spectators and played to gain access to the arcade venue where they could meet and socialize with friends.

Action Seekers and Escape Artists—the former are drawn by the excitement and the thrill of winning money, while the latter sought to escape problems at home.

Ironically, in spite of evidence that age controls are not enforced adequately for casinos (Frank, 1990; Lesieur & Klein, 1987) and lottery ticket sales (Harshbarger, 1994; Radecki, 1994), there is no ethnographic field research on teen gambling in the United States. Research like Fisher's should be encouraged in North America. It is imperative that researchers conduct intensive interviews and ethnographic observations of teen gamblers. What is most important is a style of research that places teens within the context of social settings and social groups. While it is easier to do research among "captive" populations in schools and treatment facilities or in disembodied contexts like telephone interviews, research conducted in the field may prove to be fruitful and innovative.

The Range of Teen Gambling Problems

According to researchers, problematic gambling among teens involves some of the following characteristics: a sudden drop in school work, nightly outings and evasions regarding whereabouts, personality changes, missing money, expensive possessions sold, loss of interest in other activities, lack of concentration, a "don't care" attitude, and poor appearance or hygiene (Griffiths, 1995).

While Griffiths and others (see Haubrich-Casperson & Van Nispen, 1993) observed these behaviors, additional behavior patterns have been documented in surveys: 3 percent to 4 percent of teens argued with their parents over gambling; 4 percent to 5 percent sneaked bets; 2 percent to 6 percent hid betting slips, lottery tickets, and other signs of gambling; 9 percent to 17 percent used their lunch money for gambling; 7 percent sold personal possessions; 2 percent to 5 percent stole from someone in their family; 3 percent to 5 percent cut classes; 1 percent to 7 percent stole from nonrelatives; and 2 percent to 6 percent borrowed from someone and had not paid them back (Evans, 1989; Huxley & Carroll, 1992; Insight Canada Research, 1994; Ladouceur & Mireault, 1988; Lesieur, Klein, & Rimm, 1985; Omnifacts Research Ltd., 1993; Winters, Stinchfield, & Fulkerson, 1990; see table 12.2 for complete connection between references and data cited).

Gambling problems (among adults as well as teens) fall within six basic dimensions: loss of control, emotional problems (including personality changes), family problems, vocational (job/school) problems, financial problems, and legal problems; and data have focused on financial, family, school, and legal dimensions. The extent to which these dimensions are examined individually varies from researcher to researcher. Most attempt to combine these into an overall measure of problem gambling.

Measuring Gambling Problems Among Teens

The epidemiological picture for problem and pathological gambling is clouded by a lack of conceptual and methodological consistency in research. Researchers have de-

Table 12.2 Signs of Problematic Gambling Documented

Problem	Evans 1989 (%)	Huxley & Carroll 1992 (%)	Insight Canada 1994 (%)	Ladouceur & Mireault 1988 (%)	Lesieur, Klein, & Rimm 1985 (%)	Omnifacts 1993 (%)	Winters, Stinchfield, & Fulkerson 1990 (%)
Argue with parents over gambling	—	—	3.0[a]	3.0	4.0	—	3.9
Sneak bets	—	—	—	4.0	5.0	—	—
Hide betting slips, lottery tickets, etc.	—	—	5.0[a]	5.0	6.0	4.4	2.1
Gamble with lunch money	17.0	24.0[b]	16.0	9.0	14.0	—	—
Sell possessions	—	—	7.0	—	—	—	—
Borrow and not pay back due to gambling	—	—	6.0	2.3	—	6.0	4.4
Steal from family	—	12.0	3.0	5.0	2.2	—	—
Steal from others	7.0	—	<1.0	2.5	4.0	—	—
Any illegal activity paid for by gambling	—	—	—	8.9	10.0	—	—
Cut classes	—	14.0[b]	3.0[a] (including work)	5.4	5.0	3.8 (including work)	2.7
Work problems	—	—	—	1.7	—	—	—

[a] Last 12 months only.
[b] Fruit machine gambling only.

fined and measured problem gambling by using the Gamblers Anonymous (GA) twenty questions, the American Psychiatric Association's DSM-III, DSM-III-R, and DSM-IV criteria, the South Oaks Gambling Screen (SOGS), a modification of the SOGS called the SOGS-RA (revised for adolescents), the Diagnostic Interview Schedule (DIS), and the Massachusetts Gambling Screen (MAGS). The full range of studies and the different measures of problem gambling used by researchers are summarized in table 12.3.

The earliest efforts at measuring adolescent gambling problems were rather crude, in that they took the adult criteria and applied them to teens. Using a modification of the DSM-III criteria for pathological gambling among youths, Lesieur and Klein (1987) found that 5.7 percent of eleventh and twelfth graders in New Jersey high schools were "probable pathological gamblers." Using a French translation of the same questionnaire, Ladouceur and Mireault (1988) found that 3.6 percent of Quebec City teens satisfied the same criteria, while 1.7 percent satisfied a more stringent version of these criteria.

At approximately the same time as the above studies, Jacobs, Marston, Singer, Widaman, and Little (see Jacobs, 1989), using the Gamblers Anonymous twenty questions, found that 4 percent of high school students were compulsive gamblers. However, because the GA 20 questions and the DSM-III criteria are worded differently, there is no way of knowing whether the same individuals would have been classified as problem gamblers if they had been asked the youth version of the DSM-III and the GA twenty questions at the same time. The issue is clouded even further by the fact that neither the DSM-III nor the GA twenty questions has been validated with adolescent subjects.

Steinberg (1988, as cited in Jacobs, 1989) increased the complexity of this issue by using a combination of Diagnostic Interview Schedule (DIS), DSM-III, and DSM-III-R criteria. Rates achieved using these measures were 5.1 percent (DIS), 4.6 percent (DSM-III), and 13.3 percent (DSM-III-R), with a "composite" across all three measures of 7.7 percent.

Four studies have used the South Oaks Gambling Screen (Ladouceur, Dubé, & Bujold, 1994b; Lesieur et al., 1991; Oster & Knapp, 1994; Zitzow, 1993), a validated and reliable screening instrument developed for use with adults (Lesieur & Blume, 1987). While three of these studies (Lesieur et al., 1991; Ladouceur, Dubé, & Bujold, 1994b; Oster & Knapp, 1994) were done with college students, Zitzow's study included younger adolescents. Although the SOGS has been validated for use with adults (Lesieur & Blume, 1987), there is no validation for adolescents. In addition to the use of the adult SOGS, Insight Canada Research (1994) used a nonvalidated adolescent version of the SOGS in Ontario.

In an effort to resolve the confusion, Winters, Stinchfield, and Fulkerson (1993a) modified the South Oaks Gambling Screen. Using what they called the SOGS-RA (South Oaks Gambling Screen Revised for Adolescents) and indicators of daily or weekly gambling in combination, Winters et al. (1993b) determined that 8.7 percent of Minnesota youths between 15 and 18 were problem gamblers. In a follow-up study conducted 18 months later with more stringent criteria, Winters and Stinchfield (1993) found that the rate of "potentially pathological" gamblers had remained approximately the same, that is, the rate increased nonsignificantly from 2.9 percent to 3.5 percent.

In what at first glance appeared to be replications of the Winters and Stinchfield studies, Volberg (1993) and Wallisch (1993) conducted statewide surveys of problematic gambling among youths in Washington and Texas, respectively. Unfortunately, while both used what appeared to be the SOGS-RA, each made new and untested modifications to this scale. Volberg's measure was more conservative and, not surprisingly, yielded a lower level of problem gambling than the scale used by Winters and Stinchfield. Wallisch also made modifications to the SOGS-RA, but these modifications were different from Volberg's. Thus, the results are not comparable with either Volberg's study or the Minnesota studies.

Researchers in Nova Scotia (Omnifacts Research Ltd., 1993) surveyed three hundred adolescents aged 13 to 17. These researchers found that 8.7 percent of these youths had a possible gambling problem, while 3 percent had a possible pathological gambling problem. However, the Omnifacts researchers ignored developments in scale construction and altered the South Oaks Gambling Screen, making it no longer a validated and reliable instrument in the process (Lesieur, 1994, pp. 388–89).

Going in a different direction and moving researchers from the DSM-III criteria to the DSM-IV criteria, Fisher (1993b, 1995) developed the "DSM-IV-J" as a screening device to use with teen gamblers in the United Kingdom. This instrument, based on the developing DSM-IV criteria for pathological gambling (Lesieur & Rosenthal, 1991), used nine separate dimensions of pathological gambling. Fisher found that 5.7 percent of the United Kingdom teens she studied were probable pathological gamblers.

In Massachusetts the DSM-IV criteria were used again in the development of yet another adolescent gambling screen—the Massachusetts Gambling Screen (MAGS) (Shaffer, LaBrie, Scanlan, & Cummings, 1994). The prevalence rates found with this instrument (6.4 percent for the DSM-IV and 8.5 percent for the MAGS) are comparable to those found in other studies. The MAGS, while originally designed to be a simpler instrument than the SOGS, requires complicated scoring. However, both computerized scoring and hand-scoring sheets are available.

Adding to the complexity in defining gambling problems are the issues of subclinical levels of problem gambling and at-risk gambling. Some researchers have used subthreshold scores on the SOGS to classify respondents as problem gamblers. Most of these studies (Ladouceur, Dubé, & Bujold, 1994b; Lesieur et al., 1991; Oster & Knapp, 1994; Zitzow, 1992) use a score of 3 or 4 (the threshold is 5 or more), while one (Insight Canada Research, 1994) uses a score of 1 to 4. Omnifacts Research

Table 12.3 *Epidemiological Studies of Problem/Pathological Gambling Among Adolescents*

Researcher	Report Publication Year	Location	Sample size	Youth Age Range	Percent subclinical/"at-risk" (%)	Percent problem/pathological gamblers (%)
Fisher	1993b	UK	460	11–16 yrs.	—	5.7[a]
Insight Canada	1994	Ontario	400	12–19 yrs.	33.0[b]	4.0[c]
Jacobs et al.[q]	1985	Calif.	843	9–12 grade	—	4.0[d]
Jacobs et al.[q]	1987	Calif.	257	9–12 grade	—	4.0[d]
Ladouceur et al.	1994b	Québec	1,471	college students	5.8[e]	2.8[f]
Ladouceur & Mireault	1988	Québec	1,612	9–11 grade	—	1.7[g] (3.6[h])
Lesieur et al.	1991	5 states	1,771	college students	15.0[e]	5.7[f]
Lesieur & Klein	1987	N.J.	892	11–12 grade	—	5.7[h]
Omnifacts Research	1993	Nova Scotia	300	13–17 yrs.	8.7[i]	3.0[j]
Oster & Knapp	1994	Nev. 1992	544	college students	23.7[e]	11.2[f] 5.1[k] 4.2l[l]
Oster & Knapp	1994	Nev. 1994	350	college students	17.4[e]	8.0[f] 5.7[k]
Shaffer et al.	1994	Mass.	856	13–20 yrs.	—	6.4[l] 8.5[m]
Steinberg	1988	Conn.	573	high school	—	7.7[n]
Volberg	1993	Wash.	1,054	13–17 yrs.	9.0[o]	0.9[o]
Winters et al.	1990	Minn.	1,094	15–18 yrs.	19.9[p]	6.3[q]
Winters et al.	1993b	Minn.	702	15–18 yrs.	17.1[p]	8.7[q]

Winters et al.	1995	Minn.	532	16–20 yrs.	14.7[p]	9.5[q]
					9.3[r]	3.5
Wallisch[s]	1993	Tex.	924	14–17 yrs.	12[t]	5.0[t]
Zitzow	1992	Minn.	161/115	14–19 yrs.	10.5/14.8[e,u]	5.6/9.6[t,u]

[a] DSM-IV, modified for adolescents (DSM-IV-J).
[b] SOGS (South Oaks Gambling Screen) score of 1–4.
[c] SOGS modified for adolescents.
[d] Gamblers Anonymous 20 questions.
[e] SOGS score of 3–4.
[f] SOGS.
[g] DSM-III stringent criteria.
[h] DSM-III less stringent criteria.
[i] Modified SOGS score of 3–4.
[j] SOGS modified.
[k] DSM-III-R.
[l] DSM-IV.
[m] Massachusetts Gambling Screen (MAGS).
[n] Combination of DIS, DSM-III, and DSM-III-R.
[o] Multifactor method—Washington version.
[p] Weekly gambling and SOGS-RA (South Oaks Gambling Screen revised for adolescents) formula.
[q] SOGS-RA.
[r] SOGS-RA score of 2–3.
[s] SOGS-RA but different formula for determining rate.
[t] Multifactor method—Texas version.
[u] Non–American Indian numbers are listed first, American Indian numbers listed second.

(1993) altered the SOGS in a different fashion and used a modified SOGS score of 3 or 4.

A second set of scholars uses an at-risk formula that looks at the frequency of gambling and/or scores on different problem dimensions. However, the method for calculating the formula varies with different researchers. Winters and colleagues (1990, 1993b, 1995) use weekly gambling plus any SOGS-RA score or less-than-weekly gambling and a SOGS-RA score of 2 or more to classify respondents as at-risk gamblers. In another set of calculations (1995) they rely on scores of 2 or 3 on the SOGS-RA. Volberg (1993) and Wallisch (1993) use a "multifactor method" that involves a combination of gambling frequency (weekly gambling automatically qualifies the respondent as at risk), scores on behavioral or borrowing dimensions, and amount of money spent on gambling. The levels of subclinical or at-risk gambling found in these and other studies are presented in table 12.3.

None of the above screening instruments has been validated with a criterion group of adolescent problem gamblers, a difficulty that has yet to be resolved by researchers. It is my guess that the search for a screening instrument is not over, but where we go from here is anyone's guess. In research with methadone patients, Spunt, Lesieur, Hunt, and Cahill (1995) have used the "SOGS-Plus." This instrument involves the SOGS along with additional questions that create a six-dimension[1] set of items that taps the loss of control and the family/social, work/school, financial, emotional, and illegal-activity aspects of pathological gambling. There are advantages to a multiple-dimension approach. If youths go in and out of problem gambling, as many of us suspect, a unified image of pathological gambling may prove to be a barrier to understanding progression in contrast with fluctuation.

Teen Gambling: Risk Factors

Why do teens gamble? Why do some teens gamble heavily? Why do some teens develop gambling problems? Answers to these questions have relied on survey research in the United States. More in-depth research has been done in the United Kingdom, but this research has typically been restricted to fruit-machine play.

Some researchers have examined the interconnection between "regular" gambling and "nonregular" gambling using primarily teen subjects. For example, Griffiths (1994b) has found that regular fruit-machine players are more skill-oriented than nonregulars (hence, verifying Fisher, 1993a). However, regular players are also more likely than nonregular players to use irrational verbalizations while playing (Griffiths, 1994b). By eliciting player strategy (that is, interviewing players about their use patterns), Bentall, Fisher, Kelly, Bromley, and Hawksworth (1989) found that habitual use clustered around frequency of visiting arcades, amount of money spent, overspending, and time spent on each visit. Social class was not a strong predictor of habitual play; perceived luck and length of history of play were not related to habitual play. Young males were overrepresented in this population.

Griffiths (1995), relying primarily on studies of adolescent fruit-machine players in the United Kingdom, outlined risk factors in problem gambling among teens. Using Griffith's ideas as a base, I have added references and risk factors to his original list to come up with the following analysis:

Problem and pathological gamblers

1. Are more likely to be male (Fisher, 1993b; Griffiths, 1990c; Insight Canada Research, 1994; Jacobs, 1989; Ladouceur, Dubé, & Bujold, 1994b; Lesieur & Klein, 1987; Lesieur et al., 1991; Omnifacts Research Ltd., 1993; Shaffer et al., 1994; Steinberg, May 1988; Volberg, 1993; Wallisch, 1993; Winters, Stinchfield, & Fulkerson, 1990).

2. Have parents who have gambling or other addiction problems (Insight Canada Research, 1994; Jacobs, 1989; Lesieur et al., 1991; Lesieur & Klein, 1987; Omnifacts Research Ltd., 1993; Steinberg, May 1988; Wallisch, 1993). The only study showing no relationship is Ladouceur, Dubé, and Bujold (1994b); alternatively, parental gambling alone (without taking parental problems into account) is associated with gambling problems in their children (Volberg, 1993; Winters, Stinchfield, & Fulkerson, 1990, 1993b).

3. Live in larger households (Volberg, 1993; Wallisch, 1993).

4. Are slightly more likely to come from lower social classes (Fisher, 1993b). Note: This factor is not supported by many studies but has support in surveys where researchers phrase the question of socioeconomic status in terms of coming from a neighborhood "worse off than most" (Lesieur et al., 1991; Lesieur & Klein, 1987; Steinberg, May 1988).

5. Are more likely to be nonwhite (in the United States) (Lesieur et al., 1991; Wallisch, 1993; Zitzow, July 1993); for example, Zitzow found that 9.6 percent of American Indian youths and 5.6 percent of non–American Indian youths were probable pathological gamblers.

Gambling-related characteristics of those identified as problem gamblers:

1. They began playing at an early age (Fisher, 1993b; Griffiths, 1990c; Huxley and Carroll, 1992; Jacobs, 1989; Shaffer et al., 1994; Steinberg, May 1988; Wallisch, 1993).

2. They began playing with parents or alone, in contrast to beginning with friends (Griffiths, 1990b).

3. They have had a big win (Griffiths, 1990b, 1990c).

4. They get excited during play (Griffiths, 1990a, 1990b, 1990c).

5. They are depressed before playing (Griffiths, 1993).

6. They view fruit-machine activity as skillful (Fisher, 1993b; Griffiths, 1990c, 1994b).

The following variables are associated with adolescent gambling:

1. Illegal drug use (Amati, 1981; Griffin-Shelley, Sandler, & Lees, 1992; Griffiths, 1994a; Ladouceur, Dubé, & Bujold, 1994b; Lesieur et al., 1991; Lesieur & Heineman, 1988; Omnifacts Research Ltd., 1993; Volberg, 1993; Wallisch, 1993; Winters, Stinchfield, & Fulkerson, 1990).

2. History of delinquency (Huff & Collinson, 1987; Ladouceur, Dubé, & Bujold, 1994b; Lesieur et al., 1991; Maden, Swinton, & Gunn, 1992; Wallisch, 1993; Winters, Stinchfield, & Fulkerson, 1993b).

3. Poor grades in school (Ladouceur, Dubé, & Bujold, 1994b; Lesieur et al., 1991; Lesieur & Klein, 1987; Wallisch, 1993; Winters, Stinchfield, & Fulkerson, 1990).

4. Truancy (All of the following asked about truancy in order to gamble: Barham & Cormell, 1987, as cited in Griffiths, 1989; Griffiths, 1990b, 1990c; Huff & Collinson, 1987; Huxley & Carroll, 1992; Lesieur & Klein, 1987; National Housing and Town Planning Council, 1988, as cited in Griffiths, 1989; Roberts & Pool, 1988, as cited in Griffiths, 1989. One study related problem gambling to an overall pattern of truancy: Wallisch, 1993).

5. Eating disorders (Ladouceur, Dubé, & Bujold, 1994b; Lesieur et al., 1991).

6. Suicide attempts (Ladouceur, Dubé, & Bujold, 1994b; Lesieur et al., 1991).

Teen Gambling and Related Problems

In studies of adults, researchers have uncovered the interconnection of chemical dependency and gambling (Lesieur, Blume, & Zoppa, 1986). More recently, similar patterns have been found among adolescents as well (Griffin-Shelley, Sandler, & Lees, 1992; Griffiths, 1994a; Lesieur et al., 1991; Lesieur & Heineman, 1988). Amati (1981), in a study of delinquent boys in India, notes: "Some senior delinquent boys stated that the use of alcohol makes them bold and courageous and raises their stamina in crime and gambling. According to these boys, it enhances their capacity for betting in gambling—a quality that is highly appreciated by the delinquents in general" (pp. 407–408).

Griffin-Shelley and colleagues (1992) used the GA twenty questions and found that 14 of 76 adolescents (18.4 percent) in a dual-diagnosis unit of a psychiatric hospital were compulsive gamblers. Researchers diagnosed 69 of the 76 (91 percent) as chemically dependent. Lesieur and Heineman (1988) found that 8 percent of 75 patients aged 18 or younger in a therapeutic community were pathological gamblers. A similar pattern of cross-usage was found among college students, where pathological gambling was significantly correlated with illegal drug use and drunkenness (Lesieur et al., 1991). While the results in these studies are quite variable, they all point in the same direction: There is an overlap among excessive behaviors including gambling.

Gambling is associated with crime in many studies; among them is Amati's (1981) research. For example, 100 male trainees (aged 16 to 21) in a youth custody center were surveyed (Huff & Collinson, 1987); 60 of them gambled. Of the gamblers, 14 (23 percent) admitted committing a criminal offense to finance their gambling; 8 (14 percent) admitted to theft. Another study of young offenders (Maden, Swinton, & Gunn, 1992) found that 12 percent (48 out of 404) were excessive gamblers. The gamblers were more likely to have been in care (under state supervision) or in children's homes and were more likely to have received psychiatric treatment than other offenders. Whether these other factors are antecedents or consequences of the teens' gambling is uncertain.

Gambling can be seen as part of a behavioral complex that includes other deviant forms of behavior. Youths who gamble are also likely to smoke, drink, use other drugs, be truant, and engage in crime. For example, Wallisch (1993) found that compared with nonproblem gamblers, adolescent problem gamblers were more likely to have skipped school, were sent to the principal more often, and were more likely to have the school call home about them. Furthermore, problem gamblers were more likely to have committed illegal acts and been arrested, and they were more likely to have friends who carry weapons and belong to gangs. However, while these relationships exist, most teen problem gamblers do not exhibit a pattern of serious delinquency (Wallisch, 1993).

Because of the extensive overlap of gambling with other troublesome behavior, it is difficult to evaluate studies that report theft committed to finance gambling (Barham & Cormell, 1987, as cited in Griffiths, 1989; Evans, 1989; Fisher, 1993b, 1994; Griffiths, 1990b; Huff & Collinson, 1987; Huxley & Carroll, 1992; Ladouceur, Dubé, & Bujold, 1994b; Ladouceur & Mireault, 1988; Lesieur & Klein, 1987; Lesieur, Klein, & Rimm, 1985; National Housing and Town Planning Council, 1988, as cited in Griffiths, 1989; Roberts & Pool, 1988, as cited in Griffiths, 1989; Winters, Stinchfield, & Fulkerson, 1990). No one can assess whether these deviant behaviors are actually caused by gambling, whether gambling is the consequence of these behaviors, or whether the behaviors are associated with gambling in some other way. This is particularly the case for those who report prostitution and drug sales to finance gambling (Barham & Cormell, 1987, as cited in Griffiths, 1989; Lesieur, Klein, & Rimm, 1985).

Studies of gambling and delinquency are correlational and do not establish a clear causal relationship between crime (or even using lunch money for gambling) and a need to gamble. This situation has its parallel in the world of drug studies, where the "enslavement" hypothesis has been contrasted to the "criminal turns to drugs" hypothesis (Inciardi, 1986). The causal sequence—whether individuals are slaves to drugs or whether crime comes first—has been investigated by numerous scholars (see Tonry & Wilson, 1990). An alternative "intensification" hypothesis has received support. According to this view (Inciardi, 1986), drugs intensify crime.

The causal sequence for gambling, while studied among adults (Blaszczynski & McConaghy, 1994; Lesieur, 1984), has yet to be thoroughly investigated among teens.

A related issue, particularly in the United Kingdom and Hong Kong, is whether video arcades with gambling machines are, as some say, "breeding grounds for drug use and violent crime" (Karp, 1992, p. 33), or whether these venues are representative of places that attract adolescents who would get into trouble in any event (Agnew & Petersen, 1991, as cited in Abbott, Palmisano, & Dickerson, 1995). In all probability, as with similar cultural phenomena, the two patterns interact. Until researchers conduct studies that factor in these complex interactions, we must be content with the notion that we do not know how these patterns connect.

Parents and Teen Gamblers

Parents of Young Gamblers is a program developed in the United Kingdom in response to teen gambling (Moody, 1989). When children have problems, their parents are frequently at a loss as to what to do. Other than Moody's description in the *Journal of Gambling Behavior*, no research has been done on this program. In addition, the experiences of parents who attend Gam-Anon have not been investigated.

Teens and Parent Gamblers

The alternative issue of teens living with adult gamblers has been only sparsely addressed in two studies that are now more than five years old (Jacobs et al., 1989; Lesieur & Rothschild, 1989). These studies found that adult gambling problems are associated with a wide range of difficulties for youths that go beyond the issue of teen gambling. According to Jacobs et al. (1989),

> One cannot resist the conclusion that without early and competent intervention, children of problem gamblers (a) will be seriously disadvantaged when attempting to solve their present and future problems of living, and (b) as a consequence are, themselves, high-risk candidates for developing one or another form of dysfunctional behavior, including one or another addictive pattern of behavior. (p. 267)

There are many parallels between being a child of a compulsive gambler and being a child of an alcoholic or drug addict. Research here is so sparse and preliminary, however, that replication and further development are sorely needed.

Gambling and Attraction

Children frequently learn about gambling from their parents. For example, some researchers note that more than half of teens have gambled with their parents (Ladouceur & Mireault, 1988; Lesieur, Klein, & Rimm, 1985; Winters, Stinchfield, & Kim, 1995). Parents are more likely to gamble with their teens than to object to their teen's gambling. Ladouceur and Mireault (1988) revealed that 61 percent of adolescents gambled with their parents, and only 16 percent of parents objected to this gambling. Winters et al. (1995) found that almost 73 percent of underage teens who gambled with scratch tabs, pull tabs, or lottery tickets got them from their parents.

Teens are attracted to gambling. Should anyone doubt this statement, the Casino Control Commission in New Jersey gathers data on the number of teens removed from the casinos and the number refused entry. In 1993, 178,000 underage gamblers were stopped at the door and another 15,000 were escorted from the buildings ("The serious problem of high school gambling," 1995). These data contrast with data from 1987, when 200,000 were refused entry and 35,000 were ushered from the floor (Bruner, 1989). These data suggest the possibility of two different scenarios: Either 20,000 fewer underage gamblers are entering (security is stronger upon entry) or fewer are being caught (security is weaker). Without an objective assessment we cannot tell which scenario is more accurate.

While some age controls are evident in some casino locations, they appear to be virtually nonexistent at lottery ticket sales outlets. In two studies using similar methods (Harshbarger, 1994; Radecki, 1994), underage youths attempted to purchase lottery tickets. With parental consent, the Massachusetts attorney general's office (Harshbarger, 1994) used young people to purchase lottery tickets (with staff from the attorney general's office present). In 80 percent of the cases, these youths were successful. The youngest purchaser was 9 years old. Only 40 percent of the stores investigated in this study posted the signs for help with compulsive gambling that are required by Massachusetts state law. In Illinois, a 16-year-old successfully purchased lottery tickets at 49 out of 50 lottery ticket sales locations (Radecki, 1994).

More recently, casinos in Las Vegas have been targeting families, a tactic that seems to be working. "In 1987, children under 21 made up 5 percent of Las Vegas's 16.2 million annual visitor volume. In 1993, the junior slice grew to 7.9 percent of the rising 23.5 million visitor pie" (Kaplan, 1994, p. 6A). As inducements to bring children, casinos provide day-care centers, amusement parks, carnival games, and other activities. The carnival games are particularly interesting, as they actually are gambling games. Arnie Wexler, the past director of the Council on Compulsive Gambling of New Jersey, calls the children in the carnival games at Circus Circus "compulsive gamblers in training" (Wexler, 1994). Whether these children are at risk is worthy of research.

Many high schools are so blind to the issue of teen problem gambling that they have promoted "casino nights" at proms and graduations (Zeigler, 1995). These events are designed primarily as a means of combating alcohol use and drunk driving. In the process, ironically, teens are taught to play games that have an addictive potential. The issue of adult promotion of gambling as a "healthy alternative" for teens is one that rarely is challenged.

While machines that cannot "card" customers are common—for example, lottery machines in Illinois and self-service machines in New Jersey racetracks (Loder, 1995)—some places have begun to limit gaming in an effort to restrict access to adults. However, this effort has been limited to video poker and slot machines. These limitations have been established in Spain (Becona, Labrador, Echeburua, Ochoa, & Vallejo, 1995) and Nova Scotia (Steeves, 1994) and have been proposed for the Netherlands (Geller, 1994). In each of these locations, gaming machines are allowed only where alcoholic beverages are sold. Given the United Kingdom's experience with extensive fruit-machine gambling problems among youths, this appears to be a wise move.

Prevention Programs

In 1989 Harrah's launched Project 21, a program to prevent those under age 21 from gambling in casinos.[2] Part of this effort is a series of advertisements claiming that teens will ruin their lives if they get arrested for gambling in the casinos. An advertisement (cosponsored by Harrah's, Trop World, and the Claridge in Atlantic City) states,

> If you're under twenty-one and caught gambling, one pull, one spin, one roll, can put you in the jackpot of your life . . . You will be arrested . . . You will be prosecuted . . . You will have a record . . . A record of conviction will definitely increase the odds against: (a) Landing a good job. (b) Attending the college of your choice.

Given the high rate of teenage gambling, it is doubtful that teens believe their lives will be ruined in this way because they gamble. No such stigma applies to underage drinking, and the Project 21 assumption that it would apply to underage gambling needs to be examined. An assessment of this statement's accuracy and believability among teens would be useful.

Project 21 now includes seven casinos and offers $10,000 in scholarships to five artists who draw posters and five authors who write articles that will be used in advertising (Wyckoff, 1995). As noted above, the number of underage youths ejected from the casino floor in Atlantic City declined from 35,000 in 1987 to 15,000 in 1993. It is possible that this decrease was a consequence of Project 21. However, since no systematic research has been conducted, the impact of the program is uncertain and has yet to be evaluated.

Curriculum Development for Schools

State councils on compulsive gambling in New Jersey, Texas, Minnesota, and Massachusetts have launched prevention programs as well. For example, representatives from the Council on Compulsive Gambling of New Jersey visit high schools to speak to students and teachers. They survey students (Belluck, 1992; Orlando, 1994) and pass out educational material including book covers ("Students get anti-gambling message," 1994). The impact of these programs appears to be positive. For example, according to staff at the Council on Compulsive Gambling of New Jersey, the public awareness efforts result in calls to statewide hotlines.[3]

Appeals have been made for systematic education about gambling in school systems. For example, a bill was introduced in the New Jersey legislature to add gambling prevention to health classes (Allee, 1995). What will be on the agenda for these courses? What issues will be addressed? What evidence is there that these courses will be effective in addressing these issues?

To date there is only one extensive curriculum for gambling education that has been disseminated in the United States (Svendsen & Griffin, 1994). The curriculum focuses on choices about whether, when, and how much to gamble. While it is a "teacher-developed" and "student-tested" program, it has not yet been evaluated.

Those in prevention may learn a lesson from drug education programs. The effectiveness of drug education programs has been challenged. A recent meta-analysis of the effectiveness of Project DARE (Drug Abuse Resistance Education) (Ennett, Tobler, Ringwalt, & Flewelling, 1994), for example, found increases in overall student knowledge about drugs but extremely small-effect sizes of change in student drug use (the weighted mean of .06 was not statistically significant). The small effects were attributed to possible reductions in tobacco use. Changes in alcohol use were not statistically significant, and marijuana use was unaffected. Other programs (Tobler, 1992) have been shown to be more effective. In other words, the most widely used drug programs have questionable effects and may be a waste of taxpayer dollars.

The message for gambling education is clear. Caution is essential. Programs can educate individuals about gambling-related problems, but these programs may be of limited effect in reducing teen gambling. Teen gambling prevention programs that are developed must be evaluated for effectiveness. Researchers should determine whether reported gambling and problem gambling increase, decline, or remain the same as a result of these efforts. Gaboury and Ladouceur (1993) evaluated one prevention program in Quebec. Knowledge about gambling, coping skills, attitudes about gambling, and the gambling behavior of 134 experimental and 155 control subjects were evaluated before and after a high school gambling prevention program. Knowledge about gambling and coping skills improved after the program, but coping skills returned to baseline levels. Neither gambling attitudes nor behavior were changed as a result of the program.

Treatment—A Data Lacuna

Other than single case studies (Griffiths, 1993) and descriptions of possible treatment strategies (Pursley, 1991), there is sparse discussion, in the literature, of the treatment of adolescent gamblers. Pursley, for example, advocates adapting a treatment model used for chemically dependent youths. We have no way of knowing whether this program effectively transfers to youthful gamblers.

Accounts exist of teens in Gamblers Anonymous (Griffiths, 1993; Moody, 1989). Because their problems are "early stage" (or because of other yet unspecified reasons), it appears the teens are not able to identify with adult gamblers with significantly more problems. To increase identification, three meetings of Young Gamblers Anonymous have been formed in New Jersey (Zeigler, 1995). Given the sparse nature of treatment for pathological gambling, meetings such as Young Gamblers Anonymous need to be fostered elsewhere as well.

Ladouceur, Boisvert, and Dumont (1994) have conducted the only study evaluating treatment effectiveness. They studied the effectiveness of cognitive-behavioral treatment of four adolescent male pathological gamblers. The treatment combined cognitive interventions (for example, focusing on irrational thinking, illusions of control, and automatic thoughts), problem-solving training, assertiveness training, and relapse-prevention training. All four subjects were abstinent at one- four- and six-month follow-ups.

Research: What Next?

Griffiths (1989) has outlined an Antecedent Behavior Consequence (ABC) model of research that can serve as a useful guide for research into youthful gambling behavior. To place this model into a broader social context, we should examine the antecedents, behaviors, and consequences within five major spheres: individual, peer group, family, school, and community. These spheres are outlined in figure 12.1.

Individual influences can be divided into basic demographic characteristics (gender, age, race/ethnicity, and socioeconomic status) and personality structure (including conditioning experiences, level of sensation seeking, and extent of depression). Only some of these factors have been studied in the context of gambling behavior. Demographic characteristics tend to influence gambling behavior, while the personality structure can both influence and be influenced by gambling. For example, males are more likely to gamble than females, and individuals from different ethnic groups gamble differently. On the other hand, personality variables like depressive personality style are related to problem gambling. Researchers have hypothesized that some gamblers gamble to relieve depression. Yet other researchers have found that gambling increases depression.

Some family influences have been studied as well. However, we know more about

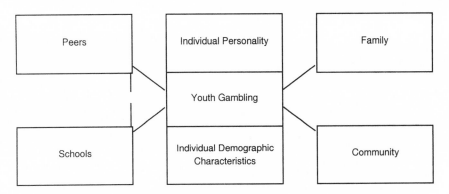

Fig. 12.1. Influences on Youth Gambling and Areas of Impact

the impact of family on gambling than of gambling's impact on the family. We know, for example, that parental gambling attitudes and behavior are reflected in their children. Children of problem gamblers are at greater risk than children of nongamblers of becoming problem gamblers themselves. The precise nature of the path from teen in a troubled family to problem teen gambler should be studied in more detail over time. In addition, we should not ignore the impact of teen gambling on other family members.

Peer influences have been examined only in a cursory way in surveys (with the notation that gamblers are likely to have gambling friends, but the nature and makeup of those friendships is unclear) and in ethnographic studies conducted in England. Fisher's studies (1993a, 1993b) find that most adolescent gamblers participate in gambling as a peer-oriented activity. The nature of these peer groups needs to be investigated. "Betting rings" are likely to be male oriented and sports centered. The extent to which teens who participate in betting rings are also involved in gambling at casinos, racetracks, and other ventures is currently unknown.

The impact of schools on adolescent gambling (from "Las Vegas nights" to school raffles) is uncertain and not yet investigated. We know more about students cutting classes in order to gamble than we do about the use of the school as a setting for gambling-related activities. Schools can be meeting places for teen gamblers, collection points for gambling debts, and venues for card games and gaming pursuits.

Community is the final area emphasized in figure 12.1. In addition to representing the availability of gambling, this box reflects the impact of the community on problem gambling and of problem gambling on the community. The legalization of gambling is reflected in increased gambling. The relationship is reciprocal. With increasing gambling come increasing problems for the community. To the extent that youths borrow or steal to finance their gambling, there are consequences for the community at large. These consequences should not be ignored.

In addition to an ABC model to better understand youthful gambling, an Assessment Prevention Outcome (APO) agenda for adolescent treatment research is needed.

ASSESSMENT

There is currently a plethora of comparable assessment instruments available, with no one instrument dominant. These instruments are the Gamblers Anonymous twenty questions, the DSM-III, DSM-III-R, and DSM-IV (APA, 1994), the DSM-IV modified for adolescents (DSM-IV-J; see Fisher, 1993b), the SOGS, the SOGS-RA and its modifications, and the MAGS. Ironically, none of these has been validated with a known population of problem-gambling teens. Such a validation is essential. In addition to devising a method of identifying teen problems, researchers need to develop more complete assessment instruments—instruments, for example, to question the parents and significant others of youth gamblers.

PREVENTION AND OUTCOME

Both primary and secondary prevention programs are needed. These should be implemented with an outcome component built in, for without it, we will be less sure we are building a better world for the next generation.

Toward More Global Thinking

Teen gambling exists not only within the individual, peer group, family, school, and community contexts, but also within a larger, global context. Gambling is both produced by and productive of the larger socioeconomic system. Social forces such as government fiscal crises generate pressures to legalize gambling. The legalization of gambling produces increased teen gambling. Increased teen gambling feeds into gambling problems, which have adverse consequences for family, school, and community. These consequences must be evaluated and the problems prevented, assessed, and treated. In turn, treatment outcome should be assessed. Research is needed in all of these realms.

Notes

Portions of this chapter were presented at the North American Think Tank on Youth Gambling Issues, Harvard Medical School, Boston, April 6, 1995. The information in this chapter dates to that conference.

1. The term *dimension* is being used on a preliminary basis; no assumption of mathematical dimensions is being made.

2. The author is a member of the Council on Compulsive Gambling of New Jersey Advisory Board.

3. For a more detailed review of Project 21, see chap. 9, "Youth Gambling: The Casino Industry's Responsibility," by Philip G. Satre.

References

Abbott, M., Palmisano, B., & Dickerson, M. (1995). Video game playing, dependency and delinquency: A question of methodology? *Journal of Gambling Studies, 11,* 287–301.

Allee, R. (1995, February 1). Don't wager kids' lives. *North Jersey (Passaic, NJ) Herald and News,* p. C1.

Amati, B. H. (1984). Juvenile delinquency and habit patterns. *Indian Journal of Social Work, 44,* 405–8.

American Psychiatric Association. (1994). *DSM-IV: Diagnostic and statistical manual of mental disorders.* 4th edition. Washington, DC: American Psychiatric Association.

Arcuri, A. F., Lester, D., & Smith, F. O. (1985). Shaping adolescent gambling behavior. *Adolescence, 20,* 935–38.

Becona, E., Labrador, F., Echeburua, E., Ochoa, E., & Vallejo, M. (1995). Slot machine gambling in Spain: An important and new social problem. *Journal of Gambling Studies, 11,* 265–86.

Belluck, P. (1992, August 16). Starting too young, getting in too deep. *Philadelphia Inquirer,* A1, A10.

Bentall, R. P., Fisher, D., Kelly, V., Bromley, E., & Hawksworth, K. (1989). The use of arcade gambling machines: Demographic characteristics of users and patterns of use. *British Journal of Addiction, 84,* 555–62.

Blaszczynski, A. P., & McConaghy, N. (1994) Antisocial personality disorder and pathological gambling. *Journal of Gambling Studies, 10,* 129–45.

Bruner, K. (1989, May). High stakes: The number of teen gamblers in the United States is rising at an alarming rate. *Employee Assistance,* 26–28.

Decision Sciences, Inc. (1993). *Gambling activities and attitudes of Multnomah County juveniles.* Multnomah County, OR: Author.

Ennett, S. T., Tobler, N. S., Ringwalt, C. L., & Flewelling, R. L. (1994). How effective is drug abuse resistance education? A meta-analysis of Project DARE outcome evaluations. *American Journal of Public Health, 84,* 1394–1401.

Evans, A. (1989). Gambling machines and young people: The result of a national survey. *The Society for the Study of Gambling Newsletter, 15,* 15–17.

Fisher, S. (1993a). The pull of the fruit machines: A sociological typology of young players. *Sociological Review, 41,* 446–74.

Fisher, S. (1993b). Gambling and pathological gambling in adolescents. *Journal of Gambling Studies, 9,* 277–87.

Fisher, S. E. (1995). *Gambling in children and adolescents residing in a southwest seaside town.* Report for Channel 4 News. London: Author.

Frank, M. L. (1990). Underage gambling in Atlantic City casinos. *Psychological Reports, 67,* 907–12.

Gaboury, A., & Ladouceur, R. (1993). Evaluation of a prevention program for pathological gambling among adolescents. *Journal of Primary Prevention, 14,* 21–28.

Geller, R. (1994). Dutch move to restrict gaming machines. *Gaming & Wagering Business, 15,* 1, 4.

Griffin-Shelley, E., Sandler, K. R., & Lees, C. (1992). Multiple addictions among dually diagnosed adolescents. *Journal of Adolescent Chemical Dependency, 2*, 35–44.

Griffiths, M. D. (1989). Gambling in children and adolescents. *Journal of Gambling Behavior, 5*, 66–83.

Griffiths, M. D. (1990a). Psychobiology of the near-miss in fruit machine gambling. *Journal of Psychology, 125*, 347–57.

Griffiths, M. D. (1990b). The acquisition, development, and maintenance of fruit machine gambling in adolescents. *Journal of Gambling Studies, 6*, 193–204.

Griffiths, M. D. (1990c). Addiction to fruit machines: A preliminary study among young males. *Journal of Gambling Studies, 6*, 113–26.

Griffiths, M. D. (1993). Factors in problem adolescent fruit machine gambling: Results of a small postal survey. *Journal of Gambling Studies, 9*, 31–45.

Griffiths, M. D. (1994a). Co-existent fruit machine addiction and solvent abuse in adolescence a cause for concern. *Journal of Adolescence, 17*, 491–98.

Griffiths, M. D. (1994b). Cognitive bias and skill in fruit machine gambling: A reevaluation. Unpublished paper, University of Plymouth, UK, Psychology Department.

Griffiths, M. D. (1995). Towards a risk factor model of fruit machine addiction: A brief note. *Journal of Gambling Studies, 11*, 343–46.

Harrah's Casinos. (1995). *Harrah's survey of casino entertainment.* Memphis: Author.

Harshbarger, S. (1994, July). *Report on the sale of lottery tickets to minors in Massachusetts.* Boston: Attorney General, Commonwealth of Massachusetts.

Haubrich-Casperson, J., & Van Nispen, D. (1993). *Coping with teen gambling.* New York: Rosen Publishing Group, Inc.

Huff, G., & Collinson, F. (1987). Young offenders, gambling, and video game playing. *British Journal of Criminology, 27*, 401–10.

Hugick, L., & Saad, L. (1994, January/February). America's gambling boom. *Public Perspective,* 6-13.

Huxley, J., & Carroll, D. (1992). A survey of fruit machine gambling in adolescents. *Journal of Gambling Studies, 8*, 167–79.

Ide-Smith, S. G., & Lea, S. E. (1988). Gambling in young adolescents. *Journal of Gambling Behavior, 4*, 110–18.

Inciardi, J. A. (1986). *The war on drugs: Heroin, cocaine, crime and policy.* Palo Alto, CA: Mayfield Publishing Co.

Insight Canada Research. (1994). *An exploration of the prevalence of pathological gambling behavior among adolescents in Ontario.* Report prepared for the Canadian Foundation on Compulsive Gambling. Willowdale, Ontario: Author.

Jacobs, D. F. (1989). Illegal and undocumented: A review of teenage gambling and the plight of children of problem gamblers in America. In H. J. Shaffer, S. A. Stein, B. Gambino, & T. N. Cummings (Eds.), *Compulsive gambling: Theory, research, and practice* (pp. 249–92). Lexington, MA: Lexington Books.

Jacobs, D. F., Marston, A. R., & Singer, R. D. (1985). *Study of gambling and other health-threatening behaviors among high school students.* Unpublished manuscript. Loma Linda, CA: Jerry L. Pettis Memorial Veterans Hospital.

Jacobs, D. F., Marston, A. R., Singer, R. D., Widaman, K., & Little, T. (1987). [Study of gambling and other health-threatening behaviors among high school students]. Unpublished raw data. Loma Linda, CA: Jerry L. Pettis Memorial Veterans Hospital.

Jacobs, D. F., Marston, A. R., Singer, R. D., Widaman, K., Little, T., & Veizades, J. (1989). Children of problem gamblers. *Journal of Gambling Behavior, 5,* 261–68.

Johnston, L. D., O'Malley, P. M., & Bachman, J. G. (1992). *Smoking, drinking, and illicit drug use among American secondary school students, college students, and young adults, 1975–1991.* Rockville, MD: National Institute on Drug Abuse.

Kaplan, L. F. (1994, August 31). Casinos wager on families for the future. *USA Today,* 6A.

Karp, J. (1992, January). Video bandits: Gambling machines deemed a menace to youth. (Taiwan). *Far Eastern Economic Review, 155,* 33.

Ladouceur, R., Boisvert, J. M., & Dumont, J. (1994). Cognitive-behavioral treatment for adolescent pathological gamblers. *Behavior Modification, 16,* 230–42.

Ladouceur, R., Dubé, D., & Bujold, D. (1994a). Gambling among primary school students. *Journal of Gambling Studies, 10,* 363–70.

Ladouceur, R., Dubé, D., & Bujold, D. (1994b). Gambling among college students in the Quebec metropolitan area. *Canadian Journal of Psychiatry, 39,* 289–93.

Ladouceur, R., & Mireault, C. (1988). Gambling behaviors among high school students in the Quebec area. *Journal of Gambling Behavior, 4,* 3–12.

Lesieur, H. R. (1994). Epidemiological surveys of pathological gambling: Critique and suggestions for modification. *Journal of Gambling Studies, 10,* 385–98.

Lesieur, H. R., & Blume, S. B. (1987). The South Oaks Gambling Screen (SOGS): A new instrument for the identification of pathological gamblers. *American Journal of Psychiatry, 144,* 1184–88.

Lesieur, H. R., Blume, S. B., & Zoppa, R. (1986). Alcoholism, drug abuse, and gambling. *Alcoholism: Clinical and Experimental Research, 10,* 33–38.

Lesieur, H. R., Cross, J., Frank, M., Welch, M., White, C. M., Rubenstein, G., Moseley, K., & Mark, M. (1991). Gambling and pathological gambling among university students. *Addictive Behaviors, 16,* 517–27.

Lesieur, H. R., & Heineman, M. (1988). Pathological gambling among multiple substance abusers in a therapeutic community. *British Journal of Addiction, 83,* 765–71.

Lesieur, H. R., & Klein, R. (1987). Pathological gambling among high school students. *Addictive Behaviors, 12,* 129–35.

Lesieur, H. R., Klein, R., & Rimm, M. (1985). Pathological and problem gambling among New Jersey high school students. In W. R. Eadington (Ed.), *The Gambling studies: Proceedings of the Sixth National Conference on Gambling and Risk Taking, vol. 5* (pp. 165–75). University of Nevada, Reno: Bureau of Business & Economic Research.

Lesieur, H. R., & Rosenthal, J. (1989). Children of Gamblers Anonymous members. *Journal of Gambling Behavior, 5,* 269–81.

Lesieur, H. R., & Rosenthal, J. (1991). Pathological gambling: A review of the literature. (Prepared for the American Psychiatric Association Task Force on DSM-IV Committee on Disorders of Impulse Control Not Elsewhere Classified.) *Journal of Gambling Studies, 7,* 5–40.

Lesieur, H. R., & Rothschild, J. (1989). Children of Gamblers Anonymous members. *Journal of Gambling Behavior, 5,* 269–82.

Levine, A. (1990, June). Playing the adolescent odds. *U.S. News & World Report, 108,* 51.

Loder, C. M. (1995, January 19). Union workers push limits on betting machines. *(Newark, NJ) Star-Ledger,* p. 2.

MacFarquhar, N. (1995, March 3). New hotbed of bookies: High school. *New York Times,* p. A7.

Maden, T., Swinton, M., & Gunn, J. (1992). Gambling in young offenders. *Criminal Behavioral and Mental Health, 2,* 300–308.

Misseck, R. E. (1994, November 28). Gambling resurfaces in Union high schools. *(Newark, NJ) Star-Ledger,* p. 14.

Moody, G. (1989). Parents of young gamblers. (Special issue: Gambling and the family.) *Journal of Gambling Behavior, 5,* 313–20.

Murphy, S. (1994, January 23). Teen-age gambling rampant. *Boston Globe,* pp. 1, 34.

Omnifacts Research Limited. (1993). *An examination of the prevalence of gambling in Nova Scotia.* Research report no. 93090 for the Nova Scotia Department of Health, Drug Dependency Services. Halifax, Nova Scotia: Author.

Orlando, A. (1994, December 4).The wagers of sin snare young people. *(Newark, NJ) Sunday Star-Ledger.*

Oster, S., & Knapp, T. J. (1994, June). Casino gambling by underage patrons: Two studies of a university student population. Paper presented at the Ninth International Conference on Gambling and Risk Taking, Las Vegas.

Pursley, W. L. (1991). Adolescence, chemical dependency, and pathological gambling. *Journal of Adolescent Chemical Dependency, 1,* 25–47.

Radecki, T. E. (1994). The sales of lottery tickets to minors in Illinois. *Journal of Gambling Studies, 10,* 213–18.

The serious problem of high school gambling. (1995, March 6). *The Record* (New Jersey), p. A12.

Shaffer, H. J., LaBrie, R., Scanlan, K. M., & Cummings, T. N. (1994). Pathological gambling among adolescents: Massachusetts Gambling Screen (MAGS). *Journal of Gambling Studies, 10,* 339–62.

Spunt, B., Lesieur, H. R., Hunt, D., & Cahill, L. (1995). Gambling among methadone patients. *International Journal of the Addictions, 30,* 929–62.

Steeves, B. M. (1994). Video lotteries in New Brunswick. In C.S. Campbell (Ed.), *Gambling in Canada: The bottom line.* Burnaby, British Columbia: Simon Fraser University, Criminology Research Centre.

Steinberg, M. (1988, May). Gambling behavior among high school students in Connecticut. Paper presented at the Third National Conference on Gambling, New York.

Students get anti-gambling message. (1994, December 1). *Linden (NJ) Leader.*

Svendsen, R., & Griffin, T. (1994). *Improving your odds: A curriculum about winning, losing, and staying out of trouble with gambling.* Anoka, MN: Minnesota Institute of Public Health.

Tobler, N. S. (1992). *Meta-analysis of adolescent drug prevention programs: Final report.* Rockville, MD: National Institute on Drug Abuse.

Tonry, R., & Wilson, J. Q. (Eds.). (1990). *Drugs and crime. Crime and justice: A review of research, 13.* Chicago: University of Chicago Press.

Volberg, R. (1993). *Gambling and problem gambling among adolescents in Washington state.* Report to the Washington State Lottery. Albany, NY: Gemini Research.

Wallisch, L. S. (1993). *Gambling in Texas: 1992 Texas survey of adolescent gambling behavior.* Austin: Texas Commission on Alcohol and Drug Abuse.

Waterman, J., & Atkin, K. (1985). Young people and fruit machines. *Society for the Study of Gambling Newsletter, 7,* 23–25.

Wexler, A. S. (1994, June). Personal communication.

Winters, K. C., & Stinchfield, R. D. (1993). *Gambling behavior among Minnesota youth: Monitoring change from 1990 to 1991/1992.* Minneapolis: University of Minnesota, Center for Adolescent Substance Abuse.

Winters, K. C., Stinchfield, R. D., & Fulkerson, J. (1990). *Adolescent survey of gambling behavior in Minnesota: A benchmark.* Report to the Department of Human Services Mental Health Division. Duluth, MN: University of Minnesota, Center for Addiction Studies.

Winters, K. C., Stinchfield, R. D., & Fulkerson, J. (1993a). Toward the development of an adolescent gambling problem severity scale. *Journal of Gambling Studies, 9,* 63–84.

Winters, K. C., Stinchfield, R. D., & Fulkerson, J. (1993b). Patterns and characteristics of adolescent gambling. *Journal of Gambling Studies, 9,* 371–86.

Winters, K. C., Stinchfield, R. D., & Kim, L. G. (1995). Monitoring adolescent gambling in Minnesota. *Journal of Gambling Studies, 11,* 165–83.

Wyckoff, P. L. (1995, March 7). Casinos ante up for anti-gambling messages. *(Newark, NJ) Star-Ledger.*

Zeigler, A. (1995, January 11). Critics say adults gamble on the future of their children: Teens may bet on elder's example. *Washington Times,* p. A2.

Zitzow, D. (1992, July). Comparative study of compulsive gambling behaviors between American Indians and non-Indians within and near a rural reservation. Paper presented at the Seventh National Conference on Compulsive Gambling, New London, CT.

Juvenile Gambling in North America
Considering Past Trends and Future Prospects

Durand F. Jacobs

Introduction

As this volume reveals, the citizens of the United States and Canada now have at their disposal a broad, representative, and empirically derived database that describes the parameters of juvenile gambling in North America. This research provides information about the relationship between juvenile gambling and attending factors attributable to personal, family, peer, school, and broader community influences. Notable among these topics is the expansion of legally sanctioned forms of gambling throughout the United States and Canada over the past decade and a half.

This rapidly accumulating body of knowledge provides sometimes disturbing new insights into, first, the surprisingly early age of onset for gambling among our children; second, where, with whom, on what, and how much juveniles gamble; and third, juveniles' self-reports on the short-term negative consequences they have experienced as a result of their gambling. Several studies also have illuminated the underlying motives that lead juveniles to gamble, and revealed the unusual psychological reactions, while gambling, that sharply differentiate problem from nonproblem gamblers. These latter findings suggest new directions for further inquiries about the predisposing causes and course of problematic gambling among juveniles. These findings in turn have the potential to lead to new and improved outreach and educational, assessment, treatment, and prevention strategies.

The intent of this epilogue is to summarize and focus information about juvenile gambling in order to facilitate the attainment of four major goals:

1. To increase public awareness of the nature and extent of gambling activities among juveniles, and of the prevalence of serious gambling problems among these legally underage youth.
2. To build appropriate outreach and treatment programs for juvenile problem gamblers, staffed by specially trained education, social service, and health professionals.
3. To approach high schools and middle schools with self-screening tools and programs that will facilitate secondary prevention through early identification of, and appropriate education and counseling for, juveniles who are beginning to experience gambling-related problems.
4. To establish primary prevention programs within the curricula of both elementary and middle schools that will reduce the likelihood of children acquiring *any* addictive pattern of behavior, including pathological gambling, as they approach adolescence.

Concurrently, it also is necessary to obtain the active collaboration and financial support of the gaming industry, both public and private, in pursuit of these goals.

Background

There is reason to believe that most legally underage youth throughout North America have gambled for money during the past year. Yet, there is insufficient public recognition of, or concern with, juvenile gambling. The apparent unwillingness of adult society to acknowledge the extent of gambling behaviors among its children may reside in the belief that legal sanctions are sufficient to discourage any "really serious" gambling among those under 18 years of age . . . so, not to worry. Perhaps it could also reflect the reluctance of adult society to face up to its own role in fostering childhood and teenage gambling, since the overwhelming majority of young people who gamble report that they were introduced to this recreational diversion by their parents and older relatives. Could it be that underage gambling is simply dismissed as harmless fun and games? Alternatively, is it a delayed awareness about this new component of current adolescent experience on the part of schools, churches, government authorities, and the gaming industry? And, finally, how big a problem can it be?

A series of independent survey studies of middle school– and high school–age youth conducted between 1984 and 2000 in several states and provinces spanning North America suggests that between 40 and 90 percent of these youth (varying somewhat from locale to locale) has gambled for money during the previous year. In other words, this research indicates that within the past year, as many as 14 million 12- to 17-year-old juveniles in the United States have been gambling for money with or without adult awareness or approval. Since the overwhelming majority of these juveniles are under their state's legal gambling age, they have been gambling illegally. Furthermore, research suggests that almost 2 million of these juveniles are experiencing serious gambling-related problems. There is equal reason to believe that in Canada, 1.3 million juveniles have been gambling for money in the past twelve months, with most doing so without adult awareness or approval, and more than 200,000 of these young Canadians also are experiencing serious gambling-related problems (Jacobs, 2000).

Prevalence of Juvenile Gambling in the United States and Canada
TRENDS (1984–2000)

Numerous studies conducted in the United States between 1984 and 2000 provide support for the frequently voiced impression that the gambling involvement of middle school–age to high school–age youth has tended to increase over the past decade and a half.

Earliest prevalence studies on juvenile gambling (those conducted between 1984 and 1988) reveal a median level of 45 percent participation by high school–age students in gambling activities during the previous twelve-month period (Jacobs, Marston, & Singer, 1985; Jacobs, Marston, Singer, Widaman, & Little, 1987; Kuley & Jacobs, 1987; Lesieur & Klein, 1987; Steinberg, 1988). More recent juvenile gambling studies (those conducted between 1989 and 2000) reveal the median level of gambling participation by these juveniles to be 66 percent (Kuley & Jacobs, 1989; Shaffer, LaBrie, Scanlan, & Cummings, 1994; Volberg, 1993; Volberg & Boles, 1996; Volberg & Moore, 1999; Wallisch, 1993, 1996; Winters, Stinchfield, & Fulkerson, 1990; Westphal, Rush, Stevens, & Johnson, 1998; Proimos, DuRant, Pierce, & Goodman, 1998). These figures leave little doubt that the median level of juvenile gambling throughout the United States has increased during the past decade.

Studies conducted in Canada between 1988 and 2000 reveal an equivalent rate. During this period, the median prevalence rate for juvenile gambling in Canada was 67 percent (Govoni, Rupcich, & Frisch, 1996; Insight Canada Research, 1994; Ladouceur & Mireault, 1988; Omnifacts Research Ltd., 1993; Wynne, Smith, & Jacobs, 1996; Wiebe, Cox, & Mehmel, 2000; Adlaf & Ialomiteanu, 2000; Noonan, Turner, & Macdonald, 1999). Thus, the dominant trend over the past decade and a half indicates a progressive increase in juvenile gambling throughout North America. Based on these combined findings, one can reasonably assume that in 2000 at least six out of ten middle school–age and high school–age students throughout North America had gambled for money during the past year (Jacobs, 2000).

GAMES PLAYED BY JUVENILE GAMBLERS

A consistent finding across all studies of youthful gambling in the United States and Canada is that juveniles 12 to 17 years of age have managed to participate to some degree in every form of social, government-sanctioned, and illegal gambling opportunity available in their communities, and in places where they travel (Jacobs, 2000). To the casual observer, the range of activities on which these youth have gambled for money is quite startling. It ranges from betting on cards, dice, and board games with family and friends to betting on games of personal skill, such as pool and bowling; playing arcade or video games for money; buying raffle tickets; sports betting with friends, or at off-track betting parlors; wagering at horse and dog racetracks; gambling in bingo and card rooms; betting on jai alai games; playing slot machines and table games in casinos; buying pull-tabs and lottery tickets from vendors at lottery counters, or playing at free-standing video lottery terminals; playing the stock market; placing bets with a bookie; and gambling on the Internet. Juveniles manage to gamble on every form of wagering available to adults in a given community. Naturally, communities will differ regarding the local availability of one or another kind of gambling outlet. Some have readily accessible casinos, others have lotteries, and still others have nearby racetracks.

Surveys done over the past decade throughout North America show that, notwithstanding local availability, the four most popular games among juveniles are (1) cards, dice, and board games with family and friends, (2) games of personal skill with peers, (3) sports betting, usually with peers in school settings but also with a bookie, and (4) bingo (Shaffer, Hall, & Vander Bilt, 1997). However, where a state or provincial lottery had been operative *before* the survey was completed, lottery games typically usurp first or second ranking among the games favored by juvenile gamblers. Indeed, introducing a state or provincial lottery invariably produces an increase in the numbers of both adults and juveniles who gamble in that jurisdiction. After completing the first study ever done on gambling in America, Kallick, Suits, Dielman, and Hybels (1976) concluded that, when a state (or other government body) promotes one form of gambling, all forms of gambling—both legal and illegal—tend to increase. Studies conducted in states that operate lotteries tend to reveal higher estimates of juvenile gambling than studies conducted in states without lotteries (Jacobs, 1994, 2000).

Although no direct causal effect can be shown between the operation of a lottery and a corresponding increase of gambling among juveniles in that locale, the circumstantial evidence clearly points in that direction. Few would contest the fact that using advertising to introduce and promote a lottery creates the most widespread, plentiful, and locally accessible vehicle for gambling throughout that province or state. Certainly, far more lottery sales outlets are readily at hand than any other form of gambling. For instance, in 2001 the California lottery had 19,000 individual sales outlets and 1,200 self-serving terminals (SSTs) strategically located throughout the state. On average, this makes one sales outlet available for every 1,500 residents in the neighborhoods surrounding those sales sites. A similar, carefully planned distribution pattern prevails in other lottery venues throughout North America. Moreover, a government-supported and government-promoted lottery also fosters a more affirmative and socially acceptable community attitude toward wagering ("playing") than is enjoyed by any other form of legalized gambling. The impact of this general climate of "it's OK to play" does not escape the attention of juveniles, who, though legally underage, quickly find the purchase of lottery tickets a minor adventure, seldom discouraged by vendors, and often aided and abetted by parents and older relatives (Ladouceur & Mireault, 1988; Jacobs, 1989a; Winters, Stinchfield, & Fulkerson, 1990).

Findings from studies investigating underage participation in the lottery (Kuley & Jacobs, 1989; Jacobs, 1994; Westphal et al., 1998; Volberg & Moore, 1999) support the following two hypotheses: (1) Active promotion of a state or provincial lottery accompanied by ready availability of outlets for the sale of lottery tickets is correlated with increased rates of lottery ticket purchases by youth under the legal age of 18 years, and (2) Once a state or province legalizes and actively promotes this form of gambling, participation by juveniles in all forms of gambling—both legal and illegal—will tend to increase (known as the "Pied Piper Effect"). These issues have significant implications for lottery advertising, enforcement of laws prohibiting minors from gambling, and the accountability of elected officials and appointed lottery commissioners for contributing to juvenile gambling in general and to gambling-related problems among juveniles in particular.

GENDER DIFFERENCES AMONG JUVENILE PLAYERS

Over the past decade and a half, gambling has revealed itself to be a male-dominated activity, both among juveniles and their adult models. Like their adult counterparts, male juveniles tend to gamble on more games, gamble more often, spend more time and money, and experience more gambling-related problems than do female juveniles. The preferred games on which male juveniles gamble may differ from those females play along a skill/knowledge to pure luck continuum. Research shows that boys tend to cluster more at the skill/knowledge end, with card and board games, games of personal skill, and sports betting most popular among them. Alternatively, female juveniles have been more oriented to games of chance like raffles, bingo, lotteries, and pull-tabs (where available). However, in places where horse and dog races and machine games, such as video lottery terminals and slot machines, are locally accessible, researchers have observed juvenile participation in these activities to be divided equally between the sexes. All of these findings may reflect the social context and historical moment within which these young people have gambled. More research is necessary to clarify these matters.

AGE OF ONSET FOR GAMBLING AMONG JUVENILES

Children throughout the United States and Canada report their first gambling experience at a surprisingly early age, ranging from 10 to 13 years. By the time children in North America are 12 years old, one can expect that the majority have already gambled for money. As a general rule, one can assume that the earliest gambling experiences among children tend to occur under a set of circumstances where: (1) opportunities to wager even small amounts of money are readily accessible, (2) the social climate of the home and local environment is conducive to, and accepting of, such behavior, and (3) the rules of the games to be played are within the child's capacity to understand. How these circumstances emerge is straightforward: Children simply become involved in social and recreational activities (including gambling) that have already been going on around them, and to which they are welcomed as new players by family members, other adults, and older peers in the local community.

As has long been the case with juvenile drinking, adults throughout North American societies appear to overlook their role as "accessory before the fact." They seem to conclude that children somehow invented gambling on their own, rather than having learned it from them (Milgram, 1982). Indeed, when queried, the overwhelming majority of youth who gamble reply that they were introduced to gambling by their parents and older relatives. A case in point: the results of a questionnaire distributed to more than 1,000 students in an Atlantic City, New Jersey, high school (Arcuri, Lester, & Smith, 1985). Sixty-four percent of these legally underage students (average age below 17 years) reported they had gambled in the nearby casinos. Nine percent said they had done so at least once a week during the preceding month. Here again, the paradox of ambivalent parental attitudes is encountered: 79 percent of these students said their parents knew that they had gambled.

Ladouceur and Mireault (1988) reported a similar situation was reported a few years later. Their study involved more than 1,600 students from nine high schools in the region of Quebec City, Quebec. Sixty-six percent of these students said they had gambled once in their lifetime, with 65 percent reporting they had placed a bet in the previous year and 24 percent reporting they had gambled at least once a week. Ninety percent of these students said their parents knew they gambled, and 84 percent said their parents did not object. Indeed, 61 percent of these adolescents said they wagered in the company of their parents; 57 percent wagered with their brothers and sisters, and 15 percent with other members of the family. More than 25 percent reported they had borrowed money from parents or other relatives either to bet or to pay their gambling debts.

When youths report that their parents have experienced gambling problems, the age of onset for their own gambling occurs much earlier. For instance, Jacobs et al. (1989) reported that 75 percent of high school–age youth who described one or both of their parents as "having a problem with compulsive gambling" had first gambled before age 11, while only 34 percent of their classmates without such disordered-gambling parents had first gambled before age 11. As is the case with other potentially health-threatening pursuits of juveniles, such as smoking and alcohol and drug use, an earlier age of onset may presage later and greater problems with a given substance or activity (Proimos et al., 1998). Winters et al. (1990) observed a significantly negative relationship between the grade at which an adolescent first gambled and later severity of problem gambling. A similar situation was reported in a recent Canadian study (Wynne, Smith & Jacobs, 1996).

The majority of youth-gambling prevalence studies involves middle school and high school subjects. To this writer's knowledge, only two Canadian studies investigated lifetime prevalence rates for gambling among primary school students. Ladouceur, Dubé, and Bujold (1994) found that 81 percent of fourth graders, 84 percent of fifth graders, and 92 percent of sixth graders in their Quebec City sample had gambled sometime in the past. The lottery was by far their favorite wager, followed by cards and sports betting. Similar findings emerged from a second independent Canadian study completed in Montreal (Gupta, Derevensky, & Cioppa, 1996). In this study, 57 percent of fourth graders and 85 percent of sixth graders reported they had gambled in the past. Moreover, 48 percent of the fourth graders and 61 percent of the sixth graders said they had engaged in gambling activities at least once a week. This set of Canadian findings clearly indicates that a substantial majority of the primary-school children sampled in Quebec province had gambled well before they were 11 years of age.

Prevalence of Serious Gambling-Related Problems Among Juveniles
TRENDS (1984–2000)
Studies that estimate the prevalence of youth problem gambling reveal that the dominant trend over the past decade and a half has been an increase in the aggregate amount of gambling-related problems reported by juveniles in both the United States and Canada. In addition, these studies also show a substantial increase in the proportion of juveniles who have gambled at all during the previous year. These parallel developments lead to the conclusion that, *as increasing numbers of juveniles participate in an expanding array of gambling opportunities around them, an increasing number of them will experience serious gambling-related problems.* Moreover, this rate remains two to four times higher than the rate of problems evidenced by their adult counterparts (Jacobs, 1989a, 2000).

COMORBIDITY AMONG THOSE REPORTING SERIOUS
GAMBLING-RELATED PROBLEMS
Studies of adult pathological gamblers have reported levels of alcohol and drug abuse as high as 50 percent among those who present for treatment (Jacobs, 1984; Lesieur & Blume, 1991; Ramirez, McCormick, Russo, & Taber, 1983). Similarly, studies have shown that patients seeking substance-abuse treatment have levels of pathological gambling ranging from 9 percent to 20 percent (Lesieur & Blume, 1990; Jacobs, 1992; Lesieur, Blume, & Zoppa, 1986; Spunt, Lesieur, Hunt, & Cahill, 1995). Findings of this sort support the expectation for comorbidity among people struggling with addictive behavior patterns. That is, persons experiencing a given addictive or poten-

tially addictive pattern of behavior are often found to be engaging in other potentially addictive activities, as adjunctive methods of reducing their stress levels, and for escaping from reality problems (Jacobs, 1988c, 1990, 2000).

Many juvenile studies have sought to determine the relationship between the presence of *"serious gambling-related problems"* among youth (i.e., reporting three or more problems on gambling screens) and their concurrent use of psychoactive substances (e.g., tobacco, alcohol, and illicit drugs). It was consistently found that adolescents experiencing three or more gambling-related problems also reported twice the rate of frequent tobacco use and twice the weekly or more-often rate of alcohol use than was reported by their nonproblem classmates. Among all psychoactive products noted, alcohol was the substance of choice among all juvenile groups, closely followed by tobacco (Proimos et al., 1998). Use of marijuana and other illicit drugs was seldom reported for this population. However, when these drugs were reported, those reporting serious gambling-related problems showed use patterns two to four times greater than those with no gambling-related problems (Jacobs, 2000).

Another comorbid condition noted in the history of adult compulsive/pathological gamblers has been the presence of excessive parental gambling (Custer & Custer, 1978; Jacobs, Marston, Singer, Widaman, & Little, 1987; Taber & McCormick, 1987). When this relationship was explored by youth studies, those reporting gambling-related problems reported consistently higher levels of both parental gambling and excessive parental gambling than did their nonproblem peers by ratios of 3 to 2. In the studies reviewed by this author, overall rates of excessive parental gambling reported by juvenile subjects range from 1 percent to 13 percent in the United States, and from 1 percent to 10 percent in Canada, with median levels slightly higher in Canada (Jacobs, 2000).

Still another comorbid condition noted among adult compulsive/pathological gamblers is a high level of illegal activity (60 percent to 80 percent), resulting in trouble with the police (Custer & Milt, 1985; Lesieur, 1987). Several studies of youth gambling have explored this possible relationship among juveniles. Overall, findings revealed that while about 10 percent of the total sample reported recent involvements in illegal activities and/or problems with the police, those experiencing gambling-related problems were at least twice as likely to admit being so involved. These adolescents also emerged as more likely to report poorer school performance, truancy, higher levels of unhappiness with their lives, and more anxious and depressed feelings than those experiencing no gambling-related problems (Jacobs, 2000).

Among the twelve to twenty questions of the South Oaks Gambling Screen (SOGS) (Lesieur & Blume, 1987), several researchers using the original or some revised form of this instrument found that the six items most frequently cited by those experiencing three or more gambling-related problems were:

- When you gamble, how often do you go back another day to win back money you lost?

- Have you ever claimed to be winning money gambling, but weren't really? In fact, you lost?
- Did you ever gamble more than you intended to?
- Have you ever felt guilty about the way you gamble, or what happens when you gamble?
- Have money arguments with your family ever centered on your gambling?
- Have you ever borrowed from someone, and not paid them back, as a result of your gambling?

Despite the relatively high total of SOGS items chosen, the question garnering the *least* affirmative responses across juvenile studies was "Do you feel you have ever had a problem with gambling?" In one juvenile study (Wynne, Smith, & Jacobs, 1996), this item was deliberately placed as the last question among the SOGS items. Nonetheless, the result was essentially the same as found in other studies: 96 percent of the 225 juveniles experiencing serious gambling-related problems answered "no." This denial—on the part of adults and juveniles alike—that gambling has ever been a problem, side by side with their own reports confirming numerous problems that are a direct consequence of their gambling, leaves family members and neophyte health providers confused and uncertain while gamblers move toward the nearest exit. This finding begins to explain why so few juveniles who score high on standard screening instruments seek help for gambling problems on their own volition. It also underscores the need for public education targeted to increase self-awareness on the part of juveniles that gambling can become as addictive as alcohol (Jacobs, 1995).

A COMPOSITE PROFILE OF THOSE REPORTING "SERIOUS GAMBLING-RELATED PROBLEMS"

The following profile is drawn from frequently reported demographic, behavioral, and psychological features that have characterized adolescents experiencing three or more gambling-related problems, as described in studies of youth gambling.

DEMOGRAPHIC FEATURES
Age of onset

While current age among 12- to 17-year-olds does not consistently differentiate juveniles with very few gambling problems from those with many, age of onset for gambling does. Much earlier age of onset, that is, well before 12 years of age, consistently distinguishes adolescents with several gambling-related problems from those experiencing no gambling-related problems.

Gender Differences

Males dominate the ranks of juveniles with gambling-related problems by ratios ranging from 3 to 1 to ratios as large as 5 to 1.

Parental Gambling

Growing up in a home where parents gamble, especially when one or both are perceived by the child as gambling too much, is a situational factor found much more among adolescents with gambling problems than among those without gambling problems. The same trend is true for reports of gambling problems among other relatives or close friends.

Regional Differences

Adolescents with gambling-related problems are more likely to live in a metropolitan area than an outlying suburban or rural area. American Indians living on reservations or reserves are the exception.

Ethnic Group Membership

For a number of reasons, sampling procedures in studies of adolescent gambling have not included any sizable numbers of ethnic minority subjects. Therefore, one is impressed by two reports that relate an unusually high prevalence of gambling-related problems among Native American youths in both the United States and Canada. Zitzow (1996) completed the first. He compared Native American juveniles (N = 115), living on a reservation in Minnesota, with their non–American Indian counterparts (N = 161), living in the surrounding community. He found that the American Indian sample showed significantly higher SOGS scores than the non–American Indian sample for both "potential" pathological gambling (15 percent versus 10 percent) and "probable" pathological gambling (10 percent versus 6 percent). Parenthetically, the non-Indian youth in Zitzow's sample showed prevalence rates for problems with gambling comparable with those reported by Winters et al. (1990) for other non–American Indian Minnesota youth.

A second study, conducted by the Nechi Institute (1995) in the province of Alberta, involved assessment of gambling problems among more than 900 aboriginal youths in grades five through twelve. Fifteen percent of these First Nations youths scored in the at-risk range on the SOGS-RA. This was the same level as was found in a recent, but independent, province-wide study of Alberta juveniles, 12 to 17 years of age (Wynne, Smith, & Jacobs, 1996). However, 13 percent of the Nechi group reported an even greater number of serious gambling-related problems, compared with 8 percent of the more general Alberta sample. Readers are reminded that the rates for gambling-related problems among non-aboriginal juveniles in Alberta province were among the highest in Canada.

Studies of adults have found those in minority ethnic groups to be more at risk for gambling problems than their Caucasian counterparts (Elia & Jacobs, 1993; Volberg, 1996). Consequently, there is an urgent need for additional studies of gambling behaviors focused on American Indians (Wardman, el-Guebaly, & Hodgins,

2001), Hispanics, American blacks, Asians, and youths in other minority groups in North American to more clearly define the nature and the importance of the ethnic variable among juveniles.

BEHAVIORAL FEATURES
Games Played
Juveniles reporting gambling-related problems are distinguished by their preference for rapid, continuous, and interactive games. These include video-arcade games, card games like poker, games of personal skill, like bowling or pool, sports betting, and machine games in and out of casinos. These youth are significantly more likely than nonproblem groups to have gambled on more different games, wagered weekly or more often on two or more different games, spent more time gambling, and bet greater amounts of money, whether on one occasion, weekly, or monthly.

Sources of Gambling Money
Adolescents experiencing gambling-related problems differed from nonproblem gamblers by ratios larger than 10 to 1 in the manner in which they acquire money to gamble. This was particularly apparent in their greater use of lunch money, selling personal belongings, "borrowing" someone else's property to sell (without their knowledge), using bank cards or credit cards, and stealing or other illegal means to obtain money to gamble or to pay gambling debts. They are also more likely to work, and to work longer hours in part-time jobs.

Comorbidity
Adolescents experiencing gambling-related problems were found to be more involved in frequent and heavy use of alcohol and psychoactive drugs than their nonproblem peers. They also report more illegal activities and problems with the law, poorer school performance, and more truancy. They are many times more likely than nonproblem groups to seek help for alcohol or drug problems (of which they have more). However, very few acknowledge or seek help for their gambling-related problems. This underscores the importance of incorporating a gambling screen in the routine initial assessment of juveniles who present with substance abuse or delinquency problems.

Attitudes About Gambling
Problem-gambling adolescents are more positive in their attitudes and expectation regarding gambling than the nonproblem groups. They tend to agree with such statements as: Gambling should be legal for teenagers; if teenagers want to bet money they should be able to; lotteries are useful and a good idea; winning a big lottery jackpot is not very rare; luck or fate plays a big part in my life; gambling is a

harmless pastime; there are tricks to gambling; betting for money is not harmful; I can make a lot of money playing games of chance.

PSYCHOSOCIAL FEATURES
Reasons for Gambling
Researchers have observed a number of psychosocial factors that are more often reported by problem-gambling adolescents than nonproblem-gambling adolescents. These motives and psychological states (in concert with other influences) may predispose juveniles to become gamblers, trigger returns to gambling, or otherwise maintain gambling involvement by reinforcing gratifications obtained by a gambling activity (Jacobs, 1989b; Winters & Stinchfield, 1993). Reasons for gambling found to be more prevalent among problem-gambling juveniles include gambling for excitement; to win money; because of skill at it; to escape from everyday problems; because of boredom, loneliness, sadness, or depression; to feel more powerful; to be in control of social situations; to feel less shy; and to make friends.

Dissociative Reactions While Gambling
Studies by Jacobs (1982, 1988a, 1989b) and by Kuley and Jacobs (1988) were the first to identify extremely high rates of dissociative reactions while gambling. These higher rates for dissociation significantly differentiated adult compulsive/pathological gamblers from adult social gamblers and from normative controls of adults and adolescents who also gambled. More recent studies, comparing dissociative reactions among juveniles who reported three to five or more gambling-related problems with juveniles reporting no problems have shown results strikingly similar to those reported for adult pathological gamblers (Gupta & Derevensky, 1998a). The five items chosen by Jacobs to identify dissociative reactions while gambling were:
- A blurring of reality testing ("feeling like one is in a trance")
- A sense of depersonalization ("feeling like a different person")
- An out-of-body sensation ("feeling like being outside oneself—watching oneself"),
- Deep engrossment in an activity that obscures other reality demands ("losing track of time")
- Having an amnesiac episode ("a memory blackout for things that happened while gambling")

Three independent Canadian studies (Insight Canada Research, 1994; Wynne, Smith, & Jacobs, 1996; Gupta & Derevensky, 1998b) document how juveniles who report progressively more gambling-related problems also report a progressively increasing presence of each of these five dissociative experiences while gambling. These replicated findings for problem-gambling groups are remarkably different from the very low prevalence reported by the nonproblem groups. Winters et al.

(1990) included only two of these dissociative measures in their Minnesota study, but revealed a similar pattern.

The ability of the above set of dissociative items to sharply distinguish juveniles reporting some to many gambling-related problems from those reporting few if any such problems strongly recommends their inclusion in future screening instruments. Jacobs (1989b) has found that casually inserting these dissociative items during assessment of those alleged to have an addiction can be very useful in clinical and forensic situations, particularly when one is required to discriminate between those who truly have an addiction to gambling and those who are excessive indulgers or possible malingerers. By the same token, one cannot overemphasize the possible value of these items for obtaining much earlier identification of potentially at-risk youth than is possible with current gambling screens (Jacobs, 2000).

These findings of high rates of dissociation while indulging are entirely consistent with Jacobs's General Theory of Addictions (Jacobs, 1982, 1989b, 1998, 2001a). They strongly support his position that all addictive patterns of behavior (including pathological gambling) basically represent a person's chosen "vehicle" that he or she deliberately uses (a) to escape from highly stressful internal and external reality conditions and (b) to experience an altered, much more pleasant state of consciousness while indulging. This direct *problem-solving* paradigm gains further support from the sampling of reasons for gambling (noted above) given by youth who report numerous serious gambling-related problems. Consequently, future gambling screens for both juveniles and adults must go beyond phenotypic behavioral indices and tap into the deeper motives and the psychosocial rewards anticipated by those who find gambling so rewarding that they doggedly persist and accelerate their involvement in this activity, despite increasingly punishing consequences for themselves and others.

Future Prospects
PROSPECTS FOR CHANGING PREVALENCE RATES

Since the early 1980s, when the first studies of juvenile gambling began in the United States (Jacobs, Marston, & Singer, 1985; Lesieur & Klein, 1987), the dominant trend has been a progressive increase of juvenile participation in all forms of gambling. It would appear that the extent and nature of juvenile involvement in any given jurisdiction varies directly as a function of (1) the length of time legalized forms of gambling have been available in that state or province and (2) the ready accessibility of various gambling opportunities—particularly lottery outlets—in the local community where the juvenile resides.

North America has not yet reached its saturation point for per capita expenditure on gambling. Consequently, during the next five years the numbers and variety of gambling outlets readily accessible to adults (and juveniles) in states and provinces will continue to increase, as will the numbers of adult and juvenile players and the gross revenues gratefully accepted by cash-hungry governments. Throughout

North America, casino-style operations will continue to appear and to expand on state, provincial, federal, and native-held lands and waters. And they will continue to be infiltrated by underage players. Expanding opportunities for gambling on the Internet and on home television are certain to attract juvenile players, who are becoming increasingly technology literate and who will seek and find ingenious ways to join the fun.

Unfortunately, there is little of substance on the immediate horizon that promises any large-scale interventions by government or the private gaming industry to reduce underage gambling dramatically. Therefore, it is more than a safe bet that juvenile gambling on accessible games will continue to increase over the next five years, so that by the year 2007 the median prevalence levels for juvenile lifetime gambling can be expected to approach 80 percent throughout North America.

PROSPECTS FOR CHANGES IN FAVORED GAMES PLAYED

Strongly influencing the kinds of games juveniles play is the ever-expanding menu of state and provincial lottery offerings. Future prospects are for bigger payouts, plus more interactive, "skill-appearing" games like Sports Select and more continuous, rapid-outcome machine games like scratch-offs, keno, and video lottery terminals. While these games are designed to increase the expenditures made and the range of games adults play, the new interactive lottery games also can be expected to result in increased participation and expenditures by juvenile players.

Male adolescents likely will prefer the Sports Select–type games. Males as well as females will be drawn to the more passive, but more rapid-action, machine-type games. These continuous fast-action machine games will compete for preferential status with games of personal skill for males and with bingo for females. Coming up fast among male adolescents is increased sports betting among students while in middle school and high school settings, along with relatively high-stakes poker games in home settings. Juvenile involvement in both these kinds of games will continue to increase, so long as school personnel and parents remain less than fully aware of what transpires on their respective premises.

PROSPECTS FOR INCREASED GAMBLING BY FEMALE ADOLESCENTS

The changing gender representation in this still largely male-dominated activity is rapidly moving gambling toward a unisex recreational and diversionary pursuit. Studies over the past decade and a half note an increasing proportion of girls in the ranks of juvenile gamblers. This increase reflects the rapidly disappearing moral, social, and economic constraints against their participation. Paralleling and enhancing the effects of the changing social climate is the increasing availability of lottery, high-stakes bingo, pull-tabs, slots, and video lottery terminal games that appeal more to the youthful (and adult) female player. As this trend continues, it will accelerate the gender leveling among tomorrow's gamblers.

PROSPECTS FOR CHANGES IN AGE OF ONSET

Among the more than a score of studies reviewed by this author, the mean reported age of onset for an adolescent's first gambling experience ranged from 11 to 13 years of age, depending on local conditions, with an overall median at year 12, i.e., seventh graders. In past studies of representative adult populations in North America, average age of onset for 20- to 35-year-old groups typically occurred during their high school years (15 to 18 years of age), while the first gambling experience reported by older adults, aged 46 through 70 plus, did not occur until their early 20s. These differing "cohort effects" reflect the answer to an unasked, but very relevant, question: What was the nature, extent, ready availability, and social acceptability of legalized gambling when you were growing up?

Today's juveniles are the first generation to grow up in a society where an increasing number of socially acceptable and readily accessible forms of legalized gambling exist all around them. Therefore, it is not surprising that their age of onset is much younger than previous generations. The age of onset can be expected to continue to get progressively younger among juveniles over the next five years. The reason for taking this position is twofold. First, more and more of their parents and older relatives will be gambling. These adults are the principal channel through which children are introduced to gambling. Second, because of permissive social attitudes toward gambling by these adults and society at large, 10- to 17-year-old juveniles will continue to find ways to participate in all forms of gambling around them, in addition to gambling even more among themselves on cards, games of personal skill, and sports betting.

As early as 1976—long before the first juvenile gambling study was conceived—Kallick et al. (1976) observed that among adults, participation in gambling peaked in the age range of 18 to 24 years, and then declined. Recent studies indicate that gambling now peaks in the mid-30s, and tends to decline thereafter. For example, Volberg and Boles (1996) revealed that of the weekly gamblers in their adult sample, only 20 percent were under 30 years of age. Kallick et al. also noted that increased exposure and accessibility to gambling, and the varied forms of gambling, produced new gamblers. They concluded: "Gambling is a young person's pursuit . . . making it probable that subsequent generations which are exposed to gambling early and start early may not have a rate of decline as steep as we observe now" (Kallick et al., 1976, p. 7).

The growing body of evidence in the field of adolescent gambling challenges any a priori expectation that juvenile gamblers, who already show serious gambling-related problems, will somehow "mature out" in short order—particularly in environments where ever-expanding gambling continues to be socially acceptable, actively promoted by governments, and readily accessible (cf. Shaffer et al., 1997). Only a series of longitudinal research studies will provide definitive answers regarding the age at which today's cohort of juvenile gamblers will peak and then decline (Jacobs, 1989a; Shaffer et al., 1997). Meanwhile, we cannot wait and see. We must intervene now to marshal and promote appropriate services to assist those youths beginning to experience serious gambling-related problems, when and wherever they are encouraged to present themselves for help.

To further stimulate our efforts, we need only to recall that the prevalence rates for serious gambling-related problems among juveniles consistently are found to be 2 to 4 times those for adults in the same communities (Jacobs, 1989a). This leaves little doubt about where our priorities should be. There simply is no alternative to strict enforcement of laws meant to prevent gambling by minors. Such efforts could be easily and inexpensively incorporated into ongoing campaigns, including vendors' "We Card" posters, to prevent sale of tobacco and alcohol products to underage youth.

A WORD ABOUT GAMBLING SCREENS

Existing juvenile-gambling screens, while reasonably effective for gross epidemiological purposes—that is, obtaining comparable information from large numbers of persons in a defined group—leave much to be desired when applied to clinical use (Abbott & Volberg, 1996). In the past, adaptations of instruments like the SOGS (originally designed for adults) have been provisionally accepted for use with juveniles—until something better is developed (Volberg, 1993). At this writing, however, screening instruments have not been standardized on those juveniles independently diagnosed as pathological gamblers. It is understood that the latter action would require developing some agreed-upon modification in DSM-IV criteria.

Nonetheless, we are now in a better position than ever before to move forward toward better screening instruments. After more than a score of juvenile studies, we now have sufficient relevant, field-tested items to constitute a basic pool for further modification and application. It is now time to convene the first Study Commission on Gambling Screens. The charter of the commission would be first to construct and field test a set of "gold standard" epidemiological screening instruments for adults and juveniles that could be used for gathering comparable sets of data about gambling from various jurisdictions throughout the world (Jacobs, 1988b). Such instruments also would be extremely valuable for conducting social impact studies to evaluate the influence of changes in available gambling in a given jurisdiction.

A second goal of the commission would be to develop a set of screening tools for clinical application. The latter would be standardized against groups of independently diagnosed juveniles and adults using criteria such as set forth in DSM-IV (American Psychiatric Association, 1994). As noted above, some agreed-upon modification of DSM-IV would need to be developed before it could be properly applied to juveniles. The already active Research Committee of the National Council on Problem Gambling Inc. could serve as a nucleus for staffing such a commission. Other members would be drawn from among well-known researchers in the United States, Canada, the British Isles, Australia, Europe, and Asia (Jacobs, 1988b; The Wager, 2001).

A major shortcoming in the use of current gambling screens is that the anonymity accorded subjects precludes any form of feedback to them on the import of their responses (Jacobs, 1995, 2000). All too familiar is the paradox of a subject obtaining high SOGS scores, while simultaneously denying that a problem with gambling had ever existed. This pattern strongly suggests the desirability of providing some form of direct feedback to subjects scoring within the parameters of serious gambling-related problems (Weibe et al., 2000). In larger-scale studies using computerized data input, such feedback to high scorers could be programmed to follow immediately upon completion of the telephone interview. Subjects who wish to receive such feedback could be informed of the potential significance of their responses, along with directions for obtaining more detailed information from service resources in the region of the interviewee's postal code.

Another even simpler method might be to cast a given gambling screen in a "self-test" format. Upon completion of this kind of questionnaire, subjects would be directed to a scoring section to learn where they placed in the range of scores denoting increasing levels of risk for problem gambling (Jacobs, 1995). Supplementing this scoring section could be a toll-free telephone number through which the subject could obtain further information about a potential gambling problem. Those providing such toll-free feedback opportunities might be the National Council on Problem Gambling Inc. (1-800-522-4700), a state affiliate of the National Council, the Canadian Foundation on Compulsive Gambling, the group conducting the survey, or the International Service Office for Gamblers Anonymous (213-386-8789). The opportunity to receive such feedback without risk of any embarrassment or loss of anonymity would be offered in the introductory statement, soliciting participation in the survey, and might even encourage more candid responses. The prospects for improved gambling screens between now and the year 2007 are very exciting. This author is confident that future screens will build in a "self-awareness" feature of one kind or another.

It also is likely that a set of standard instruments for epidemiological studies of gambling will be validated and gain wide acceptance among researchers. Such screens (restricted to extent, locus, and kinds of gambling) could be used for both adult and juvenile populations and across various national jurisdictions (Jacobs, 1988b).

One can expect a separate development of scales used for clinical purposes. These instruments would likely provide different scoring categories for adults and juveniles, and perhaps for males and females (Volberg, 2001). Special scales also may be developed to discriminate between "action" and "escapist" types of gamblers. Certain to be included among the special scales will be items assessing levels of dissociative experiences while gambling. A battery of these special scales will reduce the numbers of false positives and false negatives that have complicated the interpretation of more traditional screens.

PROSPECTS REGARDING PUBLIC, GOVERNMENTAL, AND GAMING
INDUSTRY REACTIONS TO JUVENILE GAMBLING

In the first review of juvenile gambling in America (Jacobs, 1989a), this author noted that

> teenage gambling was not yet conceptualized as an issue fifteen years ago, even though teenage involvement with potentially addictive substances such as alcohol, prescription, and illicit drugs were matters of serious concern and have remained the subject of systematic nationwide evaluation since 1975 (Johnston et al., 1979). Potentially harmful effects of teenage gambling simply had not been a matter for professional, scientific, governmental, or lay scrutiny, as attested to by the virtually silent literature on this topic before 1980 . . . it was not until the latter months of 1988 that the issue of teenage gambling, its extent, content, and risks first crossed the threshold of general public awareness. This was caused by a flurry of research reports and interviews with knowledgeable professionals that appeared in newspapers and magazines throughout the country, and were highlighted in radio talk shows and in national TV news and dramatic programs. Ironically, it was due mainly to the nationwide publicity surrounding the [then] largest-ever $60 million California lottery prize that led to "the dark side of underage gambling" being illuminated by the national media. (pp. 263–64)

Unfortunately, the debut of underage gambling on the public scene was short-lived. The notoriously short memory and attention span of the public and the media quickly resulted in a state of mixed ignorance, complacency, and denial. Media attention revived in early 1990, sparked by publication of *Compulsive Gambling: Theory, Research, and Practice* (Shaffer, Stein, Gambino, & Cummings, 1989). Once again, researchers, health professionals, elected officials, and gaming industry representatives were contacted for a flurry of interviews, appearances on national radio and TV, and print articles about teenage gambling. Since that time, media coverage of gambling-related problems of youth and adults has expanded steadily, albeit sporadically.

It was in the late 1980s that the casino industry first addressed the problem of teenage gambling. Led by Harrah's Casinos, Trop World and Claridge Casinos joined with the National Council on Problem Gambling Inc. to create the unique and still continuing Project 21. The objective was to make legally underage youth aware of the potential negative consequences of their gambling. Project 21 warned that "once convicted, you will have a police record and this record of conviction will remain for at least five years. This is not the kind of mark that looks good to a potential employer or on a college application." Project 21 also sponsored scholarships for high school students who competed in a poster contest to make youths more aware of the dangers of gambling.[1] Sometime later, Trump Casinos went one step further with the short video "Slammer," which vividly depicted the possibility of underage youth facing six months in jail or a stay in a detention center for slipping into a casino to gamble.

Unfortunately, these early, well-meaning efforts, advanced by several Atlantic City casino operators, received limited public attention and had a limited effect on the practices of the overwhelming majority of casino interests in the United States and Canada. However, in the recent past, what may be seen as a major breakthrough has occurred. This time an additional group of casinos broke their longstanding inattention to problem gambling, and for the first time joined to publicly decry the existence and extent of compulsive gambling, and of underage gambling in particular (American Gaming Association, 1996, 1998). Each member promised to support accredited programs of research, education, and treatment. Among those following Harrah's leadership in taking this enlightened stand were Grand Casinos, Boyd Casinos, and Caesar's World.

These overtures represent a major change from the entrenched, avoidant positions most gambling interests had previously held toward problem gambling. As a result, prospects over the next five years are cautiously positive. It is hoped that financial support from the gaming industry (e.g., the AGA-sponsored National Center for Responsible Gaming) will continue to be available, and even expand, as it seeks to collaborate actively with public, private, and voluntary entities at the state and national level to increase public awareness about problem gambling and to facilitate treatment, prevention, and research for problem gamblers, both juvenile and adult.

The continuing accumulation of scientific data, documenting the kind and extent of problems associated with gambling, will continue to impress government and industry that they have a clear responsibility to join efforts to assist those who have become, or who are at risk of becoming, casualties of gambling. In hopes of accelerating this process, this author has challenged the entire gambling industry with the issue of "product safety." A product safety issue becomes relevant when credible research reveals that a portion of the population who use a product or participate in a particular activity may be harmed. When this kind of issue arises relative to gambling, responsible public and private operators would be expected to inform potential consumers of the possible risk so that they can make a knowing choice about participating in that activity. Also, consumers who are concerned that they or someone they know might be negatively affected should be directed to a toll-free help line to obtain more information or assistance about a gambling-related problem.

Another responsibility of manufacturers and purveyors of gambling materials is to support the training of health professionals (most of whom know little about problem gambling) so that they may learn how to diagnose this condition and how to intervene appropriately with the identified patient and the family to bring the problem under control. Also, health insurance companies must provide funding to defray the costs of such treatment. Last, all elements of the gaming industry, public and private, must underwrite research into the factors that predispose persons to be at greater risk for developing serious gambling-related problems so that preventive steps may be taken to deter such an eventuality (Jacobs, 2001a, 2001b).

PROSPECTS FOR GOVERNMENTAL SUPPORT FOR THE PREVENTION OF PROBLEM GAMBLING

This brings us to the matter of government-promoted gambling. Among the thirty-eight states and the District of Columbia that in 1995 enjoyed revenues of over $32 billion from lotteries alone (Keating, 1996), only a baker's dozen provided any measure of financial support for education, treatment, prevention, or research to assist those citizens who were already experiencing, or were at risk of developing, serious gambling-related problems. To date, annual helping responses by state governments range from a few thousand dollars for brochures and billboards to more than $2 million in Texas and Oregon. The median range has been around $100,000, but even this level is subject to the vagaries of legislative priorities (National Council on Problem Gambling, 1999). Only one state (Minnesota) specifically directed funding to study and assist juveniles experiencing problems with gambling. Prospects over the next five years are uncertain as to whether state legislatures will appreciably increase funding for such purposes, particularly when faced with economic downturns. A concerted media campaign exposing the extent of juvenile involvement in legalized forms of gambling could result in more rigorous enforcement of existing laws against gambling by minors, along with a windfall of tax dollars to encourage school-based programs to include education and counseling regarding gambling hazards within their ongoing drug and alcohol prevention efforts.

At the federal level in the United States, nothing specific has been done to identify or to assist juveniles with serious gambling-related problems. Indeed, diagnosed pathological gamblers of any age were specifically excluded from consideration under the 1990 Americans with Disabilities Act, although protection was assured for recovering alcoholics and drug addicts (Pertzoff, 1990). A recent inquiry found that even the Justice Department's Office of Juvenile Justice and Delinquency Prevention had no efforts focused on teenage gambling. However, there was one harbinger of positive change at the federal level. On August 3, 1996, the U.S. Congress created the National Gambling Impact Study Commission. Among its mandated activities, the commission assessed the extent of pathological and problem gambling, including its impact on affected individuals, families, businesses, social institutions, and the economy. This assessment of the prevalence of gambling did include a small sample of 16- and 17-year-olds. Findings from such an authoritative and highly visible research effort, one hopes, will serve to greatly accelerate the educational, remedial, and preventive efforts recommended in this chapter. However, little in the way of improved services has been stimulated since the commission released its initial report in 1999 (National Opinion Research Center, 1999).

There is much better news about governmental reactions to juvenile gambling in Canada. Most of Canada's provinces and territories have set aside funding from lottery revenues to address problem gambling among its citizens. Since 1993, a growing number of provinces have financed province-wide prevalence studies of adult and juvenile gambling. The major substance-abuse agencies in Alberta, Manitoba, Ontario, and Quebec have moved decisively to expand their ongoing adult drug and alcohol programs to cover increased public awareness, educational, treatment, and prevention activities for juvenile gamblers. Other provinces are expected to follow their example.

The North American Think Tank on Youth Gambling Issues held at Harvard University in 1995 aimed to produce positive changes in governmental and private industry attitudes and programs regarding juvenile gambling issues. This event represented the first major step in what has become an accelerating effort in the United States and Canada to respond to the issue of youth gambling. While additional approaches may surface and details of implementation may change, the think tank resulted in an authoritative publication that offered a blueprint to guide progress over the following five years. That report is included in the appendix of this book. The momentum generated by the original North American Think Tank helped foster the convening of the Second International Think Tank on Youth Gambling, held at McGill University, Quebec, on May 4–6, 2001. This meeting drew a select group of invited experts from nine countries. Their primary goals were to emphasize youth gambling as a public health problem, update critical issues, and identify several areas for further investigation and application. The group's work continues to be supported by the newly established International Centre for Youth Gambling Problems and High Risk Behaviors, located in its permanent home at McGill University (The Wager, 2001).

A FINAL WORD

Someday, we may have answers to how juvenile gambling continued so long without arousing the attention and concern of the general public. It boggles the mind to try to understand how a phenomenon so pervasive, openly practiced, and patently illegal could continue during every week and in virtually every state and province across North America without drawing the attention of the media, much less the authorities.

Even more confounding is the fact that millions of legally underage youth throughout the United States and Canada have been buying lottery tickets in their own neighborhoods from thousands of state- and province-sanctioned lottery vendors, placing bets with bookies (both peer and professional) and at windows of scores of licensed state and provincial horse and dog tracks, playing at municipally registered bingo games, and (to a lesser extent) wagering at casinos, commercial card parlors, jai alai games, and legal off-track betting emporia—without being questioned, "carded," or unceremoniously ejected.

There is no consensus on how youngsters should be prepared to participate in a society where almost everyone gambles. Indeed, today's children and adolescents are the first generation to be raised in an environment where legalized gambling is so pervasive, readily accessible, government promoted, and socially acceptable.

The findings discussed above, about the surprisingly early age of onset for gambling among minors, make it imperative that policymakers introduce cautionary educational programs for children at or before their entry into middle school. Indeed, there is justification for beginning early prevention efforts at the primary school level, where preadolescents may be taught social skills of communication, stress management, and various coping skills and problem-solving strategies, including the laws of probability, that will anticipate and put them in better stead to deal with the physical, psychological, social, and occupational stresses that characterize the adolescent years. Meanwhile, prompt availability of counseling and treatment must be organized for the one in seven juveniles throughout North America who already report serious gambling-related problems. Such resources could rather quickly and economically be integrated into existing adolescent drug, alcohol, and eating disorder programs already functioning in schools, churches, drop-in centers, hospitals, and outpatient settings.

Long overdue are periodic state, provincial, and federally funded social-impact studies to identify the extent to which new and changing forms of legalized gambling contribute to increased gambling rates and, particularly, to rates of problem gambling among potentially vulnerable groups such as juveniles, females, minorities, and the elderly. The scientific literature consistently indicates that adolescents are at much higher risk than adults for developing addictive patterns of behavior involving a variety of substances and activities, including pathological gambling. The already high rates of tenuously controlled problem gambling behaviors, repeatedly documented among middle school–age and high school–age students, accentuate the need for increased general public awareness, personal self-awareness, early identification, determined outreach efforts, and enhanced educational, counseling, and preventive interventions for this high-risk group of young North Americans.

The early twenty-first century will mark the historic heyday of legalized gambling throughout North America and the world at large. Our response to this development will determine the extent to which present and future generations of youth will be placed at risk.

Note

1. For a more detailed description of Project 21, see chap. 9, "Youth Gambling: The Casino Industry's Responsibility," by Philip G. Satre.

References

Abbott, M. W., & Volberg, R. A. (1996). The New Zealand national survey of problem and pathological gambling. *Journal of Gambling Studies, 12,* 143–60.

Adlaf, E. F., & Ialomiteanu, A. (2000). Prevalence of problem gambling in adolescents: Findings from the 1999 Ontario student drug use survey. *Canadian Journal of Psychiatry, 45,* 752–55.

American Gaming Association. (1996, 1998). *Responsible gaming resource guide.* Washington, DC: Author.

American Psychiatric Association. (1994). *Diagnostic and statistical manual of mental disorders.* 4th edition, revised. Washington, DC: Author.

Arcuri, A. F., Lester, D., & Smith, F. (1985). Shaping adolescent gambling behavior. *Adolescence, 20,* 935–38.

Custer, R. L., & Custer, L. F. (1978). Characteristics of the recovering compulsive gambler: A survey of 150 members of Gamblers Anonymous. Paper presented at the Fourth National Conference on Gambling, Reno, NV.

Custer, R. L., & Milt, H. (1985). *When luck runs out.* New York: Facts on File Publications.

Derevensky, J. L., & Gupta, R. (2000). Prevalence estimates of adolescent gambling: A comparison of the SOGS-RA, DSM-IV-J, and the GA 20 questions. *Journal of Gambling Studies, 16* (2/3), 227–51.

Elia, C., & Jacobs, D. F. (1993). The incidence of pathological gambling among Native Americans treated for alcohol dependence. *International Journal of the Addictions, 28,* 659–66.

Govoni, R., Rupcich, N., & Frisch, G. R. (1996). Gambling behavior of adolescent gamblers. *Journal of Gambling Studies, 12,* 305–17.

Gupta, R., & Derevensky, J. L. (1998a). An empirical examination of Jacobs' General Theory of Addictions: Do adolescent gamblers fit the theory? *Journal of Gambling Studies, 14* (1), 17–49.

Gupta, R., & Derevensky, J. L. (1998b). Adolescent gambling behavior: A prevalence study and examination of the correlates associated with problem gambling. *Journal of Gambling Studies, 14* (4), 319–45.

Gupta, R., Derevensky, J. L., & Cioppa, G. D. (1996). The relationship between gambling and video-game playing behavior in children. Paper presented at the Ninth International Conference on Gambling and Risk Taking, Las Vegas, NV.

Insight Canada Research. (1994). *An exploration of the prevalence of pathological gambling behaviour among adolescents in Ontario.* Report prepared for the Canadian Foundation on Compulsive Gambling. Willowdale, Ontario: Author.

Jacobs, D. F. (1982). The addictive personality syndrome: A new theoretical model for understanding and treating addictions. In W. R. Eadington (Ed.), *The gambling papers, vol. 2: Pathological gambling, theory and practice* (pp. 1–55). Reno: University of Nevada Press.

Jacobs, D. F. (1984). Factors alleged as predisposing to compulsive gambling. In *Sharing Recovery through Gamblers Anonymous* (227–33). Los Angeles: Gamblers Anonymous Publishing Company.

Jacobs, D. F. (1988a). Evidence for a common dissociative-like reaction among addicts. *Journal of Gambling Behavior, 4,* 27–37.

Jacobs, D. F. (1988b). Planning for a uniform epidemiological survey of problem gambling on four continents. In W. R. Eadington (Ed.), *Gambling research: Proceedings of the Seventh International Conference on Gambling and Risk Taking* (pp. 63–68). Reno: University of Nevada.

Jacobs, D. F. (1988c). Gambling behaviors of high school students: Implications for government-supported gambling. Paper presented at the National Policy Symposium on Lotteries and Gambling, Vancouver, British Columbia.

Jacobs, D. F. (1989a). Illegal and undocumented: A review of teenage gambling and the plight of children of problem gamblers in America. In H. J. Shaffer, S. Stein, B. Gambino, & T. Cummings (Eds.), *Compulsive gambling: Theory, research, and practice* (pp. 249–92). Lexington, MA: Lexington Books.

Jacobs, D. F. (1989b). A general theory of addictions: Rationale for and evidence supporting a new approach for understanding and treating addictive behaviors. In H. J. Shaffer, S. Stein, B. Gambino, & T. Cummings (Eds.), *Compulsive gambling: Theory, research, and practice* (pp. 35–64). Lexington, MA: Lexington Books.

Jacobs, D. F. (1990). Focus on teenage gamblers. *Behavior Today, 21* (11), 1–4.

Jacobs, D. F. (1992). Prevalence of problem gambling among hospitalized adult male substance abusers. Paper presented at the Sixth National Conference on Gambling Behavior, Cleveland, OH.

Jacobs, D. F. (1994). Evidence supporting the "Pied Piper Effect" of lottery promotion and sales on juvenile gambling. Paper presented at the Eighth National Conference on Gambling Behavior, Seattle, WA.

Jacobs, D. F. (1995). A 14 year old plays cards for cash: Is it more than fun and games? *Brown University Child and Adolescent Behavior Letter, 4,* 1–3.

Jacobs, D. F. (2000). Juvenile gambling in North America: An analysis of long-term trends and future prospects. *Journal of Gambling Studies, 16* (2/3), 119–52.

Jacobs, D. F. (2001a). Compulsive gambling research: Part I of an interview with Durand F. Jacobs on the etiology of addictive behaviors, as portrayed by the General Theory of Addictions. *Lottery Insights, 2* (2), 14–18.

Jacobs, D. F. (2001b). Compulsive gambling research: Part II of an interview with Durand F. Jacobs on improved treatment and prevention strategies. *Lottery Insights, 2* (3), 6–10.

Jacobs, D. F., Marston, A. R., & Singer, R. D., (1985). *Study of gambling and other health-threatening behaviors among high school students.* Unpublished manuscript. Loma Linda, CA: Jerry L. Pettis Memorial Veterans Hospital.

Jacobs, D. F., Marston, A. R., Singer, R. D., Widaman, K., & Little, T. (1987). [Study of gambling and other health-threatening behaviors among high school students]. Unpublished raw data. Loma Linda, CA: Jerry L. Pettis Memorial Veterans Hospital.

Jacobs, D. F., Marston, A. R., Singer, R. D., Widaman, K., Little, T., & Veizades, J. (1989). Children of problem gamblers. *Journal of Gambling Behavior, 5,* 261–68.

Johnston, L., Bachman, J., & O'Malley, P. (1979). *1979 highlights: Drugs and the nation's high school students: Five year national trends.* Rockville, MD: National Institute on Drug Abuse.

Kallick, M., Suits, D., Dielman, T., & Hybels, J. (1976). *A survey of American gambling attitudes and behavior.* Washington, DC: U.S. Government Printing Office.

Keating, P. (1996, May). Lotto fever: We all lose! *Money,* 142–49.

Kuley, N., & Jacobs, D. F. (1987). [A pre-lottery benchmark study of teenage gambling in Virginia]. Unpublished raw data. Loma Linda, CA: Loma Linda University Department of Psychiatry.

Kuley, N. B., & Jacobs, D. F. (1988). The relationship between dissociative-like experiences and sensation seeking among social and problem gamblers. *Journal of Gambling Behavior, 4,* 197–207.

Kuley, N., & Jacobs, D. F. (1989). [A post-lottery impact study of effects on teenage gambling behaviors]. Unpublished research study. Loma Linda, CA: Loma Linda University Medical Center Department of Psychiatry.

Ladouceur, R., Dubé, D., & Bujold, A. (1994). Gambling among primary school students. *Journal of Gambling Studies, 10,* 363–70.

Ladouceur, R., & Mireault, C. (1988). Gambling behaviors among high school students in the Quebec area. *Journal of Gambling Behavior, 4,* 3–12.

Lesieur, H. R. (1987). Gambling, pathological gambling, and crime. In T. Galski (Ed.), *The handbook of pathological gambling* (pp. 89–110). Springfield, IL: Charles C. Thomas.

Lesieur, H. R., & Blume, S. B. (1987). The South Oaks Gambling Screen (SOGS): A new instrument for the identification of pathological gamblers. *American Journal of Psychiatry, 144,* 1184–88.

Lesieur, H. R., & Blume, S. B. (1990). Characteristics of pathological gamblers identified among patients on a psychiatric admissions service. *Hospital and Community Psychiatry, 41,* 1009–12.

Lesieur, H. R., & Blume, S. B. (1991). Evaluation of patients treated for pathological gambling in a combined alcohol, substance abuse, and pathological gambling treatment unit using the Addiction Severity Index. *British Journal of Addictions, 86,* 1017–28.

Lesieur, H. R., Blume, S. B., & Zoppa, R. M. (1986). Alcoholism, drug abuse, and gambling. *Alcoholism: Clinical and Experimental Research, 10,* 33–38.

Lesieur, H. R., & Klein, R. (1987). Pathological gambling among high school students. *Addictive Behaviors, 12,* 129–35.

Milgram, G. G. (1982). Youthful drinking: Past and present. *Journal of Drug Education, 12,* 289–308.

National Council on Problem Gambling. (1999). *National survey of problem gambling programs.* Washington, DC: Author.

National Opinion Research Center. (1999). *Overview of national survey and community database research on gambling behavior.* Report to the National Gambling Impact Study Commission. Chicago: University of Chicago.

Nechi Training Research & Health Promotions Institute. (1995). *Firewatch on aboriginal adolescent gambling.* Edmonton, Alberta: Author.

Noonan, G., Turner, N. E., & Macdonald, J. (1999). *Gambling and problem gambling among students in grades 5 to 11.* Report prepared for the Addiction Research Foundation of the Center for Addiction and Mental Health, Ontario, Canada.

Omnifacts Research Limited. (1993). *An examination of the prevalence of gambling in Nova Scotia.* Research report no. 93090 for the Nova Scotia Department of Health, Drug Dependency Services. Halifax, Nova Scotia: Author.

Pertzoff, L. (1990). Americans with disabilities act: Compulsive gamblers not covered. *Delaware Council on Gambling Problems Newsletter, 6*, 2.

Proimos, J., DuRant, R. H., Pierce, J. D., & Goodman, E. (1998). Gambling and other risk behaviors among 8th to 12th grade students. *Pediatrics, 102* (2), 1–6.

Ramirez, L. F., McCormick, R. A., Russo, A. M., & Taber, J. I. (1983). Patterns of substance abuse in pathological gamblers undergoing treatment. *Addictive Behaviors, 8*, 425–28.

Shaffer, H. J., Hall, M. N., & Vander Bilt, J. (1997). *Estimating the prevalence of disordered gambling behavior in the United States and Canada: A meta-analysis.* Boston: Presidents and Fellows of Harvard College.

Shaffer, H. J., LaBrie, R., Scanlan, K. M., & Cummings, T. N. (1994). Pathological gambling among adolescents: Massachusetts Gambling Screen (MAGS). *Journal of Gambling Studies, 10*, 339–62.

Shaffer, H. J., Stein, S., Gambino, B., & Cummings, T. N. (Eds.). (1989). *Compulsive gambling: Theory, research, and practice.* Lexington, MA: Lexington Books.

Spunt, B., Lesieur, H., Hunt, D., & Cahill, L. (1995). Gambling among methadone patients. *International Journal of the Addictions, 30*, 929–62.

Steinberg, M. (1988, May). Gambling behavior among high school students in Connecticut. Paper presented at the Third National Conference on Gambling, New London, CT.

Taber, J. I., & McCormick, R. A. (1987). The pathological gambler in treatment. In T. Galski (Ed.), *The handbook of pathological gambling* (pp. 137–68). Springfield, IL: Charles C. Thomas.

Volberg, R. A. (1993). *Gambling and problem gambling in Washington state.* Report to the Washington State Lottery. Albany, NY: Gemini Research.

Volberg, R. A. (1996). Prevalence studies of problem gambling in the United States. *Journal of Gambling Studies, 12*, 111–28.

Volberg, R. A. (2001). *Measures to track gambling rates, behaviors, and related factors.* Report prepared for the National Council on Problem Gambling, Washington, DC.

Volberg, R. A., & Boles, J. (1996). *Gambling and problem gambling in Georgia.* Report to the Georgia Department of Human Resources. Roaring Springs, PA: Gemini Research.

Volberg, R. A., & Moore, W. I. (1999). *Gambling and problem gambling among adolescents in Washington State: A replication study, 1993–1999.* A report to the Washington State Lottery. Gemini Research.

The Wager. (2001). Second International Think Tank of Youth Gambling. 6 (33). Harvard Medical School: Boston.

Wallisch, L. S. (1993). *Gambling in Texas: 1992 Texas survey of adolescent gambling behavior.* Austin: Texas Commission on Alcohol and Drug Abuse.

Wallisch, L. S. (1996). *Gambling in Texas: 1995 surveys of adult and adolescent gambling behavior.* Austin: Texas Commission on Alcohol and Drug Abuse.

Wardman, D., el-Guebaly, N., & Hodgins, D. (2001). Problem and pathological gambling in North American aboriginal populations: A review of the empirical literature. *Journal of Gambling Studies, 17* (2), 81–100.

Westphal, J. R., Rush, J. A., Stevens, I., & Johnson, L. J. (1998). Pathological gambling among Louisiana students: Grades six through twelve. Paper presented at the American Psychiatric Association Annual Meeting. Toronto, Ontario.

Wiebe, J. M. D., Cox, B. J., & Mehmel, B. G. (2000). The South Oaks Gambling Screen Revised for Adolescents (SOGS-RA): Further psychometric findings from a community sample. *Journal of Gambling Studies, 16* (2/3), 275–88.

Winters, K. C., & Stinchfield, R. D. (1993). *Gambling behavior among Minnesota youth: Monitoring change from 1990 to 1991/1992.* Duluth, MN: University of Minnesota, Center for Adolescent Substance Abuse.

Winters, K. C., Stinchfield, R., & Fulkerson, J. (1990). *Adolescent survey of gambling behavior in Minnesota: A benchmark.* Report to the Department of Human Services, Mental Health Division. Duluth, MN: University of Minnesota, Center for Addiction Studies.

Wynne, H. J., Smith, G. J., & Jacobs, D. F. (1996). *Adolescent gambling and problem gambling in Alberta.* Alberta: Alberta Alcohol and Drug Abuse Commission.

Zitzow, D. (1996). Comparative study of problematic gambling behaviors between American Indian and non-Indian adolescents within and near a Northern Plains reservation. *American Indian and Alaskan Native Mental Health Research, 7,* 14–26.

Appendix

The North American Think Tank on Youth Gambling Issues
A Blueprint for Responsible Public Policy in the Management of Compulsive Gambling

Howard J. Shaffer, Elizabeth M. George, and Thomas N. Cummings

Executive Summary

The North American Think Tank on Youth Gambling Issues convened April 6 through 8, 1995, at Harvard Medical School in Boston. Cosponsored by the Harvard Medical School Division on Addictions and the North American Training Institute, with assistance from the Massachusetts Council on Compulsive Gambling, the event brought together key leaders from throughout the United States and Canada who represented diverse fields including government, education, the gambling industry, finance, law enforcement, the judiciary, health care, and research.

The purpose of the North American Think Tank was to develop a blueprint for responsible public policy to address the issues associated with youth gambling. It was intended to remain gambling neutral, neither supporting nor opposing gambling. The event was funded by donations from private business and tribal governments.

The think tank process was a highly structured and tightly managed format, incorporating both small-group and large-group discussion and presentations by various experts on the topic of gambling and youth.

Recommendations

North American Think Tank participants developed recommendations in seven key areas.

    1. Policy Development Recommendations

        The United States and Canada should create a binational task force to coordi-

nate the development of a North American response to youth gambling and solicit the funds necessary to pay for needed programs.

2. Funding Recommendations

The task force should be structured as a not-for-profit organization to attract
funding from public and private sector sources.

3. Law Enforcement Recommendations

The gambling industry should establish industry standards for enforcement of
underage gambling prohibitions, support tougher penalties against vendors
who fail to enforce legal gambling age limits, and aggressively promote policies that prohibit payment of prizes to minors gambling illegally.

4. Research Recommendations

An international research effort should be undertaken to determine the prevalence of youth gambling and the effectiveness of prevention and treatment
programs; the findings should be disseminated via an electronic "information
superhighway" through a national or international clearinghouse.

5. Treatment and Training Recommendations

Treatment methods in North America should be inventoried and evaluated for
clinical efficacy, and professional training for youth gambling treatment providers should be tailored to meet training needs.

6. Education Recommendations

Curriculums and programs should be developed to educate children, parents,
and teachers about the issue of youth gambling.

7. Public Awareness and Media Recommendations

The public and policymakers should be educated about youth gambling
through the media and various other strategies, and the gambling industry
should develop and promote a voluntary standards program to discourage the
targeting of gambling advertising to young consumers.

Participants recommended that an interim task force be established to draft a plan
for establishment of a permanent binational organization. The Harvard Medical
School Division on Addictions and the North American Training Institute were
asked to serve as conveners of that interim task force. With the completion of this final report that process is ready to begin.

It should be emphasized that the North American Think Tank was only the first
step in what must be a long-term effort to respond to the issue of youth gambling.
While additional approaches may surface or details of implementation may change,
think tank participants, with this report, have helped to create an outline—a blueprint—from which to proceed.

Introduction

With the rapid expansion of gambling over the past ten years, forty-eight states in the United States and all Canadian provinces offer some forms of privately owned and/or government-sponsored gambling. While gambling generates obvious and important economic benefits, there is no question that it also carries certain costs, one of which is pathological gambling. While most forms of gambling are illegal for underage youth, there is compelling evidence that, in fact, youngsters are gambling in unprecedented numbers. According to recent studies, card playing, sports betting, and games of personal skill, in that order of preference, are particularly popular among juvenile gamblers. Lottery, bingo, pull-tabs, and video machines are popular in those states and provinces where they are legal.

Recent scientific studies have repeatedly suggested that children and adolescents may be at higher risk than adults of becoming pathological gamblers and suffering the tragic consequences of this powerful disorder. Studies in the United States and Canada have revealed that between 9.9 percent and 14.2 percent of adolescents are experiencing some symptoms of problem gambling, and between 4.4 percent and 7.4 percent meet the criteria for pathological gambling.[1] Moreover, the prevalence rates for pathological gambling among adolescents have consistently been found to be twice those found for adults. For this reason, the issue of youth gambling is becoming a major concern for North American communities, policymakers, and the general public.

To address this issue, the North American Think Tank on Youth Gambling Issues met on April 6 through April 8, 1995, at Harvard Medical School in Boston. The mission of the think tank was to develop a blueprint for responsible public policy in addressing the issues associated with youth gambling. The event was intended to remain gambling neutral, neither supporting nor opposing gambling. It was convened and jointly sponsored by the North American Training Institute and the Harvard Medical School Division on Addictions with assistance from the Massachusetts Council on Compulsive Gambling Inc.

The North American Training Institute is a national leader in the field of problem-gambling education, training, and prevention. In 1993 the council hosted the first Minnesota Public Policy Think Tank on Compulsive Gambling, a two-day event that served as the prototype for the North American Think Tank. In recent years, the Minnesota council has placed particular emphasis on youth-gambling issues, developing public education and prevention models for state and national distribution. One pilot program focused on prevention of youth gambling. Designed by the council in cooperation with high school students from northern Minnesota, the program has received national attention.

The Harvard Medical School Division on Addictions was established to foster education, discovery, and communication in the field of substance abuse and addiction, including gambling addiction. The work of the Division on Addictions has centered on improving health care practitioners' abilities to identify and treat addicted individuals, attracting talented researchers and scientists into the field of addiction to study risk factors, the effects of certain drugs, and the efficacy of various treatment methods. The Division on Addictions has also worked on developing effective education and prevention programs and integrating discussion of addictions into ongoing health care and drug policy deliberations at the national level.

The Massachusetts Council on Compulsive Gambling was established in 1983 and has served as a national model for effective programming in education and community awareness. In collaboration with the Harvard Medical School, it convened the nation's first think tank on compulsive gambling in 1988. The Massachusetts Council developed the Massachusetts Gambling Screen (MAGS) for use in screening adolescents for gambling problems, and in 1994 it attracted national attention when it conducted and published research on prevalence and problems associated with adolescent gambling.

Development of the Think Tank

Participants in the North American Think Tank on Youth Gambling were selected on the basis of their special interest in the topic of problem gambling among youth. They came from Canada and the United States, from government, education, the gambling industry, finance, law enforcement, health care, the judiciary, and the research community. Although their backgrounds and perspectives were widely diverse, they shared a common commitment to invest their time, energy, and considerable talents in the development of a national strategy to address the problem of youth gambling. Neither presenters nor participants were compensated for their attendance.

Funding for the North American Think Tank was provided by progressive gaming operators, bankers, insurance executives, lawyers, and tribal governments in Mississippi and Minnesota—two of America's most significant gaming markets. The fundraising effort was led by Thomas J. Brosig, executive vice-president of Grand Casinos Inc., who along with colleagues in Mississippi and Minnesota formed the National Policy Board on Youth Gambling Issues as a vehicle to raise funds for the Harvard Think Tank and for implementation of its recommendations in the future.

A complete list of volunteers, sponsors, and contributors to the North American Think Tank on Youth Gambling is included at the end of this report. Without their support, this event would not have been possible.

Definition of Terms

Many of the terms contained in this report have different meanings to different people. To ensure that think tank participants and readers of this report share a common understanding of some of these key terms, we offer the following definitions.

GAMBLING

There are many forms of gambling operated by private or public entities or a combination of both. For purposes of this report, the term *gambling industry* refers to legal, government-sponsored lotteries; charitable bingo or pull-tab games; tribal casinos, bingo halls, and card rooms; and privately owned casinos, betting parlors, racetracks, or other legally sanctioned establishments.

UNDERAGE GAMBLING

Minimum legal gambling ages vary from jurisdiction to jurisdiction and from one gambling form to another within jurisdictions. For example, in most states, the minimum legal age for purchasing lottery tickets is 18, as is the minimum for pull-tabs and pari-mutuel betting. In some states, the minimum legal age for casino gambling is 18; in others, 21. In some states, 18-year-olds may play the lottery or pull-tabs legally but may not gamble at casinos or place pari-mutuel bets. For the purposes of this report, *underage gambling* is defined as gambling by youth under the minimum legal age to place a bet in a particular venue.

PROBLEM GAMBLING

It is estimated that between 9.9 percent and 14.2 percent of children and youth may be "problem gamblers." For purposes of this report, *problem gambling* is defined as some loss of control over one's gambling behavior, leading to negative consequences.

PATHOLOGICAL GAMBLING

According to the American Psychiatric Association, and for purposes of this report, *pathological gambling* is defined as a chronic and progressive psychological disorder characterized by emotional dependence, loss of control, and accompanying negative consequences in the gambler's school, social, or family life. The distinction between "problem gambling" and "pathological gambling" is similar to the distinction most people recognize between alcohol abuse and alcoholism. As previously cited, between 4.4 percent and 7.4 percent of youth meet the criteria for pathological gamblers.

The Think Tank Process

The think tank was structured to allow for general-session presentations by leading North American experts, as well as extensive discussion among participants in breakout groups. Each presentation was placed on the agenda so that the information presented in that session would be directly relevant to the breakout sessions scheduled to follow. This process helped to ensure that each group conducted its deliberations with the same general background as a frame of reference. The text of these presentations is available upon request. General-session presenters and their topics are listed below.

General Session Presenters

- Keynote address: Philip G. Satre, president and chief executive officer, Promus Companies (parent company of Harrah's Casinos), Memphis, Tennessee. "Why Care About Youth Gambling?"
- Thomas J. Brosig, executive vice-president, Grand Casinos Inc., Plymouth, Minnesota. "The Right Thing To Do: Exercising Leadership in Youth Gambling."
- Howard Shaffer, Ph.D., associate professor and director, Harvard Medical School Division on Addictions, Boston. "An Overview of Youth Gambling in North America."
- Henry Lesieur, Ph.D., professor and chair, Department of Criminal Justice Sciences, Illinois State University, Normal, Illinois. "Adolescent Gambling Research: The Next Wave."
- I. Nelson Rose, J.D., professor of law, Whittier Law School, Los Angeles. "Underage Gambling and the Law."
- William R. Eadington, Ph.D., director, Institute for the Study of Gambling and Commercial Gaming, University of Nevada, Reno. "The Economics of Underage Gambling."
- Joseph Malone, Massachusetts state treasurer, and Eric Turner, executive director, Massachusetts State Lottery, Braintree, Massachusetts. "Youth Gambling in the Public Sector."
- Wayne M. York, director, Cape Breton Region, Department of Health, Drug Dependency Services Division, Sydney, Nova Scotia. "The Canadian Perspective."
- Durand F. Jacobs, Ph.D., clinical professor of medicine, Loma Linda University Medical School, Redlands, California. "Ten-Year Trends in Youth Gambling."

Breakout Sessions

Think tank participants were assigned to five separate groups for the breakout sessions. They remained with those groups for the duration of the conference. The process was deductive in approach, moving from the general to the specific. A set of worksheets was provided for each session to keep the groups focused on the assigned topics and tasks.

The three breakout sessions were designed to lead from a highly generalized vision to more specific themes and goals and finally to specific recommendations for action. Each session built upon the findings of the previous session. Findings were summarized in writing by the facilitator after each session and briefly reviewed with the entire assembly before the next breakout session began, to ensure that all groups had the same information gleaned from previous sessions.

Breakout session 1 was spent developing answers to the question: "What should be the goals of a national program to address problem gambling among youth?" During the session, participants were asked to define a vision for the future and to identify the key themes and goals contained in that vision. The themes and goals served as a foundation for development of specific action recommendations later in the process.

Breakout session 2 moved to the question: "What issues need to be addressed in order to achieve the goals identified?" Participants were asked to identify current trends, decide whether the trends had positive or negative implications for the future, and define the assets and obstacles inherent in the status quo. To assist in setting priorities, participants assessed each obstacle for its seriousness and its solvability.

Breakout session 3 was devoted to the question: "What actions should be taken to address the issues and achieve the goals identified?" Participants developed specific action plan recommendations to overcome the obstacles and meet the goals established in previous breakout sessions.

Breakout sessions were facilitated by group leaders, who played a vital role in the two-day process. At a briefing before the first think tank session, group leaders familiarized themselves with the worksheets to be used and received instructions for management of the discussion process. Group leaders were asked to encourage participation from all group members, to use consensus-building techniques that unite rather than divide group participants, and to discourage adversarial behavior within the group.

Following the final breakout session, all think tank participants convened in general session to review group findings and discuss the process by which the final report would be prepared and circulated for discussion.

Summary of Breakout Session 1
A VISION FOR THE FUTURE
As indicated, the purpose of breakout session 1 was, first, to develop a general vision for the future with respect to the management of youth-gambling issues and then to identify the key themes and goals contained in that vision. From those key themes and goals, more specific action recommendations would be developed. Several key themes and goals emerged from the group process.

Theme: National Policy Development
Goal: A binational or North American task force including all key stakeholders

Theme: Funding
Goal: A consistent, dedicated revenue source for youth-gambling programs

Theme: Law Enforcement
Goal: Tougher and more consistent enforcement of existing prohibitions against underage gambling

Theme: Research

Goal: A comprehensive research program to measure the prevalence (that is, extent), of youth gambling, analyze program outcomes, and help identify the "whys" of youth gambling

Theme: Treatment and Training

Goal: Proven treatment programs for underage gamblers who need them, as well as for their families

Theme: Education

Goal: An aggressive education and prevention program in schools and communities

Theme: Public Awareness and Media

Goal: A major media campaign to increase awareness and dramatize the issues associated with youth gambling

Goal: A voluntary "code of practice" among gambling advertisers to discourage ads that target young consumers

Summary of Breakout Session 2

AN INVENTORY OF ASSETS AND POSITIVE TRENDS

The purpose of breakout session 2 was to identify the issues that need to be addressed to achieve the goals defined earlier. Think tank participants were asked to identify existing assets and positive trends that might enhance the ability to achieve the desired goals. Some of the most important assets and trends that participants identified are detailed below.

ASSETS AND POSITIVE TRENDS IN THE GAMBLING INDUSTRY

- The willingness of government and private-sector gambling entities to participate in addressing the issue of youth gambling
- The economic resources generated by government-sponsored gambling and by privately owned gaming operations through taxes, economic expansion and job creation in rural areas, and charitable contributions
- Economic development of Indian reservations, enabling tribal governments to participate as full partners in community problem-solving

ASSETS AND POSITIVE TRENDS IN COMMUNITIES

- Increasing awareness of the youth-gambling issue
- Increasing involvement of community groups and religious and fraternal organizations in discussion of the potential impacts, both positive and negative, of new gambling policies

ASSETS AND POSITIVE TRENDS IN PUBLIC POLICY
- Growing inclination of elected officials to consider problem gambling issues, including youth gambling, when evaluating gambling policy decisions
- Increasing support among lawmakers for "child protection" measures
- Increasing interest among lawmakers in funding problem gambling programs, including youth-gambling programs
- Public pressure for accountability when public funds are spent; more frequent use by lawmakers of specialized research and policy analysts to formulate public policy
- Expanding technologies, such as computer modeling, to help forecast the economic and social effects of gambling policy changes

**ASSETS AND POSITIVE TRENDS IN INSTITUTIONS
AND ORGANIZATIONS**
- U.S. and Canadian universities and independent researchers conducting credible scientific research and legitimizing the study of problem gambling
- National and state compulsive-gambling councils addressing the issue of problem gambling, including youth gambling
- Corporations that contribute support to youth and problem gambling programs
- Think tank planners, sponsors, and participants

ASSETS AND POSITIVE TRENDS IN TREATMENT AND TRAINING
- A growing base of people with experience in treatment
- Increasing sophistication of training and treatment technologies
- Increasing emphasis on training, curriculum development, and skill-building for treatment providers
- Holistic health trends emphasizing wellness and treatment of the whole person, and increasing involvement of family and friends in the treatment of problem gambling among youth and adults
- Increasing availability of creative self-help programs such as Gamblers Anonymous in the United States

ASSETS AND POSITIVE TRENDS IN THE MEDIA
- Increasing media attention to youth and problem gambling
- Strong media interest in the results of the North American Think Tank, suggesting more coverage in the future
- Potential for use of entertainment media, such as youth-oriented television, to educate children and youth about problem gambling

AN INVENTORY OF NEGATIVE TRENDS AND OBSTACLES

During breakout session 2, think tank participants also noted the emergence of some negative trends and obstacles that might affect their ability to achieve the desired goals.

NEGATIVE TRENDS AND OBSTACLES IN THE GAMBLING INDUSTRY

- Linkage of gambling with family entertainment, i.e., video arcades, thrill rides, theme parks, etc.
- Gambling advertisements featuring or aimed at young consumers
- The increased dollar value of highly publicized multistate lotteries or other prizes, stimulating youth interest in gambling

NEGATIVE TRENDS AND OBSTACLES IN COMMUNITIES

- Declining economic prosperity, leading to growing demand for "get rich quick" opportunities
- Increasing demand by youth for immediate gratification and/or relief from boredom
- Growing numbers of disaffected, "disconnected" youth
- Lack of jobs, creating a real or perceived lack of economic future for youth
- Increased access to gambling by youth due to rapid expansion
- Lack of social programs targeted to diverse cultural and ethnic groups
- Dependence of churches and not-for-profit organizations on gambling for needed revenues
- Increased accessibility of credit and cash through credit cards and ATM machines
- The inclusion of free "video blackjack" games with the purchase of home computers plays into the increasing preoccupation of children and youth with computer games and technologies, enabling an easy transfer of computer skills to high-tech interactive forms of gaming
- New gambling technologies, including the potential for unregulated youth gambling at home through on-line communications and other interactive systems
- Breakdown of family unit combined with overburdened schools
- National obsession with sports and "winners," along with tendency to ignore or refuse to recognize "losers"

NEGATIVE TRENDS AND OBSTACLES IN PUBLIC POLICY

- Rapid expansion of gambling by lawmakers without analysis of potential effects—positive and negative—on society
- Failure of lawmakers to accept responsibility for consequences of gambling expansion

- Dependence of governments on gaming revenues to reduce general operating deficits, finance vital infrastructure improvements, or fund targeted programs such as education, elderly services, and environmental and economic development
- Trend to conservative, "program-cutting" political mindset

NEGATIVE TRENDS AND OBSTACLES IN TREATMENT AND TRAINING
- Proliferation of untested, unproven treatment programs
- Turf battles among treatment providers
- Lack of adequate treatment models, training, and delivery systems
- Refusal of most insurance companies to fund prevention and treatment programs or even to consider gambling addiction, including youth gambling, as a medical problem
- Potential national reduction in U.S. health care services through federal budget cuts, which either directly reduce services or reduce funds available to states for that purpose

NEGATIVE TRENDS AND OBSTACLES IN THE MEDIA
- Frequent focus on sensationalism instead of accurate reporting on scope of problem and availability of help
- Sporadic coverage concentrated in media rating periods (sweeps) rather than ongoing coverage to create an understanding of context

Summary of Breakout Session 3
AN ACTION PLAN FOR THE FUTURE
After identifying assets, trends, and obstacles during breakout session 2, think tank participants moved on to the development of action plans during breakout session 3. Although some groups emphasized certain themes over others, most groups made an effort to address each of the major themes and goals identified in earlier sessions. Each recommendation was submitted by at least two groups and received broad support unless otherwise noted.

ACTION PLANS IN POLICY DEVELOPMENT
Recommendations included:
1. Creating a binational task force to include all key stakeholders
2. Identifying potential public and private funding sources
3. Establishing staff support to begin implementation of program
4. Developing a five-year strategic plan, including programs and public-policy initiatives
5. Using research data to gain support from policymakers
6. Identifying allies in government and the private sector

DISCUSSION

Every group agreed on the need for a broad-based binational task force to coordinate a North American response to youth gambling. Think tank participants recommended that the North American Training Institute and the Harvard Medical School Division on Addictions collaborate to appoint an interim task force, drawing from the roster of think tank participants. The interim group would assume responsibility for developing and circulating to other think tank participants a plan for the creation of the proposed binational task force.

Upon establishment, this permanent binational task force would develop a five-year strategic plan. The plan would address both programmatic and public-policy goals, which might or might not include legislative proposals.

In view of the think tank's gambling-neutral position, most members felt it would be inappropriate and unproductive for the task force to engage in lobbying to change gambling laws or to tell regulators how to do their jobs. The majority of think tank participants felt it more appropriate for the task force to seek public discussion on the issue of youth gambling in the United States and Canada rather than to seek federal legislation in either country.

ACTION PLANS IN FUNDING

Recommendations included:
1. Establishing a tax-exempt charitable structure to attract donations
2. Raising seed money for the initial operation of a task force
3. Identifying and soliciting potential public and private funding sources for recommended programs in policy development, research, treatment and training, education, and public awareness

DISCUSSION

There was broad agreement among think tank participants that both public and private sector funding sources should be explored. Some state councils and private compulsive-gambling treatment providers have received funding support from state legislatures. Increasing public concern about problem gambling may create a political environment in which public funds for youth-gambling programs could be more accessible than in previous years. In most cases, however, legislative appropriations are restricted for use on programs conducted within the granting jurisdiction, so it is unlikely that programs in one jurisdiction would qualify for funding from other jurisdictions.

Recognizing the importance of an ongoing, adequate funding source, some participants recommended that a portion of existing gaming tax revenues—from taxes already levied on the gaming industry, not new taxes—be earmarked by government mandate to fund youth-gambling programs. Some government-sponsored lotteries are already required by law to devote a portion of their proceeds to problem gambling. However, this proposal may be contrary to the trend, at least in state governments in the United States. In the face of increasing fiscal pressures, many state legislatures are reducing or eliminating existing dedicated funds in an effort to maximize the revenues available for general-fund obligations. In the current U.S. political environment, the creation of new dedicated funds for social programs might be unlikely.

While there is no mechanism other than negotiated tribal-state compacts by which such contributions could be mandated from tribal governments, there is every reason to believe that many gaming tribes would be willing to contribute voluntarily to youth-gambling programs, particularly in the area of education and prevention. Some tribal governments and tribal gaming associations have already established working relationships with problem gambling organizations, offering financial and other types of support.

Think tank participants recommended that the binational task force be structured as a tax-exempt charitable organization, enabling it to solicit funds from government, businesses, and foundations. Participants agreed that foundations or other organizations with an emphasis on youth health and wellness issues might be especially appropriate targets for fund-raising efforts.

ACTION PLANS IN LAW ENFORCEMENT

Recommendations included:

1. Encouraging the establishment of industry standards for enforcement of underage gambling prohibitions
2. Supporting tougher penalties for vendors who consistently fail to enforce existing legal gambling age limits by repeatedly selling lottery tickets or pull-tabs to underage gamblers, and for vendors who do not make a good-faith effort to restrict underage gamblers from entry into casinos, racetracks, or other legalized gambling sites
3. Supporting the enactment and aggressive promotion of gambling industry policies that prohibit payment of prizes to minors gambling illegally

DISCUSSION

Although some think tank participants supported increasing the minimum gambling age to 21 years, the majority felt that the task force should focus its efforts toward more rigorous enforcement of existing age prohibitions. They felt that tougher enforcement measures, including the possible loss of license for particularly egregious violations, should be targeted to those vendors, governmental as well as private, who consistently fail to make a good-faith effort to deter underage gambling.

Participants also noted the complexity of operational issues associated with enforcement of minimum age laws. The challenge faced by a casino that handles thousands of visitors in a single day is very different from that faced by a convenience-store operator whose lottery ticket customers usually number in the dozens. Think tank participants stressed the importance of collaboration and cooperation between gaming entities, both governmental and private, and the law enforcement community.

Think tank participants also emphasized the importance of public education in this area, pointing to Harrah's Project 21 as an excellent public service campaign to discourage underage gambling. Project 21 uses a multifaceted approach that includes employee training programs, television spots emphasizing the potential consequences of illegal gambling, and a scholarship program that awards scholarships to students who develop essays on the issue of underage gambling. The program is in use at all Harrah's locations and serves as a model for gambling entities in other states.

Think tank participants agreed that effectiveness studies of prevention programs are sorely needed. As more objective, scientific information is obtained about what works and what does not, concerned businesses and organizations will be better able to target prevention programs to maximize their effectiveness with the young audiences the programs are intended to reach.

ACTION PLANS IN RESEARCH
Recommendations included:
1. Establishing a clearinghouse to disseminate research findings on youth gambling, educational materials, and information on prevention and treatment programs; establishing Internet capability for quick dissemination
2. Developing an international research agenda encompassing prevalence studies of youth gambling as well as research to assess prevention and treatment programs
3. Requesting that the Centers for Disease Control and Prevention include questions on gambling in its annual youth health survey
4. Developing a uniform methodology for prevalence studies of youth gambling

DISCUSSION
Think tank participants agreed unanimously that extensive additional research must be done on the prevalence of youth gambling, as well as on the efficacy of existing treatment methods. Since the definition of problem gambling differs depending on the screening mechanisms used, and since so many different methodologies have been used to collect and evaluate existing data, it remains difficult, even now, to get a clear sense of the scope of the youth-gambling problem. Think tank participants felt that a greatly expanded research effort is indispensable to further efforts to address the issue of youth gambling.

As a means of encouraging such research, participants suggested the establishment of several research centers at various North American universities, which would assist the task force in setting research agendas, hosting conferences, participating in joint projects, and assisting with the dissemination of research data.

Although the issue of funding had already been discussed, think tank participants noted that increased funding for problem gambling research would stimulate interest in the field and likely lead to an increase in the number and quality of researchers working in this field.

ACTION PLANS IN TREATMENT AND TRAINING

Recommendations included:

1. Developing an inventory of North American treatment settings and methods to ensure a complete range of client-centered services
2. Preparing an analysis of the efficacy of various treatment methods, based on credible research
3. Assessing treatment resource needs to facilitate professional training of treatment providers.
4. Acting as liaison with third-party reimbursement companies (insurance companies, HMOs, EAPs, etc.) and systems funded by states or provinces

DISCUSSION

Think tank participants felt that an assessment of the efficacy of existing treatment programs and methods was long overdue and must be conducted as soon as possible. They thought such an assessment would probably result in increased government funding for treatment programs, since legislators would feel more confident that the programs funded by tax dollars had been evaluated by qualified professionals and found effective.

Think tank participants emphasized the importance of the recommended inventory as a means of evaluating the range of program (that is, the continuum of care) currently available. Gaps in existing programs would be identified and corrected most efficiently through such an inventory.

On the question of training, think tank participants felt that professional training curricula should be tailored to treatment resource needs to ensure an appropriate fit between trained professionals and the treatment programs in which they intend to work.

Think tank participants also emphasized the need for liaison with third-party reimbursement companies. Participants believed that the binational task force could play a role in educating these companies about gambling disorders and in persuading them to reimburse for pathological gambling treatment as they do for chemical dependency.

ACTION PLANS IN EDUCATION

Recommendations included:

1. Establishing an ad hoc committee to develop broad-based national/international curriculum for schools
2. Developing an educational video package to be distributed through school systems
3. Involving youth role models in educational effort
4. Educating parents and teachers about youth gambling and the dangers inherent in promoting gambling events such as casino nights

DISCUSSION

Think tank participants had well-defined ideas about the type of curriculum that should be developed for schools. They felt it should be reality based, dealing with the practical consequences of excessive gambling and avoiding ethical judgments or moralizing. It was suggested that youth role models—athletes, musicians, and movie/TV personalities—might be used to deliver these messages. Participants emphasized the importance of ensuring that educational materials are multicultural, recognizing and respecting the unique perspectives on gambling held by various cultures.

The role of parents and teachers was extensively discussed. Think tank participants felt that many parents and teachers consider gambling harmless and actually encourage it through social or fund-raising events with a casino gambling theme. Group members felt that parent-teacher-student organizations should be educated about the problem of youth gambling and the dangers inherent in institutional sponsorship of events that encourage gambling.

ACTION PLANS IN PUBLIC AWARENESS AND MEDIA

Recommendations included:

1. Publicizing the findings of the North American Think Tank on Youth Gambling Issues
2. Identifying and cultivating media allies and potential partners to assist in creating public awareness of the issue
3. Establishing binational speakers' bureaus on the topic of youth gambling
4. Establishing and publicizing a National Youth Gambling Screening Week in both the United States and Canada, highlighted by a televised screening test
5. Establishing and publicizing international toll-free information and referral hotlines for teens with gambling problems in the United States and Canada
6. Assisting the gambling industry to develop and promote voluntary standards that discourage the targeting of gambling advertising to young consumers

DISCUSSION

According to think tank participants, the results of the think tank itself should be publicized aggressively to help stimulate public discussion of youth gambling. It was felt that advance publicity on the think tank had already contributed to growing awareness, as evidenced by extensive coverage in *USA Today* and interest expressed by various television news organizations.

Think tank members acknowledged the power of television as a tool to create public awareness and recommended that the U.S. and Canadian task forces explore the possibility of nationally televised youth-gambling screenings in their respective countries, perhaps followed by a town-hall type discussion of youth gambling. In view of the strong interest in this issue by some media organizations, there may be opportunities to develop partnerships with media outlets for funding such a program. The development of a binational speakers' bureau was proposed by think tank participants, who felt that civic and community groups, professional associations, and public-policy groups would welcome presentations on this topic. The speakers' bureau would require organization and administration and would probably be a function of the binational task force when established.

The issue of gambling advertising was widely discussed. Think tank participants felt the gambling industry should adopt a "code of practice" or voluntary standards to discourage gambling advertising that appear to target younger consumers. Participants acknowledged that recent efforts by casinos to position themselves as "family destinations" could complicate the task, but believed an effort should be made among industry members to establish such standards. The role of the binational task force in this effort would be to advise, consult, and assist industry members in promoting the standards within the industry and to the general public.

Conclusion

The North American Think Tank on Youth Gambling Issues was the first international event to focus on youth gambling and to develop specific recommendations for addressing the issue. Despite the wide diversity of group members, participants demonstrated an amazing commonality of purpose in the development of their recommendations. The few issues on which there were disagreements are noted in this report.

As previously mentioned, think tank members agreed during the final think tank general session that an interim task force should be established to begin implementation of the recommendations that emerged from their two-day discussions. Participants recommended that the North American Training Institute and the Harvard Medical School Division on Addictions continue to serve as joint conveners and that they assemble a small subcommittee of think tank participants to serve as the interim task force that will draft a plan for establishing and formalizing the permanent binational organization.

As meaningful as the North American Think Tank discussions were, they represent only the first step in what must be an ongoing effort to respond to the issue of youth gambling. If the binational task force is to be established and these recommendations implemented, fund-raising will be key to the effort. Both public and private funding sources will need to be tapped.

As with any major social problem, the solution lies in our collective political will. If policymakers are convinced this problem must be addressed, they will appropriate funds to address it. If the gambling industry believes it is best served by a progressive, responsible approach to this issue, it will contribute funds to that end. If the business community recognizes that problem gambling can lead to loss of productivity and criminal activity in the workplace, it will become part of the solution. If private foundations believe that young people who are addicted to gambling need help, they will provide grants for that purpose.

The North American Think Tank on Youth Gambling Issues has launched public dialogue on this issue and recommended a response. While the details of implementation may change as new ideas emerge or better ways are discovered, think tank participants have helped define a plan to guide the development of new public policy. Think tank participants and the organizations that sponsored this important event are confident that their recommendations will indeed serve as a blueprint for the development of a responsible and responsive North American approach to the management of youth-gambling issues.

Participant List

Linda Berman, MSW*
Westchester Jewish Community Services
16 Olinda Avenue
Hastings-on-Hudson, NY 10706

Tom Brosig
Vice President
Grand Casinos, Inc.
4695 Forest View Lane
Plymouth, MN 55442

James E. Butler
Vice President and General Counsel
Harrah's Hotel–Reno
P.O. Box 10
Reno, NV 89504

Judith Byrnes
Gambling Project Coordinator
DHR–Division of Mental Health
2 Peachtree St. NE, 4th Floor, Suite 550
Atlanta, GA 30303

Colin S. Campbell, Ph.D.*
Malaspina University College
900 3rd St.
Nanaimo, BC V9R 5S5 Canada

Frank Campbell, MSW
Executive Director
Baton Rouge Crisis Intervention Center
4837 Revere Ave.
Baton Rouge, LA 70808

Judy Cornelius, M.A.
Associate Director
Institute for the Study of Gambling
University of Nevada, Reno
Reno, NV 89109

Thomas N. Cummings (Co-sponsor)
Executive Director
Massachusetts Council on Compulsive
  Gambling
190 High St., Suite 6
Boston, MA 02110

Jeffrey Derevensky, Ph.D.
Director, School of Applied/Child
  Psychology
McGill University
3700 McTavish St.
Montreal, Quebec H3A 1Y2 Canada

Kathy Donovan
Research Officer
Saskatchewan Health
2106 Montague St.
Regina, Saskatchewan S4T 3J9 Canada

William R. Eadington, Ph.D.
Department of Economics/030
University of Nevada, Reno
Reno, NV 89557-0016

Judge Donald Arthur Ebbs
Ontario Court of Justice
P.O. Box 607, City Hall Square
Windsor, Ontario N9A 6N4 Canada

G. Ron Frisch, Ph.D.
Department of Psychology
University of Windsor
Windsor, Ontario N9B 3P4 Canada

Elizabeth M. George
Executive Director
North American Training Institute
314 W. Superior St., Suite 702
Duluth, MN 55802

Alan I. Gilbert
Minnesota Attorney General's Office
1200 NCL Tower, 45 Minnesota St.
St. Paul, MN 55101

Clifford Goldberg*
United Health Care Corporation/IHR
1700 Rockville Pike, Suite 500
Rockville, MD 20852

Jeannette Hargroves
Senior Public Policy Analyst
Federal Reserve Bank of Boston
P.O. Box 2076, Research Dept. T-8
Boston, MA 02106

Durand F. Jacobs, Ph.D.
Loma Linda University Medical School
432 East Crescent Ave.
Redlands, CA 92373

Robert Jones, MSW
Treatment Consultant (Addictions)
Department of Health and Community
  Services
520 King St.
Fredericton, NB E3B 5G8 Canada

David A. Korn
President and Chief Executive Officer
The Donwood Institute
176 Brentcliffe Road
Toronto, Ontario M4G 3Z1 Canada

Robert Ladouceur, Ph.D.
Universite Laval
Quebec G1K 7P4 Canada

Henry R. Lesieur, Ph.D.
Illinois State University
Department of Criminal Justice Sciences
Normal, IL 61790-5250

John McCarthy
Minnesota Indian Gaming Association
Rt. 2, Box 95
Cass Lake, MN 56633

Joseph Malone**
Office of the State Treasurer/Receiver
   General
State House Room 227
Boston, MA 02133

Beverly Martin
Executive Director
Mississippi Casino Operators Association
2555 Marshall Road, Suite B
Biloxi, MS 39531

Charles D. Maurer, Ph.D., ABPP*
President, Board of Directors
Washington State Council on Problem
   Gambling
1001 Broadway, Suite 315
Seattle, WA 98122

Luc Provost
Assistant Director–Marketing
Societe des Casinos du Quebec, Inc.
500 Sherbrooke West
Montreal, Quebec J4X 2G1 Canada

Lynn Rambeck, Psy.D., L.P.
3400 West 66th St., Suite 240
Edina, MN 55345

Jan Rasch
Gaming Advisor to the Governor
Governor's Office
P.O. Box 139
Jackson, MS 39205-0139

I. Nelson Rose
Whittier Law School
5353 West 3rd St.
Los Angeles, CA 90020

Sirgay Sanger, M.D.
Director and Founder
Early Care Center
69 East 89th St.
New York, NY 10128

Philip G. Satre**
President and Chief Executive Officer
Promus Companies
1023 Cherry Road
Memphis, TN 38117

Kathleen Scanlan, M.A.
Program Director
Massachusetts Council on Compulsive
   Gambling
190 High St., Suite 6
Boston, MA 02110

Howard J. Shaffer, Ph.D.
Harvard Medical School
Division on Addictions
220 Longwood Ave., Goldenson Bldg.,
   Rm. 231
Boston, MA 02115

Chip Silverman, Ph.D., MPH
Green Springs Health Services
5565 Sterrett Place, Suite 500
Columbia, MD 21044

Garry Smith, Ph.D.*
University of Alberta
Department of Phy. Ed. and Sports
 Studies
Edmonton, Alberta T6G 2H9 Canada

Robert Tannenwald
Senior Economist, Research Department
Federal Reserve Bank of Boston
600 Atlantic Ave.
Boston, MA 02106

Eric M. Turner
Executive Director
Massachusetts State Lottery Commission
60 Columbian St.
Braintree, MA 02184

Larry Vigil
Legislative Assistant
Sen. Ben Nighthorse Campbell's Office
634 G St. SE
Washington, DC 20003

Rachel A. Volberg, Ph.D.
Gemini Research
310 Poplar St.
Roaring Springs, PA 16673

Tom Wispinski
Program Consultant–Problem Gambling
Alberta Alcohol and Drug Abuse
 Commission
6th Floor, 10909 Jasper Ave. NW
Edmonton, Alberta T5J 3M9 Canada

Wayne Yorke
Director, Cape Breton Region
Department of Health, Drug Dependency
 Division
500 George Place, George Street
Sydney, Nova Scotia B1P 1K6 Canada

*Group Leader
**Keynote Speaker

Note

1. Shaffer, H. J., & Hall, M. N. (1996). Estimating the prevalence of adolescent gambling disorders: A quantitative synthesis and guide toward standard gambling nomenclature. *Journal of Gambling Studies, 12* (2), 193–214.

Contributors

Tom Brosig was one of the original founders of Grand Casinos Inc. and served as its president from its inception in 1991 to 1994, when he reduced his role with the company to spend more time with his family. Between 1994 and 1996 Brosig represented the company at various speaking functions and was responsible for the company's investor-relations effort. In September 1996 Brosig was appointed director and reappointed president of Grand Casinos. He is the past president of the Mid-South region for Park Place Entertainment Corporation. Brosig also served as chairman of the National Advisory Board on Youth Gambling Issues at Harvard University. In addition, he serves or has served on the board of directors of the Gaming Entertainment Research and Education Foundation, Game Financial Corporation, Famous Dave's of America Inc., G III Apparel Group Ltd., Wilson's, The Leather Experts, Junior Achievement of the Upper Midwest Inc., ASC of Mississippi, Inc., DBA Center Circle, an alternative home for children in need of supervision, and OIC's of America, an organization that deals with alternative education programs for inner-city children. Brosig has lectured throughout the United States on leadership and organizational development, the impact of youth gambling addiction, and other topics of interest to the gaming industry and investment communities.

Terry W. Crites, associate professor and chairman of the Department of Mathematics and Statistics at Northern Arizona University, received his Ph.D. in mathematics education from the University of Missouri-Columbia in 1989. His research interests include determining how school-aged students develop number sense, make mathematical connections, and learn multiple representations of identical mathematical concepts.

Thomas N. Cummings was the executive director and founder of the Massachusetts Council on Compulsive Gambling Inc. He was the author and driving force behind the Massachusetts legislation authorizing funding for the council. This funding also supports affiliated programs on treatment and research at the Harvard Medical School. Cummings, who has lectured on compulsive gambling at the Harvard Medical School, also served with distinction on the board of directors of the National Council on Problem Gambling in Washington, DC. Cummings was the treasurer and an original member of the board of trustees of the American Academy of Health Care Providers in the Addictive Disorders and was a favored and frequent consultant to national and local media on events related to the growth of legalized gambling and problem gambling. Among his accomplishments are the first report on minority concerns and views on problem gambling and the cosponsorship of the first North American Think Tank on Adolescent Gambling. Cummings passed away on January 12, 1998. This book represents his last publication.

William R. Eadington is a professor of economics and director of the Institute for the Study of Gambling and Commercial Gaming at the University of Nevada, Reno. Dr. Eadington has written more than fifty scholarly articles and edited seven books that deal with various aspects of gambling and public policy. He has organized the International Conferences on Gambling and Risk Taking since 1974 and has participated as a convener and keynote speaker at the conferences and symposia on five continents. He also serves as a consultant to private and public sector organizations on gambling-related matters throughout the world. Eadington is on the advisory board of the National Council on Problem Gambling, the Nevada Council on Problem Gambling, the Centre for the Study of Gambling and Commercial Gaming at the University of Salford (United Kingdom), and the Australian Institute for Gambling Research. Eadington holds a B.S. degree in mathematics from the University of Santa Clara and M.A. and Ph.D. degrees in economics from the Claremont Graduate School. He has served as a visiting professor for the University of Utah and Harvard Medical School. He has also lectured at the Kennedy School of Government at Harvard University and has twice been an academic visitor at the London School of Economics.

Joanna Franklin, MS, NCGC, has been working in the addictions field for more than twenty-six years and was the first clinician hired to work in the first state-funded treatment program in Maryland. Franklin has worked as a director of gambling treatment services at Taylor Manor Hospital and has provided consultation and training on the topic of pathological gambling.

Elizabeth M. George is the chief executive officer of the North American Training Institute, a Minnesota-based private, not-for-profit corporation. George serves as associate editor for program features for the *Journal of Gambling Studies*. In 1998 she was selected to serve on the Council of State Government Center for State Trends and Innovation's expert panel session on "Gambling and the States" and was invited by the National Gambling Impact Study Commission to provide expert testimony on the topic of underage gambling. George was appointed to the National Center for Responsible Gaming Advisory Committee and was instrumental in the design of three compulsive gambling–related public policy think tanks. In 1995, along with Howard Shaffer and Thomas Cummings, she co-convened the North American Think Tank on Youth Gambling Issues held at Harvard Medical School. She is the author of numerous publications and articles on the topic of underage gambling. She has provided public policy consultation to an array of gaming corporations and tribal governmental leaders. George has provided lectures on the topic of underage gambling to audiences in the United States, Canada, Australia, and Russia.

Matthew N. Hall was a research associate at the Harvard Medical School Division on Addictions and was project manager of the Division on Addictions' Project on Gambling and Health. Hall is co-author of the first meta-analytic review of the prevalence of disordered gambling in the United States and Canada, is an editorial board member of the *Journal of Gambling Studies,* and has served as co-editor of *WAGER* (the *Weekly Addiction Gambling Educational Report*). He is also co-developer of a contemporary math curriculum for middle school students that teaches critical thinking skills, probability, and number sense within the context of gambling. He currently attends the University of Massachusetts School of Medicine.

Durand F. Jacobs, Ph.D., is a diplomate in clinical psychology, American Board of Professional Psychology. He has been a professor of medicine (psychiatry) at the Loma Linda University Medical School since 1978. He was first vice-president of the National Council on Problem Gambling from 1991 to 1999. He has been involved in treating patients, training health professionals, and researching addictive behaviors for the past forty years. In 1972 he was instrumental in establishing the first inpatient treatment program for compulsive gamblers. In 1982 he published *The General Theory of Addictions.* He is a recipient of the Herman Goldman Foundation Award, as well as the award from the Harvard Medical School, Division on Addictions, for lifelong contributions to youth-gambling work. He resides with his wife in Redlands, California.

Henry R. Lesieur, president of the Rhode Island Institute for Problem Gambling, received his Ph.D. in sociology from the University of Massachusetts, Amherst. Lesieur serves on the board of directors of the National Council on Problem Gambling and the Rhode Island Council on Problem Gambling as well as on the advisory board of other organizations. He was the founding editor of the *Journal of Gambling Studies* and is the author of *The Chase: Career of the Compulsive Gambler,* as well as articles in professional journals on crime, pathological gambling, and addictions. He is also a co-author of the South Oaks Gambling Screen. Lesieur has run workshops and given numerous professional presentations on compulsive gambling and addictions. He is a currently a doctoral candidate in the Psy.D. program at the Massachusetts School of Professional Psychology. He is a research fellow in clinical psychology at Brown University/Rhode Island Hospital, Providence, Rhode Island.

Joseph D. Malone served two terms as treasurer and receiver general of the Commonwealth of Massachusetts, during which he modernized and restructured the treasury, cutting the administrative budget by approximately 50 percent. As chairman of the Massachusetts Lottery Commission, Malone reduced lottery expenses as a percentage of gross sales to the lowest of any lottery in the country.

I. Nelson Rose is an internationally known public speaker, writer, and scholar and is recognized as one of the world's leading experts on gambling law. A tenured professor at Whittier Law School in Costa Mesa, California, Rose teaches one of the first law school classes on gaming law. The author of more than two hundred books, articles, and chapters on the subject, Rose is best known for his nationally syndicated column "Gambling and the Law" and his landmark 1986 book by the same name. He incorporated the California Council on Problem Gambling and served as its vice-president. A consultant to governments and industry, Rose has testified as an expert witness in administrative, civil, and criminal cases. He has advised international corporations, major law firms, licensed casinos, Internet operators, players, Indian tribes, and local, state, and national governments, including Arizona, California, Florida, New Jersey, Texas, Ontario, and the federal governments of Canada and the United States. With the rising interest in gambling throughout the world, Rose has addressed such diverse groups as the National Conference of State Legislatures, Congress of State Lotteries of Europe, National Academy of Sciences, and the United States Conference of Mayors. He earned his J.D. from Harvard Law School.

Sirgay Sanger, director of the Early Care Center of New York, is a graduate of Harvard College and Harvard Medical School. The founder of the Parent Child Center at St. Luke's–Roosevelt Hospital in New York, has authored four books and numerous articles. Sanger is the past president of the National Council on Problem Gambling. Formerly chairman of the Venice Committee–World Monuments Fund, he is at present founder and director of the Harvard Padova Alliance for Medicine. Board certified in adult, child, and adolescent psychiatry, he has a private practice in New York City.

Philip G. Satre is chairman and chief executive officer of Harrah's Entertainment, Inc., which operates casinos in more locations than any other company in North America. He joined the company in 1980 as vice-president, general counsel, and secretary of Harrah's, at that time a brand with two Nevada casinos and a casino under development in Atlantic City. Since that time, Satre has risen through the organization, holding various operations and senior management positions within the Harrah's brand and division, and ultimately with the company's various corporate parents. He has been president and chief executive officer of Harrah's since 1984 and on the company's board of directors since 1988. In 1997, he was promoted to chairman of Harrah's Entertainment, Inc., also maintaining his prior positions of president and chief executive officer for the corporation. A native of Martinez, California, Satre graduated from Stanford University with a B.A. degree in psychology. He earned his J.D. from the University of California, Davis. In December 1990, Satre was awarded the first Robert L. Custer Award from the National Council on Problem Gambling, Inc., for Harrah's leadership role on the issue of problem gambling.

Howard J. Shaffer is an associate professor at Harvard Medical School and director of the Harvard Medical School Division on Addictions. In addition to having an active private practice, he consults internationally to a variety of organizations in business, education, human services, and government. Shaffer is licensed as a clinical psychologist in the Commonwealth of Massachusetts and is certified by the National Register of Health Care Providers in Psychology. Shaffer is founder and former president of the board of trustees of the American Academy of Health Care Providers in the Addictive Disorders, the first international credentialing body for clinicians working in the addictive disorders. Shaffer has served as chief psychologist at the North Charles Institute for the Addictions for thirteen years and as director of the Drug Problems Resource Center at the Cambridge Hospital and director of the Special Consultation and Treatment Program for Women at the Judge Gould Institute of Human Resources. Shaffer is editor of the *Journal of Gambling Studies* and is associate editor of the *Journal of Substance Abuse Treatment.* Shaffer also serves on the editorial boards for a variety of scholarly journals. His major research interests include the social perception of addiction and disease, impulse control regulation and compulsive behaviors, disordered gambling, and the natural history of addictive behaviors. Shaffer has published many articles and books. His research and extensive writing have shaped how the health care field conceptualizes and treats the full range of addictive behaviors.

Eric M. Turner is a senior vice-president of State Street Corporation. He is a member of the sales and marketing department in the bank's Global Investor Services Group. Prior to this position, he served as head of the group's financial management and planning unit, reporting to State Street's president and chief operating officer. Before coming to State Street, he served as executive director of the Massachusetts State Lottery Commission from November 1991 to October 1995. He started his tenure with the Commonwealth of Massachusetts as deputy treasurer for debt and cash management in February 1991. Prior to joining the Commonwealth, Turner was employed as a vice-president of Drexel Burnham Lambert, where he provided investment-banking services in the firm's municipal finance department. He began his professional career as a marketing representative and later was a financial analyst with IBM. Turner is a former member of the NAACP's National Board of Directors and of the board of Jet-A-Way, Inc. He has served as secretary, treasurer, and member of the executive committee of the North American Association of State and Provincial Lotteries (NASPL). He serves as a trustee and treasurer of Lasell College in Newton, Massachusetts, treasurer of the Harvard Business School African-American Alumni Association, a member of the Harvard Business School Alumni Association, and a member of the board of trustees of Catholic Charities of Greater Boston. Also, he is a member of the Parish Council of St. Philip Neri Church. He attended Harvard University, where he earned a bachelor's degree (A.B.) in economics and a master's degree (M.B.A.) in general management. He resides in Newton, Massachusetts, with his wife, Wanda Whitmore, and four children, Weslie, Candice, Jared, and Allegra.

Lisa Vagge received her B.A. degree in psychology from Harvard University, where she conducted research on initiation to gambling among youth as part of her undergraduate thesis. Her research interests include substance use, addiction, and psychopathology. At the time of this book's preparation, she worked on clinical research projects on alcohol dependence at McLean Hospital in Belmont, Massachusetts.

Joni Vander Bilt is a research associate at Western Psychiatric Institute and Clinic, Pittsburgh, in the area of mood and anxiety disorders. She holds a faculty appointment as instructor of public health in the Department of Neurobiology at Harvard Medical School. Vander Bilt was the coordinator of *WAGER* (the *Weekly Addiction Gambling Educational Report*) for three years. She is also co-developer of a contemporary math curriculum for middle school students that teaches probability, number sense, and critical-thinking skills within the context of gambling. Vander Bilt holds an M.P.H. degree in public health from Boston University.

Wayne Yorke is the director of Yorke Psychological Services, providing counseling and consultation to community, provincial, and federal agencies. He is the past director of the Eastern Region of the Nova Scotia Department of Health Drug Dependency Services in Nova Scotia and has been overseeing administrative and clinical needs of the Drug Dependency Services for the past twenty-six years. Yorke holds an M.A. degree and a Certificate of Advanced Graduate Studies in Psychology and Counseling from Assumption College in Worcester, Massachusetts, and a bachelor of theology degree from the University of Ottawa in Ontario. Yorke has been an adjunct member of the faculty of social sciences at the University College of Cape Breton for many years. He has also served as a personnel selection officer with the Canadian Forces Reserves for the past twenty-four years. He has been a member of the program design committee for the Problem-Gambling Treatment, Education/ Prevention Programs for Nova Scotia. Yorke has lectured and published a number of articles on the topic of gambling and has served on various committees dealing with problem gambling and treatment programs. Yorke also serves as a consultant and lecturer to a number of state and provincial programs and private practitioners in Canada and the United States. He is a member of the Nova Scotia Psychological Association, the Canadian Psychological Association, a Registered Psychologist of the Board of Examiners in Psychology (Nova Scotia), and a registered member of the Canadian Health Care Providers in Psychology.

Darryl Zitzow, a clinical psychologist, currently works for the Indian Health Service within the Bemidji Area Offices of Northern Minnesota. He received his Ph.D. in clinical psychology from Walden University in Florida. He has worked within

American Indian reservations for most of the past twenty-four years. Zitzow has conducted research and published numerous articles regarding the American Indian family, including issues of family time, assessing abuse, suicide, and compulsive gambling. He has worked as a gambling researcher and therapist for the past ten years.

Index

ABC. *See* Antecedent Behavior Consequence model of research
aboriginal youth gambling in Canada, 265
abuse. *See* family violence
acting out, 88
addiction: to anticipation, 87–88; gambling as object of, 10–11, 43; Jacobs's General Theory of Addictions, 268. *See also* pathological gambling
adolescence: and acting out, 88; and addiction to anticipation, 87–88; and attraction of quick solutions, 85; and belief in magic and omnipotence, 191–92, 195; developmental issues of, 58, 84–85, 146, 191–94; developmentally delayed adolescents, 86–87; and guilt and shame, 94–95; and memory and identity deficits, 87; and oppositional behavior, 97; and pseudostupidity, 86; values and attitudes of youth, 193–94, 266; violence and abuse against adolescents, 105. *See also* youth gambling
adult gambling. *See* gambling
advertising: focus of, on legal-age audiences, 205, 299; and Harrah's Project 21, 246; for lottery, 3, 26, 221, 224, 259. *See also* media
Africa. *See specific countries*
African Americans. *See* blacks
AGA. *See* American Gaming Association
age limits for alcohol use, 135, 136, 141, 147, 148, 271
age limits for gambling: and American Indian gaming, 133, 137–38, 143, 155–56, 157, 166, 169, 172, 173–74, 182*n*33; in Canada, 140, 148, 149, 150–51; casino industry's response to,

200–201; conclusion on, 146–47; considerations on setting limits, 132–34; in countries outside of U.S., 135, 148–51; and danger, 135–38, 146–47; enforcement of, 138–45, 182–83*n*43, 221, 225–26, 284, 295–96; and Harrah's Project 21, 20, 101, 201–5, 246; introduction to, 126–30; politics and history of, 134–35, 147–48; problems with, 130–32; public policy on, 195–96; state laws on, 151–80; and underage winners and losers, 139, 145–46, 183*n*43
age limits for marriage, 134, 181*n*20
age of onset for youth gambling, 35, 100–101, 260–62, 264, 270–71
Aid to Families with Dependent Children, 41
Alabama, 151, 153
Alaska, 153–54
Alberta, Canada, 56, 265, 276
alcohol use/abuse: and addiction, 11, 43; and adult gambling, 262; age limits for alcohol use, 135, 136, 141, 147, 148, 182*n*42, 271; age of onset for alcohol use, 261; and American Indians, 42, 43, 45, 209; and drunk driving, 128, 136, 147; and family violence, 111; and immediate gratification, 85; by parents, 97, 110–11; prevention programs for, 13, 14; relationship between violence, pathological gambling and, 110–11; and youth gambling, 27, 34, 243, 262, 266
Alcoholics Anonymous, 114
Amati, B. H., 230, 243
ambivalent thinking and treatment, 94
American Gaming Association (AGA), 205, 217

American Indian gaming: and age limits
for gambling, 133, 137–38, 143,
155–56, 157, 166, 169, 172, 173–74,
182n33; and alcoholism, 42, 43, 45,
209; background on, 39–40; and
compulsive gambling research, 42–46;
and crime, 41; and education and
prevention programs, 45–47; flaws in
research on, 45–46; future research on,
46; and Internet and telephone
lotteries, 159; law on and legal
categories of, 40, 42, 63–64; negative
consequences of, 41–45; and New
Mexico gambling laws, 171; and New
York gambling laws, 171–72; and
Oregon gambling laws, 173–74;
positive consequences of, 40–41, 46;
prevalence studies on compulsive
gambling, 43–45, 241;
recommendations on, 46–47;
regulation of, 40, 42; and risk factors
for compulsive gambling, 42–43, 209;
statistics on and revenue from, 40,
63–64; traditional forms of, 39, 40; and
Washington gambling laws, 178
American Psychiatric Association, 4–5,
108, 110, 236
Americans with Disabilities Act, 275
Andersen, K., 63, 64
Antecedent Behavior Consequence (ABC)
model of research, 248–49
anticipation, addiction to, 87–88
Antigua and Barbuda, 148
APO. See Assessment Prevention
Outcome agenda
Arcuri, A. F., 27, 230
Argentina, 148
Arizona: American Indian casinos in, 63,
137–38; gambling laws in, 137–38, 154;
lottery in, 64
Arkansas, 155
Aruba, 148
Asia. See specific countries
Asians, 265

assessment instruments, 12, 31–32, 107,
236–37, 240, 250
Assessment Prevention Outcome (APO)
agenda, 249–50
AT&T, 205
Atkin, K., 231
Atlantic City. See New Jersey
Atlantic Lotto, 52–53
Aucoin, Preston, 128
Australia, 150, 151
Austria, 149
Autotote, 156

Bahamas, 135, 148, 149
Baldwin, James, 1
Belgium, 149
B-endorphin, 10
Bentall, R. P., 240
Bergler, Edmund, 42, 191–92, 195
Berman, Linda, 300
betting. See gambling; youth gambling
betting rings, 232–33, 249
bicycle races, 171
bingo: and American Indians, 39, 40, 43,
44; attitudes on, 181n18, 211; in
Canada, 52, 53; state laws on, 136,
151–80; and youth gambling, 206, 232,
259, 260, 269, 276
Blackjack, 27, 39, 40, 44, 140, 191, 292
blacks, 44, 266
Boisvert, J. M., 248
Boles, J., 270
Botvin, G. J., 14
Boyd Casinos, 274
branded slot machines, 143–45, 183n51
Britain. See Great Britain/United
Kingdom
British Columbia, Canada, 53, 56, 149
British Market Research, 230
Bromley, E., 240
Brosig, Thomas J., xiii, 19, 20, 200,
208–18, 288, 300, 304
Bujold, D., 241, 262
Bulgaria, 149

Butler, James E., 300
Byrnes, Judith, 300

Cabazon Band of Mission Indians, 155–56
Caesar's Atlantic City, 140, 183n43
Caesar's Palace casino, 139, 140, 146, 183n43
Caesar's World, 274
Cahill, L., 240
California: age limits for gambling in, 133, 143; American Indian gaming in, 133, 143; gambling laws in, 155–56; gambling research from, 230, 238; lottery in, 259, 273
Campbell, Colin S., 54, 300
Campbell, Frank, 300
Campion, Ab, 140
Canadian Foundation on Compulsive Gambling, 57, 272
Canadian gambling: aboriginal youth gambling in, 265; age limits for, 140, 148, 149, 150–51; charitable gaming industry, 53–54; conclusions and recommendations on, 59–60; economics of, 52–54; enforcement of age limits in, 140; funding to address problem gambling, 276; gambling problems among adolescents, 55, 57–59, 236, 237, 258, 263, 265, 267; gambling problems among adults, 54–56; history of, 50–51; horse races, 52, 53; illegal gambling, 53; lotteries, 50, 51–54, 57, 150–51; nature of, 51–52; overview of, 49–50; pathological gambling, 54–59; prevention program on, 247; research on, 60, 230–31, 236, 238; social context of, 49; statistics on, 50, 52–54, 236, 258, 261, 262
card playing, 8, 34, 50, 137, 206, 259, 262, 266, 269, 270, 276–77
Carroll, D., 230, 235
casino gambling: age limits for, 133, 137, 139–40, 147, 148, 200–201; and American Indian gaming, 40, 44,

63–64; casino industry's response to youth gambling, 199–218, 273–74; in countries outside of U.S., 148–51; as family activity, 102, 245, 299; and fines for underage gambling, 140, 183n43; and Harrah's Project 21, 20, 101, 201–5, 246, 273, 296; riverboat casinos, 63, 127, 137, 145, 159–60, 163, 167, 168, 205; state laws on, 127, 137, 151–80; statistics on, 63; teens removed from or denied entry to, 245, 246; and unattended children in casinos, 205; by youth, 27, 101, 228, 232, 259, 261, 276. *See also* American Indian gaming
casino industry. *See* gaming industry
Casino Niagara, 140
"casino nights" in schools, 245–46, 249
Centers for Disease Control and Prevention, 296
change, stages of, 119–20
charitable gaming industry: in Canada, 53–54; state laws on, 151–80. *See also* bingo
Cherokee Tribe, 133, 172
child abuse and neglect, 105, 106–7, 118–21
children: age-appropriate honesty with, in therapy, 114–15; amusement games for, 136–37; curfews for, 129; family therapy for children of compulsive gamblers, 113–15; industrialization and childhood, 181n22; and Internet, 129–30; of multiple-problem families, 110–11; neglect of, 121; of pathological gamblers, 102, 103, 105–7, 113–15, 118–21; and slot machines with cartoon characters, 143–45, 183n51; television viewing by, 129; unattended children in casinos, 205; violence and abuse against, 105, 106–7, 118–20. *See also* youth gambling
Chile, 149
Chippewa Indians, 166
Chippewas, 137

cigarette smoking. *See* tobacco use
Claridge Casinos, 273
Coeur d'Alene Tribe, 159
Cohen, Debra Kim, 140
Collinson, F., 230
Colorado, 156
communities: in ABC model of research,
    249; assets and positive trends in, 290;
    negative trends and obstacles in, 292
competence versus incompetence and age
    limits, 130–31, 133–34, 181*n*12
compulsive gambling. *See* pathological
    gambling
Connecticut: American Indian gaming in,
    63–64, 156, 157; gambling laws in,
    156–57; gambling research from,
    231, 238
Constitution, U.S., 126–27, 134, 135, 147
Cornelius, Judy, 301
counseling. *See* treatment of youth
    gamblers
craps, 40, 44, 72–75, 81–82
crime: by adult gamblers, 109–10; and
    American Indian gaming, 41; and
    delinquent gambling, 91–92, 242–44,
    263, 266; organized crime, 41, 222;
    stealing by youth gamblers, 234,
    235, 243
"criminal turns to drugs" hypothesis of
    drug abuse, 243
Crites, Terry W., 16, 18, 63–82, 304
Croft, Clary, 50
Cummings, Thomas N., xi–xii, 221,
    283–300, 301, 304–5
curfews, 129
Custer, Robert, 112

danger and age limits for gambling,
    135–38, 146–47
Dardenne, Jay, 180*n*3
David, Gray, 155
Decision Sciences, Inc., 230
DeGroot, M. H., 74
Delaware, 157

delegation doctrine, 145
delinquent gambling: connection between
    crime and gambling, 242–44, 263, 266;
    treatment for, 91–92
denial. *See* dissociation
Denmark, 149
depression, 27, 43, 241, 263
Derevensky, Jeffrey, 150, 301
developmental issues of adolescence, 58,
    84–85, 146, 191–94
developmentally delayed, treatment of,
    86–87
Diagnostic and Statistical Manual
    (DSM), 4–5, 108, 236, 237, 271
Dielman, T., 259
DiGregorio, Ernie, 225
dissociation: by parents, 97; by youth
    gamblers, 86, 88, 94–96, 264,
    267–68, 272
District of Columbia, 158
Dixon, Sandi and Toni, 142–43
Dobson, James, 145–46, 183*n*51
domestic violence, 103–12, 118–19, 120
Donovan, Kathy, 301
dopamine D2 receptor gene (DRD2), 10
dopamine release, 10–11
DRD2. *See* dopamine D2 receptor gene
drug abuse: and addiction, 10, 43; and
    adult gambling, 262; age of onset for,
    261; and American Indian gaming, 42;
    "criminal turns to drugs" hypothesis
    of, 243; decriminalization of marijuana,
    129, 136; "enslavement" hypothesis of,
    243; and family violence, 111; and
    immediate gratification, 85;
    "intensification" hypothesis of, 243;
    methadone patients, 240; by parents,
    97, 110–11; prevention programs for,
    13, 14, 247; relationship between
    violence, pathological gambling and,
    110–11; smoking as "gateway" risk-
    taking activity for, 36*n*4; and youth
    gambling, 27–31, 34, 101, 242–44,
    263, 266

Malta, 150

Manitoba, Canada, 56, 276

marijuana, decriminalization of, 129, 136

marriage age limits, 134, 181*n*20

Marston, A. R., 236

Martin, Beverly, 302

Maryland, 164–65

Mashantucket Pequot Tribe, 157

Mashantucket tribe, 63–64, 157

Massachusetts: advertising for state lottery in, 3, 221, 224; education and prevention programs in, 220–21, 225, 247; enforcement of age limits for gambling in, 221; family violence in, 111; gambling laws in, 165; illicit activities among youth in, 11, 34, 101; instant-ticket vending machines in, 225; prevalence of youth gambling in, 228, 231, 238; state lottery in, xii, 28–35, 211, 219–26, 226*n*1, 245; youth gambling on lottery in, 28–35, 101, 245

Massachusetts Council on Compulsive Gambling, 286

Massachusetts Gambling Screen (MAGS), 4, 31–32, 107, 236, 286

Massachusetts General Hospital, 217

mathematics of gambling: craps, 72–75, 81–82; in education programs for youth, 15–16, 35, 63–82, 197; keno, 69–71, 76–79; lottery, 64–68, 75–76, 79, 80–81; roulette, 71–72, 73, 79–82

Maurer, Charles D., 302

Mauritius, 150

McCain, John, 183*n*51

McCarthy, John, 302

McCormick, R. A., 27–28

McGervey, J. D., 66

McGill University, 150, 276

McLean, Gene, 34

media: assets and positive trends in, 291; coverage of youth gambling by, 273; and Harrah's Project 21, 202, 203; and lottery, 220; negative trends and

obstacles in, 293; recommendations on, by North American Think Tank on Youth Gambling Issues, 284, 298–99; and youth attitudes and values, 193. *See also* advertising

Melius, David, 127

memory deficits, 87

mental illness, 27

methadone patients, 240

Michigan: American Indian gaming in, 41; funding for education and prevention in, 218; gambling laws in, 165–66; unemployment in, 41

Minnesota: American Indian gaming in, 41, 44, 63, 166, 216; casino industry's response to youth gambling in, 208–18; drug abuse and youth gambling in, 27; funding in, 275; gambling laws in, 147, 166–67; gambling research from, 44, 231, 237, 238–39; prevalence of youth gambling in, 228, 231, 232, 237, 265; prevention programs in, 247

Minnesota Council on Compulsive Gambling. *See* North American Training Institute

Minnesota Indian Gaming Association, 216

Minnesota Public Policy Think Tank, 20, 213–14, 216

minority ethnic groups. *See* American Indian gaming; ethnic groups

minors. *See* youth gambling

Mirage casino, 139

Mireault, C., 230, 235, 236, 238, 245, 261

Misseck, R. E., 233

Mission Indians, 143, 155–56

Mississippi, 167, 216, 218

Missouri, 167–68, 205, 218

Montana, 168–69

Moody, G., 244

Moon, P., 50

Mothers Against Drunk Driving (MADD), 136

multiple-problem families, 110–11

instruments, 12–13; specificity of
screening measures, 12; subclinical/
"at risk" gambling, 238–40; teens and
parent gamblers, 244–45, 261, 263;
treatment programs, 248; video
gambling, 233; youth gambling,
228–50
resistance to treatment, 92, 93–94
restitution plan, 112
Rhode Island, 175
Rimm, M., 235
Rincon Band of Mission Indians, 143
risk factors: for pathological gambling,
42–43, 60; for youth gambling, 240–42
riverboat gambling, 63, 127, 137, 145,
159–60, 163, 167, 168, 205
role modeling, 115, 193
Rose, I. Nelson, 19, 126–80, 288, 302, 307
Rosenthal, R. J., 109
Roston, R., 42, 43
roulette, 40, 44, 71–72, 73, 79–82
Royer, V. H., 72
Rupcich, Nicholas, 57
Russo, A. M., 27–28

Sanger, Sirgay, 18, 84–98, 302, 307
Saskatchewan, Canada, 56
Satre, Philip G., 19, 20, 199–207, 217,
226, 288, 302, 307
Scanlan, Kathleen, 302
schizo-affective disorder, 28
schools: drug education programs in, 13,
14, 247; gambling education programs
in, 15–16, 35, 63–82, 197, 247; as
setting for gambling-related activities,
245–46, 249; truancy from and poor
school performance, 242, 243, 249, 263,
266. *See also* education programs on
gambling; prevention programs;
prevention programs on gambling
scratch tabs, 44, 269
screening instruments, 12, 31–32, 107,
236–37, 240, 250, 263–64, 271–72, 286
Sechellus, 151

self-help groups. *See* Gam-Anon; Gama-
Teen; Gamblers Anonymous (GA)
self-knowledge, 92–93, 96–97
self-regulation, 96–97
Seminole Tribe, 39
serotonin, 10
sexual intercourse: age of consent for,
181*n*20, 182*n*25; with minors, 182*n*25
Shaffer, Howard J., xiii, 1–21, 25–36, 59,
221, 231, 238, 283–300, 302, 308
shame of youth gamblers, 94–95
Shuttlesworth, D. E., 105
Silverman, Chip, 302
Singer, R. D., 236
"Slammer," 274
slot machines: age limits for, 127, 140,
147, 148; American Indian gaming law
on, 40; with cartoon characters and
branded slot machines, 143–45,
183*n*51; fines for underage use of, 140;
regular versus nonregular gamblers on,
240; state laws on, 151–80; statistics on,
27, 229; in United Kingdom, 229, 240,
246; and youth gambling generally,
259, 266, 269
Slovenia, 151
Smith, F. O., 27, 230
Smith, Garry, 303
smoking. *See* tobacco use
social class and youth gambling, 241–42
social consequences. *See* psychosocial
consequences of excessive gambling
social gambling, 137, 259
socialization of males, 195
SOGS. *See* South Oaks Gambling Screen
"SOGS-Plus," 240
SOGS-RA. *See* South Oaks Gambling
Screen Revised for Adolescents
South Africa, 151
South Carolina, 145–46, 175
South Dakota, 176
South Oaks Gambling Screen (SOGS), 4,
43–44, 55, 107, 236, 237, 240, 263–64,
265, 271, 272